KT-366-079

COMMUNITY CARE: A READER

Edited by

Joanna Bornat, Charmaine Pereira
David Pilgrim and Fiona Williams

at The Open University

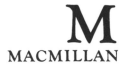
MACMILLAN in association with
The Open University

Editorial matter, selection, commissioned articles
© The Open University 1993

All rights reserved. No reproduction, copy or transmission of
this publication may be made without written permission.

No paragraph of this publication may be reproduced, copied or
transmitted save with written permission or in accordance with
the provisions of the Copyright, Designs and Patents Act 1988,
or under the terms of any licence permitting limited copying
issued by the Copyright Licensing Agency, 90 Tottenham Court
Road, London W1P 9HE.

Any person who does any unauthorised act in relation to this
publication may be liable to criminal prosecution and civil
claims for damages.

First published 1993 by
THE MACMILLAN PRESS LTD
Houndmills, Basingstoke, Hampshire RG21 2XS
and London
Companies and representatives
throughout the world

ISBN 0–333–58714–6 hardcover
ISBN 0–333–58715–4 paperback

A catalogue record for this book is available
from the British Library.

Printed in Great Britain by Mackays of Chatham PLC,
Chatham, Kent

Reprinted 1993

Sarah CB

COMMUNITY CARE:
A READER

This Reader forms part of the Open University course *Community Care* (K259), a core course for the Diploma in Health and Social Welfare. The selection of items is therefore related to other material available to students. It is designed to evoke the critical understanding of students. Opinions expressed in it are not necessarily those of the Course Team or of The Open University. If you are interested in studying the course or working towards the Diploma, please write to the Information Officer, Department of Health and Social Welfare, The Open University, Walton Hall, Milton Keynes MK7 6AA, UK.

Also published by Macmillan in association with The Open University

HEALTH AND WELLBEING
Edited by Alan Beattie, Marjorie Gott, Linda Jones and Moyra Sidell

Contents

IV Practice

Acknowledgements

The author and publishers wish to thank the following for permission to use copyright material:

Association of Community Workers for material from Jenny Finch, 'A Women's Health Group in Mansfield' in *Women in Collective Action*, eds Anne Curno *et al* (1982); British Sociological Association for material from Sara Arber and Nigel Gilbert, 'Men: the Forgotten Carers', *Sociology*, vol.23, no.1 (1989); Cambridge University Press for material from Janet Finch and Jennifer Mason, 'Filial obligations and kin support for elderly people', *Ageing and Society*, vol. 10 (1990), from Peter Townsend, 'The structured dependency of the elderly: a creation of social policy in the twentieth century', *Ageing and Society*, vol. 1, no. 1 (1981), and from Tim Dant and Brian Gearing, 'Key workers for elderly people in the community: case managers and care co-ordinators', *Journal of Social Policy*, vol. 19, no. 3; Centre for Policy on Ageing for material from *Community Life: A Code of Practice for Community Care* (1990); Confederation of Health Service Employees for material from *Community Care: Which Way Forward* (1990); Community Care for material from Ann Macfarlane, 'The Right to Make Choices', *Community Care* (1.11.90), and Susan Goff, 'Hurdles for Social Workers', *Community Care* (18.1.90); Critical Social Policy and the authors for material from a paper by Harriet Cain and Nira Yuval-Davis, *Critical Social Policy*, vol. 10, no. 2, 1990; Disabled Peoples' International for the statement issued at the end of their conference, 12–14 April, 1989; Free Association Books for material from Joanna Ryan (with Frank Thomas), 'Concepts of Normalization' in *The Politics of Mental Handicap*, 2nd revised edition (1987); Good Practices in Mental Health for 'Defining Good Practice'; Guardian News Service Ltd for material from Kate Cooney, 'Carers may be angels but does that make their dependants devils?', *Guardian* (2.1.91), and John Palmer, 'Expanding Community may find itself tongue-tied', *Guardian* (19.3.91); Harlow Council for its Charter for

Citizens' Rights; The Controller of Her Majesty's Stationery Office for material from R. Snaith, ed., *Neighbourhood Care and Social Policy* (1989), *Residential Care: A Positive Choice* and *Community Care: Agenda for Action*; Joint Unit for Social Services Research on behalf of Social Services Monographs for material from Jane Hubert, 'At Home and Alone: families and young adults with challenging behaviour' in *Better Lives: Changing Services for People with Learning Difficulties*, ed. Tim Booth (1990), Social Services Monographs: Research in Practice, Sheffield; King's Fund Centre for Health Services Development for 'A ten-point plan for carers' and material from Andrea Whittaker, 'Involving people with learning difficulties in meetings' in *Power to the People*, ed. Liz Winn (1990); Macmillan Education Ltd for material from Gillian Dalley, 'The Principles of Collective Care' in *Ideologies of Caring* (1988); MIND for material from *Waiting for Community Care* (1990); Jenny Morris for an edited version of material from *Pride Against Prejudice: Transforming Attitudes to Disability*, The Women's Press (1991); National AIDS Trust for an extract from the Declaration of Rights for People with HIV and AIDS, UK Declaration Working Group; National Council for Voluntary Organisations for 'Rural Voluntary Action Needs: A Ten Point Plan', and material from Margaret Simey, 'Reflections of a voluntary worker' in *Active Citizens: New Voices and Values*, eds N. Fielding, G. Reeve and M. Simey (Bedford Square Press, 1991); National Council for Civil Liberties for material from '50,000 Outside the Law' (1951); National Pensioners Convention Steering Committee for their Declaration of Intent; The Observer Ltd for abridged material by Mukti Jain Campion, *Observer* (14.7.91); Random Century for material from Margaret Foster, *Have the Men had Enough?* (Chatto and Windus, 1989); Routledge for material from Eileen and Steven Yeo, 'Community as Service' in *New Views of Co-operation*, ed. Steven Yeo (Routledge, 1988), from Joan Busfield, *Managing Madness: Changing Ideas and Practice* (Unwin Hyman, 1986), from Jocelyn Cornwell, *Hard-Earned Lives: Accounts of Health and Illness from East London* (Tavistock, 1984), and from Martin Bulmer, *The Social Basis of Community Care* (Unwin Hyman, 1987); The Royal Association for Disability and Rehabilitation for material from their 1991 Policy Statements; Sheil Land Associates Ltd on behalf of the author for material from Cherril Hicks, *Who Cares? Looking After People at Home* (Virago, 1988); Southwark Council, Social Services Department for their Charter of Rights; Survivors Speak Out for their Charter of Needs (1987); Values Into Action for an extract from their promotional material.

Every effort has been made to trace all the copyright-holders, but if any have been inadvertently overlooked the publishers will be pleased to make the necessary arrangement at the first opportunity.

Introduction

'Community care' as a term can be approached from a multitude of directions. It has a long and shifting history. It has been shaped and determined by policy changes. At the same time as it is a distinctive range of professional practice, it is also some people's everyday experience of life, the inspiration of a movement away from institutional care and towards supported life in the community, a euphemism for women's labour in the home, and the focus for intense debate and controversy. It is in fact a slippery concept, used as a slogan by the political left and right. This collection of articles, accounts, statements and quotations brings together as many different perspectives on community care as can be managed in one book.

Community Care: a Reader reflects these many differing meanings and conflicting perspectives. The book stands on its own as a collection of writings on key issues of contemporary debate. Readers who are interested in following up more of the issues with practical examples and debates may like to know that it links to the Open University course and pack K259 *Community Care*, for which it is the set text. For more information on the course and pack contact: The Information Officer, Department of Health and Social Welfare, The Open University, Walton Hall, Milton Keynes, MK7 6AA. Students on the course are directed to read, make notes and analyse these articles and excerpts as part of their study.

There are four parts to this Reader, each compiled by a different editor. 'Community', 'Care', 'Policy' and 'Practice' are each organised along similar lines, juxtaposing new thinking with some of the 'classics' of community care policy and thought. Each is introduced by an anthology illuminating its facets and furrows through literary quotations, personal accounts, commentaries, policy statements and charters and declarations. While some of the articles in each section may be familiar to readers with knowledge of the field, others are new, written especially for this volume.

The four editors worked collectively but divided their responsibilities between the four sections. Charmaine Pereira's section on 'Community' highlights issues of place, control, representation, identity and agency. Fiona Williams's section on 'Care' links debates around gender, race, citizenship and provision. In 'Policy', David Pilgrim includes articles and excerpts that reflect the shifts and turns of policy development through the twentieth century as care moved from large institutions into the community. Finally, Joanna Bornat's 'Practice' section, with a selection of articles and charters written by experienced practitioners and users, draws on examples of care and support highlighting issues for carers, both paid and unpaid, and for users of services.

The editors would like to thank Sonia Morgan for her meticulous checking and chasing up, and for resisting and indulging, in their proper places, editorial whims. We would also like to thank Gillian Parker for her help in editing articles in the 'Care' section and Serena Stewardson for her careful work in word-processing the manuscript.

Part I

COMMUNITY

1

Introduction

What do we mean by 'community' and who, or what, is the 'community' in 'community care'? In this section of the Reader, we bring together a number of writings that focus in different ways on the diverse aspects of 'community'. Some of the texts are autobiographical or reflective in form, others are articles discussing issues of policy and of action. There are writings too that address the ways in which 'community' is 'presented' to us and its inherent complexities and contradictions.

The senses in which the word 'community' can be used are notably wide-ranging. The range of usage is reflected in the edited anthology: 'The breadth of community', a collection that highlights the elusive meanings of 'community'. Some of these meanings and their associated values – solidarity, interest and identity – are the focus of Joanna Bornat's chapter on 'Representations of community'. She discusses questions of representivity and exclusion, reflecting on the place of myth within this – which communities are we talking about and how are they remembered?

What is the significance of 'community' for women? Fiona Williams argues that community and women are interconnected in complex and contradictory ways: *which* women and *which* communities are of central importance. By understanding 'community' as women's *space* – the space that belongs to women and within which they can begin to determine some of its conditions – as well as women's *place* – the place to which they are relegated and over which they are denied control – we can begin to make sense of some of the contradictions. In her case study of a women's health group in Mansfield, Jenny Finch draws attention to what community involvement means in practice and, in particular, what kinds of processes are involved.

Social change has brought with it, among other things, changes in the social relationships of modern urban communities. The implications of this for neighbouring form the focus of the extracts from 'Neighbourhood care and social policy'. Philip Abrams and his colleagues (authors of the writings edited by Ray Snaith) are keen to emphasise the limita-

3

tions of informal care among neighbours who may only know each other in passing. Neighbourliness, if it were to play any part in neighbourhood or community care, would have to be *organised*. The ways in which neighbours may get drawn into caring are the subject of the chapter by Suzy Croft and Peter Beresford in which they describe their personal experience of caring for their next-door neighbour, an older person with senile dementia.

We conclude this section with two views of community service. The first extract is by Margaret Simey, reflecting on her past as a voluntary worker. The second, by Eileen and Stephen Yeo, places this piece in context by reflecting on the social forces behind such work. The writing touches on contradictory currents underlying community involvement: charitable work by middle-class women and working-class struggles to improve living conditions.

In focusing on the diverse and elusive senses of 'community', our aim is not solely to raise questions about what exactly we mean by the word but to deepen our understanding of any action based on the premise of 'community'.

2

Anthology: The Breadth of Community

Compiled by CHARMAINE PEREIRA

The word 'community' is, nowadays, a ubiquitous term. It crops up in all kinds of situations though its meaning remains elusive. 'Community' has been used in senses that include the personal, political, cultural, geographical, historical, national and international. This anthology brings together a number of writings on 'community', the aim being not so much to clarify the meaning as to illustrate the breadth of its usage. The choice of extracts is not intended to be comprehensive and has been, necessarily, selective. Diversity of style and presentation, not to mention content, have been the criteria for selection.

An extract from Jocelyn Cornwell's sociological text **Hard-Earned Lives: Accounts of Health and Illness from East London**, *Tavistock, London, 1984, pp. 40–50.*

Thirty years ago, Young and Willmott's (1957) description of social life in Bethnal Green established that place as the model of 'community' in modern urban settings. [. . .] By 'community' they meant two things: the existence of some kind of collective life that residents identify with, and a social life and social relationships based on reputation rather than status (i.e. on *who* people are to each other rather than *how much* they own or possess).

The definition of 'community' became stronger and more exaggerated in the course of their research careers. Originally Young defined 'community' simply as 'a sense of solidarity with other people sharing a common territory' (Young, 1955: 33). In *Family and Kinship*, Young, with Willmott, began to develop the idea that 'community' is collective life, lived on the streets and in public places, but at the same time they acknowledged the central importance of privacy and of 'your home being your own' to people surrounded at very close quarters by many

5

others. [. . .] By the time they wrote *Family and Class in a London Suburb* (Willmott and Young 1971), they were making the straightforward assertion that collective life was more important than life in the home. [. . .]

The other aspect of community, of people knowing one another because of who they are to each other rather than how much they own, relies on them having lived together and known one another a long time, but there is also something more to it. Young and Willmott saw relationships in Bethnal Green as finer, more moral and essentially *more human* than relationships on the new housing estate they called Green-leigh, because they did not involve questions of money and status. [. . .]

Young and Willmott's romantic vision of harmony and friendliness in Bethnal Green is not supported by reports of social life in 'face-to-face' communities, either in our own society in the past, or in other societies. In these studies [. . .] attention is more commonly paid to what Bailey (1971) calls the 'small politics' of everyday life which encourage enmity as much as friendship, and in which gossip and flattery, one-upmanship and ostracization are all powerful weapons. [. . .]

It is not novel to criticise Young and Willmott for romanticising Bethnal Green. [. . .] However, it is especially intriguing in the context of the present study because the interviews for the study contain public accounts of community that present a similarly romanticised version of 'community' life in Bethnal Green. [. . .] They were statements addres-sed to 'the public' in the sense that they reiterated old themes that people knew were acceptable; in some instances they could be best described as extended cliches. [. . .]

Neighbourliness, friendliness and concern for others (in the past), in contrast with selfishness, competitiveness and snobbery (in the present) were the main themes of the public accounts of community. [. . .] The dominant elements [. . .] were the fact of *similarity* between people and the shared experience of poverty or near-poverty. Again and again people said that money had introduced a new materialism and had undermined the trust in others that provided the basis for the relation-ships they had with their neighbours:

> Ann Cullen: 'I knew when I lived in Golden Row that I could walk out my front door and leave it open and no one was going to rob me, because I was the same as them. But I couldn't do that here. Not for the people in here. [. . .]'

Having money, they said, not only makes people mistrust one another's motives, it also gives individuals the means *to purchase* their own necessities and allows them to become less dependent on communal life. Private washing machines replaced the public laundry; private cars replaced weekends spent in the market or working on the garden;

private televisions and videos replaced football and the local pub. [. . .]

The portrait of community life – past and present – painted in private accounts were very different. As well as the willingness to help the invalid neighbour, it included the turning of the blind eye to other people's troubles; as well as the open doors and the familiarity with others, it included the arguments, fights and brawls, particularly over children, and the petty snobberies that kept people apart from each other. [. . .] In place of the active concern for the welfare of others, the impression the private accounts of community life gave was that of the over-riding importance of looking after oneself and one's own. [. . .]

> Florrie Neagle: 'All rough people, years ago.'
> Harold Neagle: 'All stick to one another.'
> JC: 'Were you part of that?'
> HN: 'Oh, yes. I came home one day from work and she's in the middle of the flats having a fight with two women. I went up to someone and said, "What's all the bother?" He said, "It's your old woman having a fight." '
> JC: 'Doesn't sound like you were all sticking together.'
> FN: 'No, well it's kids.'
> HN: 'It's children. If you had children, and she's another tenant in the flats, and her kids are hitting your kids, you'll go down after them.'
> FN: 'You're not going to just stand there, are you?'

[The interviews] demonstrate such radical differences in the way people experience community and in what they know about it that [. . .] the idea of 'a community life' existing at *any* time, in the past *or* in the present, seems something of a fiction. [. . .] It is particularly striking when the differences are between men and women living in the same household. [. . .]

> Mick Chalmers: 'I think the world has changed since I was a kid 'cause, I mean, I remember I used to live down a turning just like this, and I can remember when I was a kid, like in the summer we used to [. . .] all the street doors would be open and there'd be chairs out in the streets, and you'd walk along and talk to them. I mean you can walk down here in the daytime and you don't even see a soul. I mean I don't know who lives two doors away from me. You'd come home and me Nan would say, "Your Mum ain't in, she's out somewhere", and I'd go along and I'd walk in all the houses looking for me Mum. And, you know, all the doors were open and you'd just walk in.' Sarah Chalmers: 'See, what it is, with Mick it's different, but with me, I can walk outside the door, walk round the shops where it would take me five minutes to walk there and back, and I'll be out about half an hour, three-quarters of an hour. Because I bump into people that I know and talk and everything else. So I think it's more friendlier when you're in an area and you know people than when you don't know them.'

Mick and Sarah do not experience 'the community' in the same way as each other, so neither of them is capable of giving a fully rounded account of 'community'. The spaces they occupy – socially as well as geographically – are different. [. . .] Nowadays, the men rarely work locally, and most of their sense of community comes from the atmosphere of the local pub (if they are drinkers). Women, on the other hand, occupy a much wider range of communal spaces – the shops, the street, the school gates, their relatives' houses – and they have a much wider variety of contacts, not only with shopkeepers and other mothers, but also in the schools, pubs and blocks of flats where many of them are employed as cleaners.

———————

From **Paid Servant**, a novel by E. R. Braithwaite, New English Library, London, 1962, pp. 84–6.

There were several other visitors there when I arrived. [. . .] It was a friendly, informal gathering, with topics of conversation varied and interesting while they lasted. [. . .]

Eventually conversation got round to current changes within the social structure in Britain, and this in turn led to discussion on the various immigrant groups in the country and their contributions to its social, cultural and economic development. [. . .] So it fluctuated, back and forth, coming now to the inevitable question of mixed marriages. [. . .]

I tried to stay on the outer edge of these discussions, hearing, feeling, remembering, recording it all in my mind, or as much as was possible; now and then a question would be put to me and I'd be compelled to say my piece. As when someone suggested that, in mixed marriages, the children were the chief sufferers as they could find no place in either camp, so to speak. To this I replied:

We seem to be ignoring one important factor. Irrespective of who his parents are, a child born into a family is part of that family, so he naturally belongs, and needs from them love, companionship, help, guidance, encouragement, advice and example in positive living. He needs these things irrespective of his parents' racial origins. If he is born into a community where tolerance prevails, then there is no special problem. However, a coloured child born in Britain, for instance, not only needs the things I have mentioned, but is severely handicapped without them, because the community considers his colour a handicap and therefore imposes special pressure and proscriptions upon him. He needs these things not as insulation against the pressures, but as sources from which to draw strength in order to meet and deal with them with wisdom, courage and resolution.

And supposing, for argument's sake, such a child didn't have parents to comfort and advise? Then he is a sitting duck for everything the community feels like throwing at him.

Community is a blanket word like 'nation' or 'club'; we can so easily wrap ourselves in it and become anonymous. It must be remembered that we contribute to those prejudices as much by not protesting against them as by deliberately acting in agreement.

---

*From **Behind the Frontlines**, by Ferdinand Dennis, Victor Gollancz, London, 1988, p. 146.*

Tiger Bay: a rainbow estate

Tiger Bay is officially known as Butetown. It is a council estate of less than a square mile. Its boundaries are so well defined that once there, a visitor could quite easily forget where he [*sic*] is. On one side is a railway line and canal. On the entrance side is the main road I'd been driven along, and beyond that an old dock wall, a high barrier of crumbling gray and black stones. A small commercial area servicing Cardiff Docks stands at one end; and at the other is Cardiff city centre.

Tiger Bay has much in common with Liverpool 8. Together they represent Britain's oldest settlement of people of African descent. Tiger Bay is not so old, though. It developed along with Cardiff Docks. From the second half of the nineteenth century, Cardiff was the paramount coal-exporting city in the world. Black sailors began arriving then, but their numbers really grew after the First World War.

Along with African and West Indian sailors, Tiger Bay also became home to Asians, southern Europeans, Filipinos and Chinese. In its heyday Tiger Bay was an exciting cosmopolitan community.

---

*Extract from an article by the political correspondent of the **Guardian**, John Palmer, 19 March 1991.*

Expanding community may find itself tongue-tied

More and more 'no-vacancy' notices are appearing on the windows of the European Community's 'Tower of Babel'. Given the lengthening queue of countries seeking to join the Community, it is not difficult to see why the EC bureaucracy believes there is no room for any more languages.

Language is an extremely complex and politically sensitive issue in the EC. The present 12 member states use nine official languages – Danish,

Dutch, English, French, German, Greek, Italian, Portuguese and Spanish: plus Irish as far as the publication of constitutional and official documents is concerned.

---

*From **The Crack**, by journalist Sally Belfrage, Grafton, London, 1987, pp. 68, 71.*

On the night of Saturday, April 3rd, a gang of armed and masked men entered two houses in Ormeau Road, shooting and wounding a youth in each house before disappearing. No organization has claimed responsibility for this act. [. . .]

As the mothers in this district, we wish to make known to those responsible, that this community, Ormeau Road, has had too much death and destruction in its midst. [. . .] We want an end to death. We want to live in peace with one another and nearby communities. We want to try to provide a better life for our young people, so that they can feel wanted, so that they have self-respect, a place in the community. [. . .]

[. . .] The way the politicians have them believing, the Catholic community in these hard-line areas thinks there's no poor Protestants, that all the Protestants are working. In the Protestant hard-line areas, they think the same of the Catholics. When you hit the Women's Information Group, you discover that we're all in poverty. Let me tell you, when I rise in the morning, my first thought's not what religion I am.

---

*By sociologists Niva Yuval-Davis and Floye Anthias, in **Woman-Nation-State**, Macmillan, Basingstoke, 1989, pp. 3–4.*

The boundaries of the state

One major issue in this context is the delineation of the boundary between 'the state' and 'the nation'. There is the further problem of delineating the state from the economy and the gamut of social institutions, social groups and relations that may be conceptualised as part of 'civil society'. [. . .] The tendency in much of the literature on the state to identify it with 'the nation' is linked to the historical fact that nationalism in the West has been a central force in the development of the nation-state. The ensuing conflation of the boundary of the state with that of the nation fails to recognise that state processes can be more delimited than national processes. There are often groups of subjects (minorities;

and sometimes as in South Africa, majorities) that are excluded from participation in the state or are a special focus of state concerns as well as national liberation struggles by minorities who reside in more than one state (like the Kurds or the Palestinians). Nor does it take account of the opposite, that is that the state can extend beyond the boundary of the nation, so that the nation-state form may be replaced by a supranational structure as, for example, potentially lies in the European Community.

---

*From **Tales of Two Cities**, by D. Murphy, Penguin, Harmondsworth, 1987, p. 68.*

I wondered then – how *territorial* is all this? Now many Bradfordians object to the cooking smells of curry; a century ago they objected to the cooking smells of bacon and cabbage, the traditional Irish dish. [. . .] The sense of being invaded, especially if your own status in society provides little sense of security, must stimulate very primitive feelings. Then, to justify the hatred you find within, it becomes necessary to build up an image of a cruel, dishonest, dirty, lazy, drug-pushing community – the sort of people it is proper to despise, if you are 'decent English'.

---

*Extract from **Home is where the Heart is: Voices from Calderdale**, by R. Rooney, B. Lewis and R. Shuhle, Yorkshire Art Circus/Continuum, Castleford, West Yorkshire, 1989.*

Caring about the neighbours as much as you care for your own house is what constitutes a good neighbourhood. You can be as friendly and as nice as pie, but if you move into a nice area and paint your house black and play music all night you won't get on. Likewise if you spend all your time caring for your house and garden and you have little time for Mr Jones next door, then you're ruining the neighbourhood. It's like everything else – you need balance.

Your closest friends were the women whose kitchens faced yours over the other side of the backs. Most of our lives revolved around kitchens. That is where the tub was and where a mess could be made without too much trouble. It was the community who looked after the children. If you were going upstairs to do a bit of vacuuming then you shouted to a neighbour and she kept an eye on your child. Later in the day you would do the same for her. If a child wanted a drink he or she didn't necessarily go home but went to the nearest door. My husband reckons that a well worn track goes from our door to the biscuits.

From the text **The Family and Social Change**, by C. Rosser and C. Harris, Routledge and Kegan Paul, London, 1965, p. 12.

A different atmosphere altogether, I tell you. The children are all over the place now, and you never know where they are going next. The Mam holds them altogether somehow, but I don't know what it's going to be like when she's gone. You want to see them get on, of course – the Mam is always saying that she doesn't want to stand in their way – but we've lost something from the old days, I can tell you. They don't *cling* as we did. Once they're married, they're off. I sometimes wonder just what we've gained, taking things all round. Not that I want to put the clock back – I remember it all too well for that – the misery and the pinching and the poverty. And when I say 'poverty' I don't just mean poor, I mean *real* poverty – and no messing about. I don't want to go back to that, but I do think we've lost a lot too when I look at the way the children seem to live, hardly ever seeing one another except when they meet here at their Mam's and hardly knowing who their neighbour is. Tell you the truth I wouldn't like to live with any one of them. We lived all together in the old days in Morriston – now they all seem to live in worlds of their own.

By B. Bryan, S. Dadzie and S. Scafe, **The Heart of the Race**: Black Women's Lives in Britain, Virago, London, 1985, pp. 159–60.

It was as a result of (their) experiences of a racist police force that Black women began to organise against specific incidents of abuse and against legislation like the 'SUS' law which legitimised police brutality.

Because it was our children and community who were victims of this law, Black mothers were in the forefront of campaigns like the 'SCRAP SUS' initiative. This began in a Black woman's front room in Deptford and eventually swept throughout the Black community, uniting the generations in a call for the law to be scrapped.

[. . .] Over the next few months, we held a series of public meetings and demonstrations, wrote to the press, organised a petition, made badges – everything we could think of to publicise the SUS issue. It was important to us that the television and newspapers should acknowledge how the SUS law was being used by the police against Black kids. Eventually they began to take a very unusual interest in our grievances and they got reported quite widely in the media. That's how people outside the Black community got to know about SUS. Black mothers covered the groundwork which made SUS into a public issue. It was only after this that the local Community Relations Council decided to get off their backsides and get involved in it too. Before that, they didn't want to know.

*Extract from **The Road to Wigan Pier**, George Orwell, cited within B. Camp-*
*bell's **Wigan Pier Revisited**, Virago, London, 1984, pp. 31, 34.*

As you walk through the industrial towns you lose yourself in labyrinths of
little brick houses blackened by smoke, festering in planless chaos round miry
alleys and little cindered yards where there are stinking dustbins and lines of
grimy washing and half-ruinous w.c.s [. . .] at their very worst the Corporation houses are better than the slums they replace. The mere possession of a
bathroom and a bit of garden would outweigh almost any disadvantage. [. . .]
If people are going to live in large towns at all they must learn to live on top of
one another. But the Northern working people do not take kindly to living in
flats.

   [. . .] If George Orwell were to return to Sheffield today he'd see the
metamorphosis from spacious if spartan semi-detached suburbias to dense
tower blocks. An epitaph to this era of modern housing stands on the crest of
the city – where once there was a slope of slums, there now stands a barrage of
flats for thousands. They were hailed in their day as 'bold' and one of the most
'uncompromising' developments of the fifties, which simply meant that they
were deliberately ugly – the genre of 'brutalism'. The only concession to the
consumers is this awful, artless building is an attempt to build community
spirit into the structure, as if this, one of the few social assets of the working
class, would otherwise be given no natural home. The architects built a system
of simulated streets in the air and presumably the people are supposed to play
their part in making it all a success by playing in those streets, which measure
three metres wide. There is nothing in the 'street' other than front doors – no
shops, pubs or laundries, cafes or telephone boxes, no places to gather. So the
only point of being in the street is to come and go, which is precisely all that
people do. The designers also wanted to provide privacy. They did this not by
providing sheltered gardens or sound insulation, they just put no windows in
the street. Blind alleys.

---

*By Colin Ward, **The Child in the Country**, Bedford Square Press, London, 1988,*
pp. 34–5.

We all have, according to temperament, two contrasting perceptions of
the village.

   One is of the ancient, unchanging community, somehow insulated
from time, meeting most of its needs from its internal economy, with its
blacksmith and farrier, carpenter, builder and undertaker, general store
and carrier (maintaining a few, if regrettable contacts with the outside
world), and its life centred around the pub and the church, with its
rectory whence the rector's wife and daughters dispensed charity to the
deserving poor.

   The other perception of the village is of the contemporary village,
inhabited by commuters, weekenders and the retired, with the indige-
nous population confined to the estate on the fringe, where the smithy
is now a petrol station, the pub is full of fake beams and pool tables,

while of the two general stores one is an antique shop and the other a wine bar and restaurant.

A whole shelf of books describes the transition from one of these perceptions to the other, dating the change from the time when the authors ceased to be children. Thus, 'During the 1940s the scene was virtually as it had been for generations, apart from one or two mechanical innovations, with men working on the land, boys following in their fathers' footsteps, and women busying themselves with the home and family. Characters who had been moulded by the hardness of life, the machinations of moneymaking, or the infidelity of the elements, lived and worked together in the village to form a real community. [. . .]

[. . .] a whole series of important points needs to be made about the view of history this represents.

The first is that far more devastating changes occurred in rural life at the time when landowners pursued their policy of enclosure; the second is that the whole thrust of the agricultural industry for 150 years has been to dispense with labour, and that the days when it was possible for us to see 'boys following in their fathers' footsteps' ended long before the author I have quoted was born, while the days when girls wanted to follow in their mothers' footsteps, not into domesticity but into domestic service, ended when they realised that there were alternatives to the exploitation involved. A new generation of domestic employers brings into English rural life servants from the poor half of the world, sending their International Postal Orders back home from the village post office just to support their families. They are villages where the crucial decision about whether a sub-post office remains viable depends on such global accidents.

The third point to be made is that villages were never hermetic communities: there always were comings and goings; and the fourth is that rural settlements have always consisted of several different communities who happened to occupy the same territorial space. The gap between them in the past was infinitely greater than the gap between different rural residents today. The class gradations of English society (and to an even greater degree in the Anglo-ascendancy in Wales, Scotland and Ireland) ensured that village people and village children lived in a world entirely different from that of their betters (*sic*).

Extract from a paper by Harriet Cain and Nira Yuval-Davis in **Critical Social Policy***, Vol. 10, No. 2, 1990, pp. 6–7.*

The 'equal opportunities' community

In early 'Race Relations' legislation the term 'community' was adopted from its common usage in British social policy of the time which tended to use it in relation to working class neighbourhoods, in a romantic and conservative fashion. However, during the 60s and 70s, the American meaning was imported, in which 'community' was used to describe ethnic minorities (Anthias and Yuval-Davis, forthcoming). This created inconsistencies and confusions which became highlighted during the 80s.

The confusion with relation to the boundaries of 'the community' is crucial in understanding some of the issues which have bogged down and have created obstructions, divisions and frustrations in anti-racist struggles. Is 'the community' everybody who lives in a certain area, is 'the community' a particular grouping conscious of itself as a grouping or is 'the community' paradoxically, all those who have been excluded from feeling part of 'the community'? We would argue that in the specific sphere of the 'race relations industry' and in the urban politics in Britain of the 80s, the hegemonic answer to 'who is "the community"' has made three conceptual jumps and the following conflations:

(a) From focusing the attention on disadvantaged sections of the population, motivated by populist and democratic aspirations, 'the community' in actuality has become to a large extent reduced to the categories of 'Equal Opportunities' – previously excluded to a large extent from definitions of 'the community'.
(b) From focusing on the 'Equal Opportunities' disadvantaged sections of the population, the politics of 'the community' have become reduced to the voluntary sector and local government sponsored organisations which aspire to represent and serve them.
(c) From focusing on the disadvantaged section of the population, 'community' has become reduced to a large extent to the 'professional community activists'.

We shall now turn to looking at some of the ways these conflations have occurred.

Social policy conceptions of 'the community' have often ignored marginal sections in the population. The intimate, close and rooted image of 'the community' implied a homogeneity composing family, neighbourhood and parish, all of whom conformed to an hegemonic culture, often English, and usually working class. It was against this mould that the 'popular planning' approach, heralded by the GLC and other radical local authorities has been developed in the late 70s and early 80s. They struggled to include in this vision of 'the community' all those previously excluded, and which, at least in some areas of the 'inner city', constitute a major part of the local population, be it single parents, gays, blacks, refugees, etc. However, in doing so, their assumption has been that all the various equal opportunities groupings, whether gay, black, refugee etc., share intrinsically common objectives. This, however, brought new contradictions in its wake, as the various groupings viewed themselves in very different and autonomous terms, often creating conflict and competition as a result of the ways the social planners had constructed them.

---

*Personal account in **Inventing Ourselves**, a collection of accounts from the Hall Carpenter Archives, Lesbian Oral History Group, Routledge, London, 1989, pp. 105–6.*

Gilli Salvat:
No-one had ever done youth work with young lesbians before, so it was all highly controversial. We were taking a hell of a risk with everything we did so we had to work very carefully and strictly, but it was a wonderful experience. For the first time as youth workers we could be entirely 'out' and feel that we were truly working for the development of 'our' young people. It's great to see them now, out and being proud and productive people.

My work is [. . .] threatened by Thatcher's government by its attack on lesbian and gay rights and local democracy. Not only has my job been at risk by the cuts in local government spending, but the introduction of Section 28 of the Local Government Act. This Section directly threatens the community that lesbians and gays have struggled so hard to build in the last twenty years.

---

*Personal accounts from **Walking After Midnight**, Hall Carpenter Archives, Gay Men's Oral History Group, Routledge, London, 1989, pp. 184, 211, 217.*

Zahid Dar:
In mid '82, I went to a weekend of gay workshops at South Bank Poly where people were saying what the gay community needed was a centre as a focus point for the community; a while after that there was talk that the GLC were willing to fund one. When I went to my first meeting, I couldn't believe my ears. You know, at County Hall in November '82, people talking about a gay centre.

Lesbians and gays support the miners

David Donovan of the Dulais mining community:
You have worn our badge, 'Coal not Dole', and you know what harassment means, as we do. Now we will pin your badge on us, we

will support you. It won't change overnight, but now 140,000 miners know that there are other causes and other problems. We know about Blacks, and gays, and nuclear disarmament. And we will never be the same.

Mike Jackson:
We obviously had a lot of political fighting to do within our own community. One cry which was always a bit hurtful was, 'Why are you doing all this for the miners? There's people dying of AIDS and the lesbian and gay community needs support.' For a start, a lot of people in LGSM did lots of things for the community anyway. We didn't support the miners with regard to whether they supported us or not. We supported them because we were socialists, but we were attempting to be 'out' to them and we hoped there would be a dialogue.

———

*Account from **Generations of Memories**, by Jewish Women in London Group, The Women's Press, London, 1989, pp. 6–7.*

For those of us who grew up in Britain, the school history we learned was the one in which English kings and one or two queens led a triumphant march from the Stone Age to the present day. It was followed by a history of the Greeks and Romans which didn't mention their occupation of the Jews' land and the consequent oppression of the Jews, or the contribution the Jews made to resistance against their empires. The rest of school history was a cosy anglocentric celebration of a past in which the other peoples of the world were by and large either subject peoples or enemies. Usually, that history stopped at the First World War. And the ordinary people of Britain were presented as a monolithically white, English-speaking mass who either lined the streets to cheer the great or erupted dangerously as mobs.

Some of us encountered Jewish history at school in the shape of scripture lessons; some of us went to *cheder* as well, where we also learned to read Hebrew. This history was largely based on Bible stories of the tribes of Ancient Israel. Where women played any part at all, they were just as likely to have been temptresses and schemers, like Jezebel and Delilah, as heroines, like Esther and Deborah.

Our mothers' stories were very different. For most of us, 'our' history was one which included flight from persecution and sometimes the threat of death, and subsequent migration from country to country. There are few of us who have grown in the same countries as our mothers, and some of them in turn had come to live in different countries from their mothers or their grandmothers. The stories they had to tell us were often of the ways of their own families as part of the

Jewish communities of Middle and Eastern Europe; of lives sometimes lived in poverty and fear, more rarely in an insecure prosperity. There were also stories of lives strong in resisting oppression, and others which told of becoming part of a middle-class establishment, which later only too readily turned its back on them.

Through these stories many of us learned that it was the women in our families who had so often been the ones responsible for taking on those movements across continents to safe homes. It was the women who kept the memory of who and what had been in the past. For those of us who came from religious backgrounds, it was often the women who found ways to give us a consciousness of Jewishness as more than a religion, a nationality, a personal identity. For them, it meant a way of life which shaped every aspect of their existence.

[. . .] The lives of those women born and brought up in Britain (let alone those born and brought up in Europe) in some respects resemble those of gentile women of the same generation, but they differ significantly in others. The terrain in which those lives have been mapped out is different. [. . .] The view from a little terraced house may be the same, but the interior view is different.

From **The Jerusalem Bible**, *edited by A. Jones, Popular Edition, Darton, Longman and Todd, London.*

Introduction to the Acts of the Apostles

Acts is in the form of a single continuous narrative. It begins with the birth and the growth of the primitive Christian community in Jerusalem and tells of the founding of the community in Antioch by Hellenist Jews and the conversion of St Paul; it goes on to show the spread of the Church outside Palestine through the missionary travels of Paul and ends with his captivity in A.D. 61–63. [. . .]

32 The whole group of believers was united, heart and soul: no-one claimed for his own use anything that he had, as everything they owned was held in common.
34 None of their members was ever in want, as all those who owned land or houses would sell them, and bring the money from them
35 To present it to the apostles; it was then distributed to any members who might be in need.

---

*Extract from **There Ain't No Black in the Union Jack**, by Paul Gilroy, Hutchinson, London, 1987, pp. 233–5.*

For the social movement of blacks in Britain, the context in which [. . .] demands have been spontaneously articulated has been supplied by a political language premised on notions of community. Though it reflects the concentration of black people, the terms refers to far more than mere place or population. It has a moral dimension and its use evokes a rich complex of symbols surrounded by a wider cluster of meanings. The historical memory of progress from slave to citizen, actively cultivated in the present from resources provided by the past, endows it with an aura of tradition. Community, therefore, signifies not just a distinctive political ideology but a particular set of values and norms in everyday life: mutuality, co-operation, identification and symbiosis. For black Britain, all these are centrally defined by the need to escape and transform the forms of subordination which bring 'races' into being. Yet they are not limited by that objective. The disabling effects of racial categorisation are themselves seen as symbols of the other unacceptable attributes of 'racial capitalism'. The evident autonomy of racism from production relations demands that the reappropriation of production is not pursued independently of the transformation of capitalist social relations as a whole. The social bond implied by use of the term 'community' is created in the practice of collective resistance to the encroachments of reification, 'racial' or otherwise. It prefigures that transformation in the name of a radical, democratic, anti-racist populism.

[. . .] Community is as much about difference as it is about similarity and identity. It is a relational idea which suggests, for British blacks at least, the idea of antagonism – domination and subordination between one community and another. The word directs analysis to the boundary between these groups. It is a boundary which is presented primarily by symbolic means and therefore a broad range of meanings can co-exist around it, reconciling individuality and communality and competing definitions of what the movement is about.

---

*Entry for the word 'community' in Raymond Williams's **Keywords**, Flamingo, 1983, pp. 75–6.*

Community has been in the language since C14. [. . .] It became established in English in a range of senses: (i) the commons or common people, as distinguished from those or rank (C14–C17); (ii) a state or organised society, in its later uses relatively small (C14–); (iii) the people of a district (C18–); (iv) the quality of holding something in common, as in **community of interests**, **community of goods** (C16–); (v) a sense of common identity and characteristics (C16–). It will be seen that senses (i) to (iii) indicate actual social groups; senses (iv) and (v) a particular quality of relationship. [. . .] From C17 there are signs of the distinction which became especially important from C19, in which **community** was felt to be more immediate than SOCIETY (q.v.), although it must be remembered that *society* itself had this more immediate sense until C18, and *civil society* [. . .] was, like *society* and *community* in these uses, originally an attempt to distinguish the body of direct relationships from the organised establishment of *realm* or *state*. From C19 the sense of immediacy or locality was strongly developed in the context of larger and more complex industrial societies. **Community** was the word normally chosen for experiments in an alternative kind of group-living. It is still so used and has been joined, in a more limited sense, by **commune** (the French *commune* – the smallest administrative division – and the German *Gemeinde* – a civil and ecclesiastical division – had interacted with each other) and with **community**, and also passed into socialist thought (especially *commune*) and into sociology (especially *Gemeinde*) to express particular kinds of social relations. The contrast, increasingly expressed in C19, between the more direct, more total and therefore more significant relationships of **community** and the more formal, more abstract and more instrumental relationships of *state*, or of *society* in its modern sense, was influentially formalised by Tonnies (1887) as a contrast between *Gemeinschaft* and *Gesellschaft*, and these terms are now sometimes used, untranslated, in other languages. A comparable distinction is evident in C20 uses of **community**. In some uses this has been given a polemical edge, as in **community politics**, which is distinct not only from *national politics* but from formal *local politics* and normally involves various kinds of direct action and direct local organization, 'working directly with people', as which it is distinct from 'service to the **community**', which has an older sense of voluntary work supplementary to official provision or paid service.

The complexity of **community** thus relates to the difficult interaction between the tendencies originally distinguished in the historical development: on the one hand the sense of direct common concern; on the other hand the materialization of various forms of common organization, which may or may not adequately express this. **Community** can be the warmly persuasive word to describe an existing set of relationships, or the warmly persuasive word to describe an alternative set of relationships. What is most important, perhaps, is that unlike all other terms of social organization (*state, nation, society*, etc.) it seems never to be used unfavourably, and never to be given any positive opposing or distinguishing term.

3

Representations of Community

JOANNA BORNAT

I am satisfied that the picture I have tried to draw was neither exceptional nor one-sided. Talking to middle-class people who did not live in working-class districts, I find that few realise how bad conditions were such a comparatively short time ago.

(Jasper, 1969, p. 127)

Everyone can write a book. We believe that by enabling people to speak for themselves we can make our own history.

(Noakes, 1975)

These two quotations come from early publications in what tends to be described loosely as 'community publishing'. Each is typical of ideas that have driven a popular literary movement since the late 1960s. Among A. S. Jasper's reasons for writing is the desire to inform, to reveal and to reach out to others distanced from him by time and class. The second quotation, champions the cause of popular self-expression and the appropriation by working-class people of a discipline, history. Groups like Centerprise and QueenSpark are representative of the most self-conscious of local publishing ventures of the 1970s and 1980s.

Among the most radical of the community publishing groups, those with membership in the Federation of Worker Writers and Community Publishers, the language used to explain aims and practice is the language of representation, empowerment, self-determination, appropriation and creativity. Other agencies, with less radical philosophies – libraries, archives, museums, schools, colleges, social services – have followed suit with locally produced accounts published in accessible formats.

This literature emerges through a variety of processes of production. Community publishers are frequently given finished manuscripts to be considered for publication. Some represent many hours of detailed individual solitary reconstruction of a personal past, or the need to commit feelings, emotions, experience into a literary form. Sometimes the final publication is the result of a lengthy and supportive collaboration between people with a professional training in writing or teaching and others who at a relatively late stage in life are discovering their ability to express themselves in written words. Whatever the origin of the account, the process of production from manuscript to printed page is one of collaborative activity. In practice the process varies from co-operative groupwork for the majority of groups affiliated to the Federation, to a form of benign editorial decision-making by one person in most other cases.

The result is usually the small booklet, its narrative drawn from first-hand experience, typically of working-class life usually located in urban areas during the early and middle decades of the twentieth century. This genre includes poetry and fiction, which is more subversive of myths of community, more critical of the individual's relations to different communities. What I want to look at here, through an examination of over 50 such narratives, is community history writing. I have excluded from consideration collections of reminiscence produced by the commercial book trade. The focus here is on booklets with origins in collective traditions of publishing or which have in the main emerged through local rather than national initiatives.

Implicitly and explicitly, the theme of community runs through these published narratives. If these accounts have such a powerful appeal then we should perhaps consider what their ideas of community comprise. I want to consider some issues which seem to me to be relevant. I want to look at solidarity, interest and identity as the values and meanings of community in community publishing and to consider the question of representivity and exclusions. Finally I want to draw out some implications for the practice of community history writing in general and reflect on the question of myth.

3.1   The values and meanings of community

In those days, too, there was real neighbourliness. You see, you might be four or five families in that house, and perhaps the one at the bottom would make some tea and she'd shout up the stairs 'I've just made a cup of tea – coming down?' And they'd more or less take it in turn each day, and if there was anyone in real dire straits, and couldn't pay their way, I've known a neighbour take their own sheets off the bed, wash 'em and pawn 'em to help them out. That's how it was in those days – real good neighbours. I mean they'd never let anyone starve. We never used to lock our front doors – not a bit of string or nothing, the house was open day and night. The gas meters were on the stairs, and we never lost a ha'penny. There were real criminals of course – but never against their own.

(White, 1988, p. 26)

It is possible to find regional variants of this passage from the Euston Road area of north London in verbal and written accounts of urban working-class communities throughout Britain. The values are explicit: communality, 'never let anyone starve'; solidarity, 'never against their own'; honesty, 'we never lost a ha'penny'; interdependency, 'take it in turn each day'. They are pinned down physically in descriptions of community as place and in the detailed restoration of domestic life. The details of the physical and spatial fabric of community life come in descriptions of house interiors, streets of leisure, entertainment, education, welfare and employment experiences. Communities are rarely mapped out with street plans or in terms of systems of administration or local politics. The elements of community described in community publishing are rooted in domestic work, farms, mills, mines and the strategies developed for survival in country and town. The accounts describe domestic skills and the interdependency which adversity requires. Elizabeth Roberts, in her study of working-class women's lives in the north-west between 1890 and 1940, argues that these routines and skills operated on a neighbourhood basis and extended further than the blood ties of family to neighbours. Drawing on oral evidence she argues that remembered communities were not areas or neighbourhoods but often 'no more than three streets' (Roberts, 1984, p. 184).

Where privacy was physically and economically a luxury, then the reality of community life is not always positively recalled:

Everybody knew everybody. They'd peep out from behind the curtains and say, 'There goes May Sleeth, she's off . . . You could imagine it, could you? 'She's off again, up to no good'. If you spoke to a boyfriend or if you let the boy bring you to the corner of the street, it was really bad. Actually, my parents did not like me to take boyfriends home.

(Davey, 1980, p. 7)

Community could be an oppressive experience if remembered from the perspective of some of its more junior members, who were without the power that economic or parental status conferred.

Community as a system of shared values and as a spatial arrangement of supportive, if sometimes intrusive, structures is well delineated in the accounts. Community as shared interest is less well described. Class interests, depicted through personal accounts of resistance and action, do recur, most usually attached to workplace and industrial life in accounts from men. The Co-operative Movement appears as a functioning interest group which was akin to community in its inclusiveness (Salt *et al.*, 1983, p. 6).

Collective interest tends to be recalled through paid work experiences or through political action. The General Strike is most vividly recalled by those who were directly involved, miners and transport workers predominantly. It is the oral account which allows the detailed workings of the strike as a process of social interactions to emerge:

> With the strike of course it meant that as a youngster of 15 I was liberated from the pit. All my pals of fifteen and sixteen – all of us – we were really liberated. It was a magnificent glorious summer so that we spent the time more or less tramping and getting into Newcastle with collecting boxes and getting support in places like Gateshead from those people who were working.
>
> (Durham Strong Words Collective, 1979, p. 58)

Community history as the retrieved history of an interest group recurs in the many accounts of individual women's lives. Accounts from children of their own mother's struggles and triumphs, managing budgets, drunken partners, credit arrangements and family crises, together construct a picture of working-class women which is not one of passive domestic isolation. Community life is described through the dimensions of family life in these accounts, consequently it is the memory of women in the family and of survival and protection which predominates. Robert William Harvey grew up in Bristol in the 1930s with his mother and half-brother:

> Mother was better; so we could go home again. How lovely, we were free again to see one another. Mother could not go away for a rest. One came out of hospital in those days, worked, and got on with it. No sick pay and whatnots. We had become poor. The rent had to be paid. We had no money coming in. It was time to sell the things we had that could be sold, while Mother got better so that she could work longer hours.
>
> (Harvey, 1976, pp. 15–16)

Communities of interest do not appear with much frequency; possibly the revival of a declared interest depends on the reconstruction of a collective experience by those who had membership in certain events, campaigns or movements. But communities of identity are strongly represented. The choice of a title may be a selling point, but it also indicates a sense of belonging: '*The Island*' (Centerprise, 1979), *Millfields Memories* (Knight, 1976), *Reminiscences of a Bradford Mill Girl* (Newbery, 1980), *Shipley Fowk Talking* (Shipley Community History Group, n.d.). A sense of identity expressed simply as belonging is used in more complex ways, however. Between older and younger members of the working class, communities of identity confirm pride in survival and resilience.

They may also induce a unity that intervening decades may have shaken. The result may be the reconstruction of a white remembered past.

3.2 Community exclusions and individual invisibility

Community publishing broadens our understanding of the past by including the experience of those whose accounts play little part in a public history of nation and state. In terms of process and outcomes it challenges the norm in publishing. But how representative of community experience are the communities portrayed? I want to go on to look at the issue of exclusions and the extent to which some members may have become invisible through the process of recall.

Within community publishing there are a growing number of examples of accounts drawing on the experience of minority ethnic and racialised groups. Early accounts published drew on work produced in literacy and English centres (Bandali, 1977; Elbaja, 1978; Gordon, 1979). Later accounts from Jewish writers in London and Manchester (Spitalfields Books, 1979; Spector, 1988; Cohen, 1989) have been followed by accounts drawn from manuscripts and from interviews, some produced in dual language text, from Polish, Greek Cypriot and Iranian people (Lin Wong, 1989; Kyriacou, 1990; Fahey, 1991). These have contributed a multicultural perspective to community publishing.

Community publishing's growing multiculturalism counteracts its tendency otherwise to present a uniquely white working-class and Western urban image of community life. Taken as a whole the literature presents a more accurately representative perspective than the literature of commercial publishing. Taken separately the books draw on strongly delineated and separated social and cultural traditions of family and community life, even when traced through the dislocations of migration and rehousing. Nevertheless, the experience of exclusion and division tends to be unevenly described even amongst those accounts drawn from the minority communities. Most can testify to the existence of discrimination or racism. Teresa Burke recalls working in London between the wars:

> On my half day, my sister would come and meet me in Lewisham and we'd go and look round the shops. My sister had a habit of looking at the boards in Lewisham, and on the poster it would say 'NO IRISH NEED APPLY'.
> (Schweitzer, 1989)

What these accounts rarely reveal is how people felt about these exclusions within that community. An exception is a collection of dual language accounts by Asian women. Mandira's story describes the experience of lived exclusion vividly:

> Though I was not fluent in my English and been home whole day with my son I tried to make friendship with my neighbour, as she was on her own, also as same age as my aunt [who spent all her] life in our family when she became widow at age 13 years. I felt concern about her well being. We used the same corridor. If I had not seen her I knocked at her door and asked about her health and whether she needs any shopping. I was shocked when she thought I am being nosey and became rude. I started to go out more meet few neighbours on the street and came to know how horrible inconsiderate noisy people we are.
>
> (Centerprise, 1984)

A Traveller from the Westway site in London turns round the idea of community, invoking it as a force for exclusion:

> The first time when this site was opened the community here broke this site up for keeping the Travellers from getting in, to settled [sic] down. The council repaired that and they broke it down again.
>
> (Kyriacou, 1990)

What frames the experience is the constraining force of an opposing community whose identity is delineated as other, by means of power and hence with the ability to determine inclusion. Division is described in separated accounts. In the memory of white working-class people, issues of race and ethnicity are in the main absent. For instance, children might earn money lighting fires for Jewish households on Friday nights. An Irish woman has fond memories of working as a maid in a Jewish household, but the interface between the experience is described in terms of observed difference, not by familiarity or awareness of experience (Centerprise, 1979, p. 23; Schweitzer, 1989, p. 62).

The accounts I have looked at so far provide a key to identifying exclusions on the basis of race or ethnicity. What all the communities of community publishing still lack are accounts from those whose participation in community life has been determined and shaped by other dominant, socially determined divisions. I want to go on to look at the experience of physical and mental impairment.

A search through more than 50 booklets produced in the community publishing tradition reveals little to indicate that physically or mentally disabled people had membership in these communities. Looking for references to disability, there are few accounts from people with either physical or mental impairment. Considering that the literature draws on a period of time when most children with disabilities either stayed at home or lived in the community (Hurt, 1988), it is surprising that neither they nor their family members appear to be included in the reconstruction of the experience of community. There are accounts of living in children's homes and in the workhouse (Harvey, 1976, pp. 22–3; Crump, 1980; Peckham People's History, 1983, pp. 85–6; Schweitzer, 1989, pp. 51–6). There are many passing references to disabled siblings, relatives and, occasionally, neighbours. However, the view of the community from the perspective of someone with first-hand experience is relatively rare. Hugh Macdonald is one of the few people who writes as someone with disabilities. He was born with spina bifida:

> I was in a pram till I was 8. Mother used to take me to Leith Links to watch the cricket. I was only at the pictures once in my life, and that was when I was 12 – in Shettlesfon to see 'Pinocchio' (1940). I remember saying, 'I'm too old to go to the pictures' so I never was back.
>
> (Griffiths and Vestri, 1985, pp. 10–11)

As with the accounts of minority ethnic experience, the opportunity for representation seems to emerge through separate reconstruction. Working with groups of people with learning difficulties has enabled stories of exclusion and personal history to emerge. Invisible people re-emerge in the telling of their own stories. Margaret remembers:

> When I was a little girl I was put away. I was 14 and a half. I went to Cell Barnes to live because they said I was backward. My dad refused to sign the papers for me to go, but the police came and said he would have to go to prison if he didn't. I cried when I had to go with the Welfare Officer.
>
> (Atkinson, 1991, p. 45)

At the time of writing, one of the first community-published account of gay and lesbian life was about to appear. Published by QueenSpark, *Daring Hearts* is an account of gay and lesbian life in Brighton after the Second World War. Once again, however, a separate approach to recall and writing has provided the basis for community history.

3.3   Community myth?

Without the separately generated accounts, the image of community that emerges through the community publishing is one that is supportive, if at times stiflingly so. It is one in which problems are resolved through changes in economic or political fortune. Family finances improved as children grew up and brought in wages. War brought a degree of social change and opportunities for new employment and housing. The community changes its shape physically as people marry, go their separate ways or die. But in the recall and the writing it persists as a remembered and indivisible whole. Raphael Samuel argues that with its devotion to place, community history has steered itself clear of those issues that suggest the complexity of human relationships (Samuel, 1979). And it seems that it takes something more akin to a secondary analysis of interview data to bring out social class differences (Werbner, 1980). For some the whole idea of community history is better avoided as a species of persistent false consciousness (The Work Group, 1976, p. 18).

If community publishing has found the representation of difference and division difficult to include, surely we need to look for explanations as to why this may be, and whether this matters or invalidates the accounts given.

The urge to represent the past in the present is understandable, but by focusing on the remembered topography of community and family life what we may be ignoring are the parallel continuities of value and perception. If memories of community seem to exclude the non-conforming experience of the person with disability or of the gay man or lesbian woman, this is because past inhibitions and prejudices are continuous, though differently expressed, with the present. Community publishing looks back to a past with an understanding that is continuous with that past. A mother in York who describes bringing up her disabled daughter may evoke strong resonances for similar mothers and children 50 years later:

> We had no idea she was handicapped for about three years . . . and it was rather hard then because . . . nobody seemed to know – they didn't do much in that way with spastics, I don't think they understood . . . right in the middle of the war. . . . If you'd anyone handicapped when Elizabeth was young there were a lot of people who feared you; they didn't mean to be but they avoided you because I think they were frightened they might get involved.
>
> (York Oral History Project, 1987, p. 56)

Monica Jules' account reminds us of the isolation of the parent of a child with learning difficulties in the 1980s:

> Afterwards I was told my son is autistic which is a kind of mental handicap. It was a great shock to me. I could not believe it. They said he is not a normal child. There was nothing I could do to help my son except try my best to look after him until I can get more help and support from the social service.
>
> (Jules, 1987, p. 41)

Her account, with others (Beaumont Writers' Group, n.d.), helps to bring out a more complete understanding, but they stand alone as separate experiences unless we are encouraged to incorporate them into a more complex community history.

To be unaware of our own prejudices and blinkered perceptions is not unusual; however, it may be that the processes of community publishing encourage such tendencies.

The generation of accounts and their assembly into either a single narrative or a collectively produced anthology may preclude reflection and individual introspection. Even when the account is not collectively produced, the author's words will, once published, be subjected to local collective scrutiny. While separately organised groups may willingly and freely discuss and disclose experiences of racism, or of discrimination on grounds of disability, it is unlikely that a mixed group could encourage similar openness (see Gray, 1984). What seems to be a quality of the membership of groups producing community publishing is their similarity of background and experience. Whether worked on alone or as a group, the result is an emphasis on particular sets of shared memories. I want to go on to look briefly at processes in collective reconstruction as a means to understanding why these patterns may be recurring.

Discourse analysis reveals the way in which collective memory is reconstructed through cues and strategies in conversation (Middleton and Edward, 1990). Those community publishing texts that have relied on the generation of accounts from discussion might find, from analysis, that there are observable patterns in the discussion, patterns that relate as much to the social interactions of the group members as they do to the content of what is being discussed (Boden and Bielby, 1983).

Another issue arises in relation to the process of interviewing or in the taking of oral accounts. Stories that are collected in a group or in one-off interviews may suffer from the lack of opportunity to improve or to amend (Jewish Women in London Group, 1989, pp. 16–17). Jocelyn Cornwell's work in Bethnal Green (Cornwell, 1984, pp. 16, 40–54) suggests that both the frequency of the interview and the way in which questions were framed determined whether or not a 'public' or a 'private' account was given to her. In public accounts, which tended to be given at an early stage, the description of community in the past was one that conformed well to that given of Somers Town, quoted earlier. Subsequently, and if people were invited to tell a story rather than to answer a direct question, they would give what she describes as a 'private' account. From this it became clear that community life also included rivalries, snobberies, fights and a willingness to ignore other people's troubles.

My final point relates to the issue of life stage and shared perspectives. In the main the contributors to community publishing are older people recalling experience from their younger lives. For family and community this has obvious implications. A child or a younger person's view of community relationships may well be limited to their knowledge, feelings and interest at the time. But when this is overlaid with a perspective from a stage in life when change and loss may be major preoccupations, the perspectives from the two periods may be difficult to relate. Dorothy Jerrome's work highlights the importance that friendships between peers have for older women (Jerrome, 1990). Using the sharing of experience to build friendships has become part of the repertoire of social-work skills in work with older people (Fielden, 1990). While the positive values of such consolidating approaches must be appreciated, it is also important to be aware of negative payoffs: the formation of closed groups, the construction of a comfortable shared perspective.

Do the underlying meanings of conversational strategies, the hazards of interviewing and the dilemmas of group management suggest that community publishing is involved in myth construction? The answer to this is almost certainly yes. At an earlier and more defensive stage in community publishing this might have been a difficult perspective to admit to. More recent work by oral historians suggests that by ignoring the creation of myth we impoverish our understanding of the past and of ourselves (Samuel and Thompson, 1990).

Constructions of community life necessarily include stories which may have the status of art or fable. At another level, the symbolism, shape and content reflects particular preoccupations of generation and opportunity, often the amalgam of perspectives from quite separate ends of the lifespan. To accept the role of mythic reconstruction is to widen the significance of the accounts. They become not only a substantive form in their own right, they are also indicators of feeling and of perspective. To understand the contribution of myth is to focus on what is neglected as much as what is included in published accounts. If community publishing neglects issues raised by the divisions and exclusions of community life then this may tell us something about those recalled communities and about the processes of community history writing today. Perhaps, as Alessandro Portelli suggests, fabulation helps us to understand what the hopes and fears of the older generation are and to recognise continuities and discontinuities in human action (Portelli, 1988).

Acknowledgement

Thanks to Al Thomson of the Federation of Worker Writers and Community Publishers for his suggestions and supportive critical approach.

References

Atkinson, D. (ed.) (1991) 'Past times' (unpublished).

Bandali, S. (1977) *Small Accidents: the Autobiography of a Ugandan Asian*, Tulse Hill School, London.

Beaumont Writers' Group (n.d.) *The Beaumont Writers' Group*, Gatehouse, Manchester.

Boden, D. and Bielby, D. del Vento (1983) 'The past as resource: a conversational analysis of Elderly Talk', *Human Development*, Vol. 26, No. 6, pp. 308–19.

Centerprise (1979) *'The Island': the Life and Death of an East London Community 1870–1970*, Centerprise, London.

Centerprise (1984) *Breaking the Silence: Writing by Asian Women*, Centerprise, London.

Cohen, H. (1989) *Bagels with Babushka*, Gatehouse, Manchester.

Cornwell, J. (1984) *Hard-Earned Lives: Accounts of Health and Illness from East London*, Tavistock, London.

Crump, J (1980) *The Ups and Downs of Being Born*, Vassall Neighbourhood Council, London.

Davey, D. (1980 *A Sense of Adventure*, SE1 People's History Project, London.

Durham Strong Words Collective (1979) *But the World Goes on the Same: Changing Times in Durham Pit Villages*, Erdesdun Publications, Whitley Bay.

Elbaja, M. (1978) *My Life*, Shoreditch School, London.

Fahey, P. (1991) *The Irish in London: Photographs and Memories*, Centerprise, London.

Fielden, M. A. (1990) 'Reminiscence as a therapeutic intervention with sheltered housing residents: a comprehensive study', *British Journal of Social Work*, Vol. 20, pp. 21–44.

Gordon, I. (1979) *Going where the Work is*, Hackney Reading Centre, London.

Gray, R. (1984) 'History is what you want to say': publishing people's history – the experience of Peckham People's History Group', *Oral History*, Vol. 12, No. 2, autumn, pp. 38–46.

Griffiths, S. and Vestri, P. (1985) *Changed Days: More Stories and Reminiscences from the Prestonfield Remembers Group*, Edinburgh University Settlement.

Harvey, R. W. (1976) *A Bristol Childhood*, WEA Western District.

Hurt, J. S. (1988) 'The inter-war years', in *Outside the Mainstream: A History of Special Education*, Batsford, London.

Jasper, A. S. (1969) *A Hoxton Childhood*, Centerprise, London.

Jerrome, D. (1990) 'Intimate relationships', in Bond, J. and Coleman, P. (eds) *Ageing in Society: an Introduction to Social Gerontology*, Sage, London.

Jewish Women in London Group (1989) *Generations of Memories: Voices of Jewish Women*, The Women's Press, London.

Jules, M. (1987) *Wesley My Only Son*, Hackney Reading Centre, London.

Knight, D. (1976) *Millfields Memories*, Centerprise, London.

Kyriacou, S. (ed.) (1989–90) *Travelling Light: Poles on Foreign Soil; The Irish in Exile: Stories of Emigration; In Exile: Iranian Recollections; The Forgotten Lives: Gypsies and Travellers on the Westway Site; The Motherland Calls: African–Caribbean Experiences; Xeni: Greek Cypriots in London*; Ethnic Communities Oral History Project.

Lin Wong, M. (1989) *Chinese Liverpudlians*, Liver Press, Liverpool.

Middleton, D. and Edward, D. (eds) (1990) 'Conversational remembering: a psychological approach', in *Collective Remembering*, Sage, London.

Newbery, M. (1980) *Reminiscence of a Bradford Mill Girl*, Bradford Metropolitan Council.

Noakes, D. (1975) From a foreword note in *'The Town Beehive': a Young Girl's Lot, Brighton 1910–1934*, QueenSpark, Brighton.

Peckham People's History (1983) *The Times of Our Lives*, Peckham People's Publishing Project, London.

Portelli, A. (1988) 'Uchronic dreams: working class memory and possible worlds', *Oral History*, Vol. 16, No. 2, pp. 46–56.

Roberts, E. (1984) *A Woman's Place: an Oral History of Working Class Women, 1890–1940*, Blackwell, Oxford.

Salt, C., Schweitzer, P. and Wilson, M. (1983) *Of Whole Heart Cometh Hope*, Age Exchange, London.

Samuel, R. (1979) 'Urban history and local history', *History Workshop*, Vol. 8, Autumn, p. vi.

Samuel, R. and Thompson, P. (1990) *The Myths We Live By*, Routledge, London.

Schweitzer, P. (ed.) (1989) *Across the Irish Sea*, Age Exchange, London.

Shipley Community History Group (n.d.) *Shipley Fowk Talking*, Bradford.

Spector, C. (1988) *Volla Volla Jew Boy*, Centerprise, London.

Spitalfields Books (1979) *Where's Your Horns? People of Spitalfields Talk About the Evacuation*, Spitalfields Books, London.

The Work Group (1976) 'A critique of "community studies" and its role in social thought', University of Birmingham, Centre for Contemporary Cultural Studies.

Werbner, P. (1980) 'Rich man poor man – or a community of suffering: heroic motifs in Manchester Pakistani life histories', *Oral History*, Vol. 8, No. 1, pp. 43–8.

White, M. (1988) *And Grandmother's Bed Went Too: Poor but Happy in Somers Town*, St Pancras Housing Association in Camden, London.

York Oral History Project (1987) *York Memories at Home: Personal Accounts of Domestic Life in York*, York, Oral History Project.

4

Women and Community

FIONA WILLIAMS

It is now a common observation that the invisible threat in government reports and policy documents that ties the notion of 'community' to that of 'care' is, by and large, women (see, for example, chapters 11, 14 and 18). It is mainly, though not entirely, women who form the focus for the dynamics of care and support. But what of 'community'? Are women principal actors here, too? And what does 'community' mean for women? In this chapter I suggest that community has different and contradictory meanings for women. Community may represent the space where women can begin to define and determine their own needs and conditions for existence. At the same time it may also represent the outer limits of women's restriction to domestic duties and limited access to an independent income and way of life – where women 'know their place'.

4.1 Space and place

Community has a particular significance for many women. It is the point of negotiation over public provision; it is a site of organisation and struggle over welfare issues; and it is the arena of paid, unpaid and low-paid work. As such, community represents an overlap of the public world of production and politics with the private world of home and care. It is the point at which women's private business becomes translated into public issues – from dependant into claimant; from unpaid to paid worker; from personal into political.

The notion of community, though, is complex, and can mean different things to different women. When women organise collectively for better child-care provision, for safer roads and streets, or when they organise to provide some of these things themselves, then community becomes women's *space*. That is, community becomes the space, in terms of both territory and opportunity, in which women can begin to determine and redefine some of its conditions. On the other hand, community may be defined and constructed in a way that limits women's control and choice. State community care policies often represent this restricted sense of community in the way they assume the responsibility of women to provide unpaid care in the community. In this way, community becomes women's *place*, the place to which they are relegated and belong: a place that represents not so much a bridge from the private to the public, but an extension of the private.

This distinction between 'space' and 'place' has its roots in the different meanings ascribed to community in general. The first – space – is derived from the sense of community representing a collective striving for communal values based on principles of co-operation. Early examples of this were the Utopian thinkers of the late eighteenth and early nineteenth centuries who attempted to build communities on the basis of co-operation and equality, including equality between men and women (Taylor, 1983). The second idea of community – of women's place – is derived from the community ideal that imposes harmony upon a divided, conflictual and alienated world. Far from attempting to change things, this ideal seeks to promote integration based upon people's acceptance of their 'place' as subordinate or superior in the community. Victorian religious ideas of 'the rich man at his castle, the poor man at his gate', where the world was yet 'bright and beautiful', espoused this ideal. Within this ideal not only do rich and poor know their place, but men and women too, for the hierarchical relations within the community tend to be seen as based upon, and emanating from, the hierarchical relations within the family (Davidoff *et al.*, 1976). The sense of community as harmony in the face of division and inequality has been influential in state social policy programmes of social intervention from the Community Development Programme of the 1960s to the various community schemes in policing, health and social work in the 1970s and 1980s. And the notion that at the community's core are ordered families with a traditional sexual division of labour is implicit and explicit in government reports on community care and law and order (see Langan, 1992 and Williams, 1992b). Although this distinction between space and place is significant for women, it has also to be set against how community is experienced by people today. The ideals of community described above stress both locality and unity, and they imply rurality, whereas in reality communities (based on locality) have seldom realised the unified ideal, and today are increasingly marked by urbanism, cosmopolitanism and differences of identity, as Dick Hebdige explains:

> The values and meanings attached to place and homeland remain as charged as ever but the networks in which people are caught up extend far beyond the neighbourhoods in which they're physically located or the alliances to which they are consciously committed.

The forcible immigration, enslavement or containment of populations from both Africa and Europe, for instance has created transnational identity networks. . . . Diasporic identities can link an unemployed youth in Johannesburg to a bank clerk in Brixton, or a secretary in Brooklyn to a complex web of sympathies and solidarities.

(Hebdige, 1990, p. 20)

4.2 Confined to community?

In Jocelyn's Cornwell's study of London East End working-class community (see chapter 2) she observes gender differences in the experiences of community. For women, the social relationships of the community are more significant in their lives; they 'occupy a much wider range of communal spaces – the shops, the street, the school gates, their relatives' houses' (Cornwell, 1984, p. 50). But how far does the importance of community in this sense of immediate locality actually reflect an exclusion from the outside world? How far does it reflect limited access to money, job opportunities, independent transport and time? Are women locked into community? Factors such as poverty, (lack of) time and independent transport can restrict the sphere in which people develop social relationships, and these particularly affect women.

Women figure disproportionately amongst poor people. Of the major groups in society who experience poverty – old people, single parents, low-paid and unemployed people, disabled and long-term sick people – women are over-represented (Glendinning and Millar, 1987). In terms of their access to sources of income, whether this is through paid work in the labour market, through forms of income maintenance, or through household or family income, women are disadvantaged. In the first case women's average gross weekly wage is only around two-thirds that of men. They are concentrated increasingly in low-paid and part-time work. And there are added racial dimensions to these inequalities. Black women workers have, on average, lower rates of pay than white women workers, although Afro-Caribbean women in particular are more likely to work full-time and therefore earn, in total, more. However, they do so in jobs with unsocial hours, poor rates of pay and worse conditions (Arnott, 1987). These disadvantages at work are reflected in the benefits and pensions that women receive – if they receive them, for in many cases married or cohabiting women have no eligibility to benefits in their own right, but only as a dependant of their male partner. Even so, more women than men survive on minimal state benefits and pensions. In 1984 2.3 million single women and 1 million married women were living on supplementary benefit (income support) compared with 1.2 million single men and 1 million married men

(Department of Health and Social Security, 1987). Over the 1980s social security policies have reinforced these forms of gender inequalities (Glendinning, 1987), though, historically, women have always been more likely to be poor (Lewis and Piachaud, 1987).

In terms of women's access to household income there is evidence to suggest that men maintain greater control over the household resources than women, even though women usually carry greater responsibility for managing resources for the needs of the whole family, especially where those resources are scarce. Women may not only suffer poverty, they will probably have the responsibility for managing poverty too. In the process, it is also more likely that women put the needs of others in the family before their own (Graham, 1984; Pahl, 1988). Dependency on a male wage, therefore, may be as risky as dependency on paid work or on a state benefit or pension. However, dependency upon a male wage has never really been a viable option for the majority of black women or poor working-class women whose male partners have been marginal-ised from access to decently paid work (to a 'breadwinner' wage).

Women's lack of access to resources may, then, serve to lock them more securely to home, neighbourhood and locality. This constraint may be reinforced by other factors – many women do not own a car or have access to a family car, and are therefore dependent upon public transport. Women who work, especially those who work part-time, are likely to work within their locality in order to give them greater flexibility to do their shopping, caring and other domestic work. For many women with paid work and domestic responsibilities time becomes a premium, and this again restricts their mobility (Mackenzie, 1988, pp. 34–6). Resources in the community may also be inaccessible to disabled women, intensifying their restriction.

These restrictions are compounded by unequal opportunities for women within the community. Leisure facilities are often seen as men's space – pubs, clubs, playing-fields – unless they are designated speci-fically as women's – women's nights, women's groups. In political groups or neighbourhood and community organisations men may hold the key positions of power while women raise funds and make tea. Streets may be seen as unsafe at night, and secluded areas unsafe by day for women and children. Fear of violence or sexual and racial harass-ment are particularly intense for vulnerable groups such as older women and disabled women. The threat of racial abuse or violence can also prevent black men and women from feeling comfortable outside their own immediate communities. Indeed a combination of racism and sexism, poverty and local housing resources and policies, can imprison black women into their neighbourhoods in very specific ways:

> The accumulated effects of twenty-five years of racist housing policies have ensured that growing numbers of black women are imprisoned on the upper

floors of dilapidated tower blocks in every inner-city with little hope of escape. If our white neighbours harass us, or if our men abuse us, we often have no choice but to leave, exposing ourselves and our children to the traumas of homelessness.

(Bryan *et al.*, 1985, p. 95)

The confinement of women – particularly women in poverty – to their neighbourhood has also to be set against trends in patterns of leisure and consumption. Over the 1980s consumption has become a major leisure-time activity for those who have managed to retain access to a decent and uninterrupted income. Increasingly facilities such as cinemas and shopping precincts (as well as other services such as post offices and hospitals) are not local but in city centre or out-of-town complexes. The inaccessibility of these facilities to single parents, older or disabled women (and men) represents another dimension of exclusion from a way of life experienced by the majority.

At the same time, in this way of life there seems less room for community in its collective or communal sense. Some writers see the rise of materialism as heralding the decline of communal solidarity (Seabrook, 1982; Roberts, 1984). From this viewpoint, what links the private world of the family or household today to the public world of, in this case the market-place, or to welfare provision, is its ability to *consume*. The family represents an important consumption unit, choosing its household furnishings and food along with its health care, housing and the right schools for its children. In so far as community is seen as meaningful then it is as a vehicle for the defence of property against some outside threat, as in Neighbourhood Watch schemes. However, as we detail below, new lines of solidarity have emerged across and within the bonds of frugality.

Limited access to money or transport and fear of violence are not the only factors to confine women to their locality. Middle-class married women may often find themselves in suburbs or rural villages, their lives restricted by child-care responsibilities and effectively banished from the cities where their husbands work. On the other hand, for some women the very nature of unprotected city life provides the possibility for freedom and new solidarities, as Elizabeth Wilson explains:

While women have been shifted away from urban space and *equated* with anti-urbanism, in an often subtle and indeed subliminal way, minority groups have twisted an advantage from being at the interface of urban freedom and ideological repression. Like the bohemian subcultures (to which some blacks and gays were always drawn), their emergence was in part the result of prejudice and labelling. It was also the reaction to stereotyping; urban cultures were part of a process of self-definition. Lesbians and gay men created communities or 'ghettoes' both for safety and for a sense of identity.

(Wilson, 1991, p. 120)

Confinement, marginalisation and exclusion can themselves create the bonds that turn place into space.

4.3   Women in action

In so far as many women have, for a variety of reasons, found themselves confined in particular ways to their 'place' within the community, what have they made of it? Many women, as the quotation earlier from Jocelyn Cornwell noted, develop an organic relationship with their immediate community. For mothers in particular, it is where they shop, meet other mothers and work. The development of such relationships is not, however, inevitable. Mothers of young children may be severely limited in the access to anything other than superficial relationships or may face exclusions through difference – being new to an area; being black in a white community; having a disabled child. Some women may find that they have less support than others. In a study by Ann Oakley and Linda Rajan (1991) of the support and networks of pregnant women, they found that more working-class women than middle-class women experienced isolation and lack of social support. Nevertheless it is usually women who are at the front line of negotiations over nurseries, schools, housing, health and other welfare agencies. Not surprisingly, then, women have also been central in community-based actions to organise, defend or protest about such services.

In her journey through the north of England in 1984, Beatrix Campbell commented:

> in all the towns I visited there was a plethora of women's groups fighting their local authority landlords, fighting for nurseries, for better health care for women, organising mothers' and toddlers groups, girls' rights in youth clubs and children's playschemes. They are often less insistent about expressing disappointment at men's non-cooperation because they barely expect it to be otherwise, though their criticisms are fortified by the existence of feminism in the culture at large. Women's community politics around housing, health and children – the same preoccupations as united their working class antecedents throughout the twentieth century – are a continuing indication of women's resilience.
>
> (Campbell, 1984, p. 197)

This involvement of women in local struggles has a long tradition. For example, women led 'corn riots' over the high prices and scarcity of corn in Dover in 1740, in Taunton in 1753 and in London in 1800. In 1831 women led mass demonstrations in Merthyr Tydfil against debt-collection during a period of economic depression (Beddoe, 1983). During the First World War women in Glasgow, London and Leeds organised strikes against rent increases (just as during 1988–9 women in Leeds organised successfully against the takeover of their council housing estates by housing action trusts).

Such forms of action represent women's attempts to gain greater control over the conditions in which they collectively live – their space. At the same time, however, women's involvement in struggles in the community also reflects their relative exclusion from the major traditional forms of working-class political protest – the trade unions and the labour movement. It also reflects the resistance by the labour movement to take up those issues not directly concerned with wages and conditions. This is not to minimise the importance of struggles by women trade unionists nor the occasions when the labour movement has supported women's issues – for example, trade union support in the 1970s for women's rights to abortion. It means that politically the community has been both women's space and women's place – that is, one of the few areas open to women to organise over issues of direct importance to them.

This process of marginalisation from the main institutions of political struggle applies to many groups of resistance – black people and minority ethnic groups, disabled people, poor people, many of whom, of course, are also women. The organisation of claimants' unions, of self-advocacy groups for disabled people, of Afro-Caribbean women against racist educational assessment procedures or of Bangladeshi men and women against racist immigration controls which divide their families, are often based in the community. In most cases, too, these sorts of struggles have long histories (see, for example, Rowbotham, 1974; Sivanandan, 1982), which diverge from the history of the labour movement and are also quite separate and distinct from the history of community work (as told, for example, in Craig, 1989). Nevertheless, it is significant that some of the major trade union struggles in the 1970s and 1980s gained strength from this sort of community organisation. In the 1970s the strikes by black men and women workers at Grunwick and Imperial Typewriters found support from the black community long before being recognised by the trade union movement. The 1984 miners' strike was a defence of long-established communities and the work upon which they depended using trade unionism combined with support and the collective organisation of the women in the mining communities. Interestingly, too, the very involvement of the women in such a central way challenged and, to some extent, transformed the traditional male–female relations that had been part of the culture of those communities. What had been women's place became their space to organise and to change.

The way in which involvement in 'public' issues such as workplace strikes has impacted upon women's capacity to challenge 'private' issues within the family represents an important shift in the influence of the second wave of feminism from the 1960s. The impact of the women's movement had a considerable influence upon women's issues and women's organisations in the community (Williams, 1989; Dominelli, 1990). First, it strengthened the demand that higher priority be given for issues traditionally regarded as 'women's concerns' – care of children or older relatives, for example. Second, it succeeded in turning the 'personal' into the 'political' by putting on the agenda areas of women's lives previously hidden from general concern, such as rape, abuse, violence and sexuality. Third, women's organisations and campaigns have thrown new perspectives on old issues – such as the organisation of education, training and employment opportunities geared to women's needs, or issues of physical and mental well-being. They have also challenged the assumption that work is what men do and where they organise, and home is where women's unpaid work is rewarded through men's pay and their conditions improved by virtue of men's struggles. And it is also the case that many of these campaigns have been carried out in the localities or communities, for example the setting up of refuges for battered women, or of well-women clinics or rape crisis centres.

Feminist campaigns and struggles have also been influential by incorporating their own demands for change into ways of organising. So, for example, the refuge movement for women suffering from domestic violence has attempted to organise refuges along non-hierarchical and non-bureaucratic lines involving the users of the service in the running, decision-making and caring for and counselling others in the refuge. This attempt to challenge the unequal relationship between the providers of services (often professionals) and the users of the services has also been reflected in the women's health movement. Women have campaigned not only for a recognition of their own health needs but also for greater control and say in, for example, childbirth or reproductive rights. This has also involved attempts to demystify professional, in this case medical, knowledge so that women have greater knowledge about their own bodies.

From this highlighting and development of struggles over women's issues has emerged a further important understanding: that women's interests, needs and experiences are themselves different, mediated by differences of class, race, disability, age and sexuality. For example, white women's groups have drawn attention to the lack of seriousness with which the police handle victims of rape or domestic violence. However, black women's problems in this situation are compounded by the hostility of white police towards both black women and black men (Mama, 1989). Similarly, the issue of reproductive rights affects women in different ways. Rights to abortion need to take into account rights to *have children* for infertile women or women who have been subjected to unwanted sterilisation or who have had their fertility limited – disabled women, black women, Third World women, poor working-class women. In addition, campaigns that focus on women's needs as wives and mothers can be in danger of ignoring the needs of women who may be neither – older women, lesbians, women without children (Williams, 1992a). The acknowledgement of the diversity of women's experiences has emerged through the development of groups that represent new lines of solidarity – Afro-Caribbean and Asian women, disabled women, lesbians, older women, single parents, carers. At the same time this development has been seen by some as undermining the possibility for women's *united* strength to push for general improvements in areas such as low pay and child-care provision (Adams, 1989). The challenge lies, perhaps, in the need for united action which also recognises different experiences and needs.

To conclude: in different ways community can be the space that women struggle to define as theirs, whether it be for health facilities that are responsive to their needs; for better housing, and transport; for freedom from sexual and/or racial harassment; for non-racist and non-sexist child-care provision and space to play; for collective forms of saving, buying and distribution; for equal training and employment opportunities; or for the space to celebrate and not hide their sexuality or ethnicity. At the same time community can in different ways be the place to which women are confined. This is a crucial contradiction in the lives of women and their relation to community.

Acknowledgement

My thanks to Lyvinia Elleschild for her comments on an earlier draft of this chapter.

References

Adams, M. L. (1989) 'There's no place like home: on the place of identity in feminist politics', *Feminist Review*, No. 31, pp. 22–33.

Arnott, H. (1987) 'Second class citizens', in Walker, A. and Walker C. (eds) *The Growing Divide*, CPAG, London.

Beddoe, D. (1983) *Discovering Women's History: a Practical Manual*, Pandora Press, London.

Bryan, B., Dadzie, S. and Scafe, S. (1985) *The Heart of the Race: Black Women's Lives in Britain*, Virago, London.

Campbell, B. (1984) *Wigan Pier Revisited*, Virago, London.

Cornwell, J. (1984) *Hard-Earned Lives: Accounts of Health and Illness from East London*, Tavistock, London.

Craig, G. (1989) 'Community work and the state', *Community Development Journal*, Vol. 24, No. 1, pp. 3–18.

Davidoff, L., L'Esperance, J. and Newby, H. (1976) 'Landscape with figures: home and community in English society', in Mitchell, J. and Oakley, A. (eds) *The Rights and Wrongs of Women*, Penguin, Harmondsworth.

Department of Health and Social Security (1987) *Social Security Statistics, 1984*, HMSO, London.

Dominelli, L. (1990) *Women and Community Action*, Venture Press, Birmingham.

Glendinning, C. (1987) 'Impoverishing women', in Walker, A. and Walker, C. (eds) *The Growing Divide*, CPAG, London.

Glendinning, C. and Millar, J. (eds) (1987) *Women and Poverty in Britain*, Wheatsheaf, Brighton.

Graham, H. (1984) *Women, Health and the Family*, Wheatsheaf, Brighton.

Hebdige, D. (1990) 'Fax to the future', *Marxism Today*, January.

Langan, M. (1992) 'Who cares? Women in the mixed Economy of care', in Langan, M. and Day, L. (eds) *Women, Oppression and Social Work*, Routledge, London.

Lewis, J. and Piachaud, D. (1987) 'Women and poverty in the twentieth century', in Glendinning, C. and Millar, J. (eds) *Women and Poverty in Britain*, Wheatsheaf, Brighton.

Mackenzie, S. (1988) 'Balancing our space and time: the impact of women's organisation on the British city, 1920–1980', in Little, S., Peake, L. and Richardson, P. (eds) *Women in Cities: Gender and the Urban Environment*, Macmillan, London.

Mama, A. (1989) 'Violence against black women: gender, race and state responses', *Feminist Review*, No. 32, pp. 30–48.

Oakley, A. and Rajan, L. (1991) 'Social class and social support: the same or different?', *Sociology*, Vol. 25, No. 1, pp. 31–60.

Pahl, J. (1988) 'Earning, sharing, spending: married couples and their money', in Walker, R. and Parker, G. (eds) *Money Matters: Income, Wealth and Financial Welfare*, Sage, London.

Roberts, E. (1984) *A Woman's Place: an Oral History of Working Class Women*, Blackwell, Oxford.

Rowbotham, S. (1974) *Hidden from History*, Pluto Press, London.

Seabrook, J. (1982) *Unemployment*, Granada, London.

Sivanandan, A. (1982) *A Different Hunger: Writings on Black Resistance*, Pluto Press, London.

Taylor, B. (1983) *Eve and the New Jerusalem*, Virago, London.

Williams, F. (1989) *Social Policy: a Critical Introduction, Issues of Race, Gender and Class*, Polity Press, Cambridge.

Williams, F. (1992a) 'The family: change, challenge and contradiction', in *Social Welfare and Social Work Yearbook 1992*, Open University Press, Milton Keynes.

Williams, F. (1992b) 'Somewhere over the rainbow: universality and diversity in social policy', in Manning, N. and Page, R. (eds) *Social Policy Review, 1992*, Social Policy Association, London.

Wilson, E. (1991) *The Sphinx in the City: Urban Life, the Control of Disorder, and Women*, Virago, London.

5

A Women's Health Group in Mansfield*

JENNY FINCH

The existence of a women's health group in Mansfield might come as a surprise to some people. Mansfield is not a large city, with all sorts of community groups springing up in response to the pressures of urban life; it is a mining town in Nottinghamshire with a population of 55,000.

The group was originally started by the local Community Health Council (CHC) as a pressure group to encourage the Area Health Authority to set up a well-woman clinic in Mansfield. When Islington CHC waged a successful campaign for well-woman clinics to be established in their area, they got an article in the national press, encouraging women all over the country to telephone their Community Health Council and ask where the local clinic was. Central Nottinghamshire CHC, like many others, received calls from women wanting a well-woman clinic provision and they decided to act on this.

In May 1979 the CHC held a public meeting on the issue. This was well attended – about 80 people were there. Women from Islington came to talk about their clinics. There was enthusiasm for obtaining a clinic in Mansfield and a lot of women signed a list as interested in establishing a campaign.

The CHC suggested that, if women ran advice sessions on women's health problems for six months, they could ascertain the exact nature and extent of the problems and relate these to the need for a well-woman clinic. A case could then be put to the Area Health Authority.

*This chapter was first published in Curno, A. *et al.* (ed), *Women in Collective Action*, Association of Community Workers, 1982, pp. 130–139.

5.1   How the women's health group formed: who belonged to the group

After the public meeting the CHC organised a series of meetings to plan future action. These were attended by about 20 women from the public meeting. Some were health professionals – a midwife, a qualified nurse, a research assistant attached to the CHC. Two men were also involved at this stage – an employee of a pregnancy advisory service, who provided us with statistics and information relevant to women as health service consumers in Mansfield, and the secretary of the CHC, who offered support, guidance and advice. A local consultant gynaecologist made contact with the group and offered his assistance.

The health professionals at the meetings suggested that certain tasks should be undertaken, such as gathering information on activities elsewhere, to do with women and health, and establishing contact with Leicestershire, where well-woman clinics were being set up. It then fell upon them to carry out these tasks. Other members of the group did not feel they were given the time or necessary information to make up their minds about which direction they wanted to take.

The group decided to begin advice sessions in January 1980 and the CHC made their offices available for these. For several weeks before Christmas the consultant gynaecologist came along and gave mini-lectures on the functioning of the female body, including physical changes during menstruation and the menopause. He illustrated his talks with charts, diagrams and tape recordings. These lectures provided useful information and were referred back to many times. Books on women and health were borrowed, shared around and read fast and furious.

5.2   Community worker's involvement

Mansfield Community Project – where I was employed as a community worker – had identified health as an issue that warranted specific attention, and links had been built with the CHC. I began to work closely with the group in January, when the weekly advice sessions started. By then two of the health professionals had left for domestic reasons.

This left a gap for the others, who, lacking knowledge of the health service, needed time to work out how to influence it. Most of the 10 or so women attending at this stage were not used to community or organised group activity. They were housewives in an area where women are forced into the traditional role of tending to the husband's needs. In addition to this demand on their time, Iris had a part-time job as a caretaker in a clinic, Sybil did the book-keeping for the small family business, and the others had full- or part-time jobs in local firms. Frances, a teacher, was used to organising through her union. Chris, a qualified nurse, and member of the CHC, gave a lot of support. One interesting feature of this group is that, unlike many women's groups, most of its members were in their fifties. They had had experience of the health service at several different stages of their lives – through pregnancy, as young mothers, in later years, when children left home, and through the menopause.

5.3   The community worker's role

The background of the group when I joined it meant that I was encouraged towards two roles in addition to the broad one of facilitating and supporting other members. One was as a resource person. Although other members of the group had ideas and skills to offer, they seemed to lack confidence in this new area. It appeared that they needed to feel there was someone who could go away and get things done for them. Through subsequent discussion I discovered that some members felt they had not yet had a chance to familiarise themselves with the issues. Tasks had been defined for them, and they found it acceptable for someone paid to carry out some of the work, such as finding information and contacting other agencies. I always tried to make sure we had first discussed fully, as a group, whatever was to be done.

My other role was linked to a tendency I felt within the group to lean on or look to a leading person, who in the early stages had been one of the men or the women professionals. The other members had been used to their taking on responsibility and there was uncertainty as to who would now offer leadership.

I did not give health advice to callers, since I saw this as the task of others who had chosen to run the advice sessions.

5.4   Exploring a more equal way of working

Several women in the group had skills and potential which they welcomed the opportunity to develop, but I did not think this would be possible for all if only one or two members took leading roles. Some members were making bids for leadership which were causing bad feeling.

I felt that we should get away from the familiar hierarchical model of group organisation and establish a process of group discussion and decision-making by consensus. I took a higher profile myself for a while, to exemplify this method. The rest of the group seemed to like working in this way, though it took some time to get used to. Decisions made in the group were always respected.

There was, however, something of a trap in discouraging the conventional hierarchy. Some members still felt the need for a leader, and in the effort to prevent leadership developing I did get put into some aspects of this role myself. One example concerned the agenda which I had started, in order that all the group could share in full awareness of what we needed to be doing. It was not until a visitor to the group pointed it out, that I realised that I was continuing to exercise power through 'looking after' the agenda when we could have been moving to rotating it.

I now think that much more explicit discussion needs to take place if one is to break away from the conventional model. It is essential that all members of the group understand and have worked it out if power is not to re-assert itself in ways which are even more powerful because not overt.

5.5   Other aspects of the working of the group

The administrative tasks got done very efficiently by various members. Before starting a family Sybil had taught on a secretarial course. She had good secretarial skills, but had lost her confidence in these through the years of being a housewife. As a member of this group, she was able to revive these skills.

When we had to write a letter one or two of us composed a draft and then discussed it with the others. This helped to establish the principle that communication on the group's behalf should have approval of all, was a basis for discussion on points of principle, and helped us all develop our letter-writing skills.

Frances, Jan and Sybil took joint responsibility for our funds and were signatories for our account. We had a small grant from the social services department, and opened an account in a building society, where our money would earn us interest. Frances took notes each week of major items reported and decisions taken. I worked closely with individual members of the group on particular activities. Iris and I concentrated on giving talks to other interested groups of women. We worked in a pair, but Iris delivered the talks. She felt happier to read from an agreed text to start with, and gradually got used to responding to questions and remarks from the floor.

Another member, Sybil, and I attended a two-day counselling course run by a pregnancy advisory service. We then shared what we could of our learning with other members. The course helped us to understand the importance of listening to the woman seeking help, and gave Sybil confidence in the advice sessions to draw out women's anxieties and help them find a solution to their problems.

5.6   The development and running of advice sessions

Although the initial purpose of the advice sessions was to gather evidence for the well-woman clinic campaign, the sessions took on a life of their own, and continued for longer than was at first intended.

An average of two woman per session came or telephoned for advice. These were normally connected with the menopause or premenstrual tension. Several women in the group had first-hand experience of these problems. Over the months they built up a considerable knowledge – we had books and leaflets to hand, but also prepared short notes to use when people telephoned in. These gave information about the main topics callers were likely to ask about and helped women giving advice to overcome the panic you can feel when faced with an unexpected question over the telephone.

Some women brought queries about pregnancy and the Pill. We did our best on these, but decided not to concentrate on pregnancy and birth, as we felt that these topics were already being covered to some extent by other local voluntary groups in the area. There was also quite a lot of interest in mastectomy. Several women who had had the operation, or worked in hospitals with mastectomy patients, have expressed interest in a special group. This is one of several potential groups that we could support in the future.

In time the members of the women's health group gained confidence in dealing with enquiries and giving advice, and developed a suitable way to structure the sessions. The Tuesday evening advice sessions were our only opportunity to meet together and group decisions had to be made at these. For some members this weekly commitment outside the home was already quite a departure from the norm, and they had to cope with the consequential disruption and jibes from the family. All had busy lives, as housewives and usually with a part-time job outside the home as well, so it was not possible to have an additional weekly 'business' meeting.

Every week there were decisions to be made about administration and publicity, and as the group became known we also had to respond to requests to talk to other groups. It was hard initially to separate the policy-making from the advice-giving functions of the group. We would be in the middle of discussing something, when a woman (often with a friend for company) would arrive with a problem. The newcomers would then be invited to join us and we would all listen to the woman's problem. Although this meant that we often did not deal with all the business for the week, what always followed was an excellent group discussion about the visitor's health problem and about dissatisfaction with GPs, difficulties encountered at hospitals and problems within the family.

We discussed how we could organise these evenings and decided to try a rota, whereby business meetings would be held each fortnight, when everyone would attend. Two women would be on duty each week and deal with callers in a separate room, whether or not the business meetings were on. This system collapsed immediately! Every woman found she wanted to attend each week and hardly anyone had the confidence to deal with callers separately, away from the group.

But as we all learnt more about health matters, and as those giving advice became more used to answering the telephone and dealing with newcomers, we did work out a satisfactory system. We had the group meetings every week; if the telephone rang women took turns to answer the call in another room; when a woman came for help she would be given the choice of talking to someone alone or joining in with the rest of us.

5.7   Arguing the case for a well-woman clinic

When the advice sessions were running fairly smoothly, we turned our attention once more to the campaign for a well-woman clinic. None of us had actually been to a well-woman clinic. We re-established contact with Islington CHC, who had provided speakers for the public meeting, and arranged a day-trip for four of us to visit both the CHC office and a well-woman clinic. This was one of the high-spots in the group's activities. We learnt a great deal about Islington's campaign for clinics and, at the one we visited, Iris was actually examined. We shared our findings with the rest of the group and now all had a clearer picture of what a well-woman clinic – and the campaign to get one – entailed. A well-woman clinic treats a woman as a whole person. Here, she can receive under one roof several services that she would otherwise have to 'shop around' for, at her GP's and various clinics. These services include breast examination, cervical smear and pelvic examination. One important factor is that she has a reasonable amount of time – say, 20 minutes – to talk with a female doctor, and is encouraged to raise any worries she may have about her health.

By this stage, not everyone in the group was convinced of the need for a clinic. All felt that we had discovered through our advice sessions the overriding need for women to be able to discuss their health problems with other women, and one or two felt this was more important than a well-woman clinic. However, some members still wanted to pursue the group's original aim. The CHC felt that a written case should be put to the Area Health Authority for funding a clinic in Mansfield. The women's health group did not feel able to compile the necessary information for such a document so we brought in a worker from a Nottingham research and resource centre to do this.

Research was done into the kind of well-woman clinics established elsewhere in the country, and evidence was compiled on the value of screening women for certain illnesses. The researcher worked with women academics and students on a women's health survey in Mansfield. This was carried out by women volunteers and provided factual evidence of the need for a clinic. This was added to that collected by the women's health group during the advice sessions. As a result we have a very thorough document arguing our case for a well-woman clinic. In the document, the women's health group made a clear case for the involvement of lay women in any new health provision for women in the area. They wanted to make sure that the right kind of clinic was established with a relaxed atmosphere, where women have a real opportunity to discuss their health with a woman doctor. They also saw their role as counsellors as important, and would certainly want to offer this service, and to set up special-interest groups on topics like the menopause and mastectomy, alongside the services offered by health professionals at the clinic.

5.8   What the group has achieved

Every woman who passed through the group learned something about her health. The long-standing members gained in confidence and the ability to articulate their ideas. Iris, having had some experience in talking to other groups, is now our representative on the CHC. She is putting forward arguments in the struggle for better health facilities for women – such as the need for patients to have a larger role in influencing decision-making, and the difficulty for women in gaining access to particular medical services when their GP does not think them necessary.

Frances has now taken responsibility for giving talks to other interested groups. Several women in the group have developed skills in counselling.

The advice sessions are continuing and we hope to involve more women as counsellors to keep them going. The report we produced has been presented to the CHC, who have given it their official backing. The CHC will follow the normal procedures within the health service to try to establish a well-woman clinic in the district.

Changes have taken place in the local health service as a result of the interest generated by the women's health group's activities. Professionals who wanted to improve services have gained strength from our group's existence and decision-makers can no longer be as complacent. The central cytology clinic in town has been better advertised, and leaflets explaining about breast self-examination are given out at all the clinics in the district.

Something we have all gained is a greater awareness of our position in society as women. When women in this group got to know each other, and were used to sharing their experiences of health problems, they sometimes discussed the way they were treated at home, and how they felt undermined by male relatives. We are aware of the compromises in so many women's lives.

5.9   Problems the group faced

There were difficulties built into women's health group from the start. One was that it was another body – the CHC – who focused on the need for a well-woman clinic in the area, and they who set up the group. Women who joined the group agreed with this need, and, feeling they could not put forward an alternative strategy at this stage, went along with the advice-sessions-leading-to-campaign-for-clinic as outlined for them. Having done this, and accepted the support and facilities offered by the CHC, they felt bound to stick to the tasks defined for them. This caused a dilemma for some who, having explored the realm of women's health problems, felt more committed to a counselling service than to well-woman clinics.

However, the CHC has played a valuable role. Mansfield has very little tradition of community action, and, as the population is fairly static, not many new ideas are introduced. The health service is itself steeped in hierarchy and traditions, and those hold even greater sway in a place like Mansfield. What is more, there was no women's movement in the town, and very few activist women, either middle class or working class, when the health group started.

One effective way of getting new ideas accepted in a place like Mansfield is under the auspices of a respectable organisation, like the CHC. Eventually, we would hope, having broken new ground under this umbrella, fresh developments in the field of women and health will emerge independently, though links with the CHC and other health agencies will always be useful.

I think that in starting the advice sessions so early on in the group's life we missed a stage in its development. Members needed more time and space at the beginning to explore their feelings and to familiarise themselves with health issues and health service structure. Many of our organisational difficulties at the start were because of moving forward too quickly.

For the second half of this group's year of main activity, there was a core of six members. Others were with us for several weeks and then left. One problem is transport in a semi-rural area. The health district stretches over several miles and embraces many villages. One woman came by car from a village and brought a friend with her. When her marriage broke up she lost the use of the car and they both had to stop coming. Some women got what they needed from the group and left.

Some members have been women who, having been through a bad time themselves with, for example, the menopause – and at the hands of the health service – have a genuine desire to help others in a similar situation. But other women joined because they themselves needed help. Where this was the overriding factor the woman has left. Those women experienced tremendous difficulty in dealing with the advice-giving function. Some were seen to be unreliable and 'in need of help', though members offered what support they could.

Another difficulty for group members has been in accepting that success can take a long time. Our initial approaches to the health authorities have not yet produced a well-woman clinic, but there has been movement. Some of us feel encouraged by this, but it has been hard to counter the disillusionment that others feel.

5.10   The women's health group as a means of development

I feel that health is a good starting-point for women to get involved in community action. It is something which is relevant to all women. In addition to the roles we are encouraged to take on, as the one who attends to the well-being of others (wife, mother, dutiful daughter or nurse), a woman's own health is something of which she is very aware. Having suffered, sometimes quite considerably, through inappropriate care from the health service and the absence of anyone with whom to share anxieties, many women welcome and need an opportunity to talk about their health and well-being.

Women have first-hand experience of health problems, so we often want to find out more about them and have more control over our own health. This inevitably leads to our confronting attitudes within the health service and demanding a type of provision more appropriate to our needs. The desire to move on from where we are also provides the impetus to acquire new knowledge and skills. A non-hierarchical group, where the emphasis is on sharing information and providing support for other women, is an appropriate setting for this personal development.

6

Neighbourhood Care and Social Policy: Extracts*

Edited by RAY SNAITH

[*Neighbourhood Care and Social Policy*, published in 1989, is a major comparative study of organised neighbourhood care. The research was carried out some ten years earlier by Philip Abrams, Sheila Abrams, Robin Humphrey and Ray Snaith. Towards the end of the research, Professor Philip Abrams, the head of the Rowntree Research Unit in Durham University's Sociology and Social Policy Department, died unexpectedly. He left behind him a large body of work on neighbouring and local social care. The final text was edited by Ray Snaith.

Philip Abrams and his colleagues found, as many others have found, that most caring is undertaken by members of kin. The researchers ask how it might be possible to build the equivalent of close kin relations among people who are not related. Their analysis focuses on how organised schemes can mobilise resources within the community. Different kinds of neighbourhood care schemes are studied in the wider context of their social class milieu and official welfare environment.

Publication of *Neighbourhood Care and Social Policy* came at a time when official policy interest was increasingly focusing on the contribution of informal care to community care. Promotion of the role of the voluntary sector and the use of volunteers was becoming more widespread at the same time as statutory services were being reorganised on a localised basis. But although the research was government-funded, the recommendations of *Neighbourhood Care and Social Policy* have not been widely aired. Snaith's call for 'substantial financing of public and voluntary services', a 'strong but sensitive welfare state' and a vision of neighbourhood care 'compatible with greater equality for women', came at a time of a Conservative government committed to restructuring the welfare state.]

---

*This is an abridged extract from *Neighbourhood care and social policy*, DoH/HMSO, London, 1989, pp. 2–5 and pp. 131–3.

6.1 Contexts and relationships

The activation of informal neighbourhood care [. . .] tells us little about the actual nature of the relationships between local people which generate the caring. Even in the traditional working-class community, most informal care was provided by kin *because* they were kin, rather than by neighbours as such, especially since a high proportion of relatives lived within walking distance of each other. Due to the disappearance or attenuation of the social context which produced mutual aid among non-related local people in working-class neighbourhoods, it is even more the case that, as Walker (1982) puts it, 'in practice, community care is overwhelmingly care by kin, and especially female kin, not the community'. [. . .]

The key to understanding the limitations of informal care specifically among nigh-dwellers is the realisation that the development of important reciprocity-based relationships has become increasingly problematic as a result of social change. The main factors which have affected the character of modern neighbouring are levels of disposable income for the majority, the increased entry of women into the labour market, the greater availability of state-provided care, increasingly privatised family living and increased geographical mobility. The combination of these social trends has transformed neighbouring today into being more a matter of choice than of constraint, and more influenced by the wish to define privacy than by need for help. Drawing on the exchange-theory formulations of Blau and Jackson, Abrams developed this argument as follows:

> Generally the old equation of problems, resources and closure which produced the diffuse trust and reciprocity of the traditional neighbourhood type networks, within which care in 'critical life situations' could effectively be provided for and by local residents, has plainly collapsed in the face of new social patterns. Most neighbours are not constrained and do not choose to make their friends among their neighbours. Those who do tend to be seeking highly specific solutions to highly specific problems which they cannot solve elsewhere and which make them 'expensive' people to befriend from the point of view of their neighbours.
>
> (Abrams in Bulmer, 1986)

Summing up the main arguments about neighbourhood care [. . .] informal neighbourly care is primarily a product of particular social contexts; such care is unlikely to develop spontaneously in local communities among non-related residents except in certain social contexts. A context such as a locale acts as a focus for relationships which themselves produce care, notably kinship, friendship, moral community, communities of interest and economic interdependence. Above all, a social exchange relationship which is seen as valuable, necessary and potentially reciprocal is the carrier of care. Snaith (forthcoming) has argued that felt closeness of informal relationships is what matters with regard to the reliability, extent and intensity of care and support provided; that such social closeness does not necessarily mean kinship, much less nuclear family relationships; and that even family care is close (and a genuine choice) where it is also of a mutual kind.

6.2   Organising neighbourliness

[. . .] (Significant efforts were made) by a number of voluntary and statutory agencies and, in particular, by local residents themselves to develop systems of neighbourhood care. Within this broad spectrum of groups, schemes and organisations, [. . .] [some] initiatives embodied the realisation that a process of formal organising to intervene and link with informal care was necessary, in the face of the general withdrawal and restrictiveness of modern neighbouring left to itself. The broad aim of such initiatives was one of exploiting, mobilising, augmenting and focusing the resources of informal neighbouring presumed to be latent in different localities.

We see these efforts as responses, both grass-roots and official, to a changed world, to a modern context of more impersonal and privatised local life which leaves many people isolated, their neighbourhood care needs unmet, despite the provision of certain statutory services. We also see them as *crucial experiments* in identifying and testing the capacity for neighbourliness (and, more generally, for voluntary neighbourhood care) of current British society.

The local organisations resulting from these initiatives can be termed, and were often called, Good Neighbour Schemes. [. . .] We defined a Good Neighbour Scheme [. . .] as 'any organised attempt to mobilise local residents to increase the amount or range of help and care they give to one another' and further concluded that 'the aspect of neighbourhood care that is emphasised in Good Neighbour Schemes is not so much that of delivering services more efficiently or more cheaply, but quite simply that of a more neighbourly society, a society in which the locality is a setting for help and care among local residents'. Though they are formally organised, Good Neighbour Schemes seek to develop both helping *and* everyday sociability, precisely those factors identified by Kuper (1953), Shulman (1967) and McGahan (1972) as defining informal neighbouring.

Any soundly based analysis of neighbourhood care must take into account the nature of, and the differences between, the underlying social relationships within which that care is given. Although neighbourhood care of the Good Neighbour Scheme type seeks to stimulate informal care by cultivating ordinary, everyday neighbourliness, it is very different from informal care provided by kin, friends or neighbours, relying as it does on a different social basis for generating help and friendliness. This informal sector of social care is made up kin, friends and neighbours, and care flows from these prior roles. By contrast, the formal sector of care is consciously organised, and caring roles are created by that process of organisation for people who are usually unknown to each other as well as to the recipients of their services. Abrams (1980) argued that 'much of the apparent consensus about the general desirability of more neighbourhood care that exists today exists only because those who think that neighbourhood care means more *localised formal services* and those who believe it means *stronger informal systems* have not yet appreciated the degree to which they are talking about different (and possibly incompatible) things'.

Responding to Abrams' article, Bayley (1981), while accepting the necessity for distinguishing between the two types of care, argued that to make a sharp separation in the way Abrams did was mistaken. He went on to advocate a policy of 'interweaving' informal with formal care. Analysis of this interweaving has to form a central part of any investigation of neighbourhood care; and in looking at the relative mix of different sources of neighbourhood care, and also at the relative power relationships embodied in the links between those sources, particular attention must be given to the main agent determining the overall pattern of neighbourhood care provision: the statutory sector with its overall welfare policy.

Discussion of goals aimed at by the informal sector of care raises the broader issue of the strategy adopted by the formal schemes for relating to their local catchment area or immediate service delivery needs, or also about preventive, long-term caring resources and networks? As a more radical question, what ought one to think of community development or of community politics, advocated by Abrams (1980) as a strategic option for neighbourhood care projects and the regeneration of informal networks?

6.3   The undesirability of reviving traditional neighbourliness

[One] issue concerning the informal sector which is relevant to policy-making centres on what are the realistic prospects for mobilising new community resources, i.e. for neighbours becoming volunteers on the frontiers of formal social service provision. Much of the political rhetoric which surrounds the idea of community or neighbourhood care still assumes, as the 1969 Good Neighbour Campaign did, that there are Good Neighbours waiting in the social undergrowth and simply needing an authoritative call to action. Such thinking lacks a proper understanding of how neighbours normally relate to one another in our kind of society. The myth of traditional community life as a 'densely woven world of informal strongly caring networks' serves to prop up a belief in the possibility and desirability of renewing or reinvigorating laudable, traditional ways of helping people on a local basis. Myths usually embody some truth, and the truth of the myth in this case lies in the nature of the historical context, which consisted of unpleasant conditions rendered less appalling by intense neighbouring.

Although traditional, informal social care was no doubt experienced as a matter of affective ties and cherished, trustworthy networks (as it was invariably remembered as such by the old people we interviewed, whether as clients, residents or helpers), it was in effect governed by an external setting that was essentially brutal and constraining. That context was one of poverty, insecurity, isolation and the lack of formal or welfare-state resources for satisfying needs. Under these circumstances, neighbourliness was impelled by the extreme social homogeneity of everyone being, so to speak, in the same boat. But it was also impelled by calculation. Patterns of neighbouring, then as now, were, to follow Anderson's (1971) argument, also *chosen* on the basis of available resources and in the face of particular costs and opportunities.

The modern realities of neighbourhood interaction demonstrate that in general, once the social context changes and conditions of social closure, insecurity and isolation and choicelessness cease to apply, neighbouring becomes a carefully restricted matter (Abrams in Bulmer, 1986). As involvement with neighbours increasingly becomes an option, the tendency to insure against being caught by the costs of doing so has also become increasingly evident. After all, the hallmark of being a neighbour is that it is potentially the 'cheapest' of all relationships, but it can also very easily be one of the most expensive in terms of time, commitment and foregone opportunities, precisely because of the proximity and face-to-face contact involved. It is not surprising, therefore, that modern neighbouring can be classified as implying a *managed relationship*, one which involves the maximising of certain rewards for minimal investments of time, energy or other resources. The result of this approach to neighbouring being taken is that people generally prefer and expect neighbourly tasks to be those involving emergencies and simple, localised predicaments (Litwak and Szelenyi, 1969). The modern mode of neighbouring is generally casual and guarded, whereby the Good Neighbour is almost universally defined as someone who is helpful, friendly *and* distant – there when you want him [sic] and very definitely not there when you don't. Informal relationships involving deeper commitment are made outside the locality, or with others not regarded as neighbours as such.

6.4   Where are the potential community resources?

Mobilising as sources of care people who live near each other is a policy matter, and those responsible for determining policy in this area must take into account both the true nature and the actual availability of resources that may be drawn upon as informal or voluntary bases for meeting social needs. Clearly, any formal intervention needs to be supportive of the small-scale or, exceptionally, intensive neighbour-liness that is already spontaneously taking place. There do exist some survivals of the traditional mode of intense local neighbourly relation-ships. The major instance of this is provided by neighbours who are also, in fact, kin, especially mothers and daughters (or daughters-in-law). It is family ties rather than bonds of proximity that are at work here to sustain local caring. There exist also, but in a more attenuated form than hitherto, the neighbourly resources of observation, gossip and concern. These can be used by formally provided services as linking, monitoring or preventive mechanisms, although there are inherent dangers of undesirable social control and intrusions of privacy which must be guarded against. In principle, mobilising local information systems as sources of 'referrals' represents a promising method of building bridges between the formal and informal worlds of social care, one which may serve as an alternative to more conventional visiting and helping schemes. [. . .]

Over and above the general impoverishment of informal relationships between local people, we observed a further limitation on non-kin-based informal care: the most neighbourly places were those where, objec-tively, neighbourly help was least needed, and vice versa. On our evidence, this was not only true of inner-city areas (Hayes and Knight, 1981), but of working-class areas generally, the main difference between these areas being only that there was more neighbourly friendliness, as opposed to neighbourly help, outside of the inner city: such as friendli-ness, however, was generally fairly superficial. We found that the family had much the same broad significance for all social classes, but that when it came to comparing the classes with regard to actual help given, working-class people, the unskilled working-class group in particular, felt that even the family was comparatively limited in what it was actually able to offer. Furthermore, while the middle- and upper-class groups felt to a considerable extent that they were readily able to turn to family, friends and neighbours for help, the working-class ones had much weaker links with friends and, particularly, with neighbours as sources of care. Indeed, both working-class residents *and* working-class helpers were markedly more likely to describe their locality as one where people kept themselves to themselves. The clients of neighbourhood care schemes were more isolated in working-class areas, again especially so in inner-city areas. It follows, on our evidence, that not only has the traditional model of working-class neighbouring largely vanished, but that to a considerable extent the world had been turned upside-down in that today it is more accurate to speak of middle-class than of working-class neighbourliness.

In addition to the above sources of informal care, there are the potential resources of people who can be termed possible exceptions to the modern mode of neighbouring, signified by residents having only a weak sense of attachment to a local area and weak affinities with the people who live in it. We are referring here to those categories of people who are 'compelled' to live locally. Such people, in principle at least, represent major potential sources of organised neighbourhood care, given an overall situation in which neighbours are characteristically by no means always available or willing to provide even limited kinds of informal or neighbourhood care. Powerful forces have brought it about that neighbours are unlikely to want close informal involvement with others (geographical and social mobility, class fragmentation, the sharp decline in the proportion of non-employed housewives [sic] and the increasing preference for a private, family-based mode of living are the major determinants). Nevertheless, a potential pool of neighbourly help exists among the 'exceptional' categories of residents: women confined to their home and children; elderly retired people, especially those without private transport or accessible kin or those who have lived most of their life in the neighbourhood; the unemployed, especially men in areas where unemployment is concentrated and long-term; and others – newcomers, committed churchgoers and community activists, for example – who are likely to have an interest in 'political' movements and/or voluntary associations of various kinds organised on a neighbourhood basis.

We would argue that the demographic forces affecting neighbourly help referred to above are not necessarily to be regretted, and that the negative effects they have upon informal care by neighbours have therefore to be accepted. There is little prospect of non-kin-based neighbourhood networks naturally or informally playing a major part in the provision of social care. We need, therefore, to look to formally organised methods of stimulating and providing neighbourhood care. If mobility and choice are two distinctive, though by no means universal, social effects of industrialisation, formal organisation can certainly be considered a third. Abrams (1980) has further singled out community politics or 'neighbourhoodism' as the most important example of the latter effect.

References

Abrams, P. (1980) 'Social change, social networks and neighbourhood care', *Social Work Service*, No. 22, February, pp. 12–23.

Anderson, M. (1971) *Family Structure in Nineteenth Century Lancashire*, Cambridge University Press.

Bayley, M. J. (1981) 'Neighbourhood care and community care: a response to Philip Abrams', *Social Work Service*, No. 26, May, pp. 4–9.

Bulmer, M. (ed.) (1986) *Neighbours: the Work of Philip Abrams*, Cambridge University Press.

Hayes, R. and Knight, B. (1981) *Self-Help in the Inner City*, Voluntary Service Council, London.

Kuper, L. (1953) 'Blueprint for living together', in L. Kuper (ed.) *Living in Towns*, Cresset Press, London.

Litwak, E. and Szelenyi, I. (1969) 'Primary group structures and their functions: kin, neighbours and friends', *American Sociological Review*, Vol. 34, No. 4, August, pp. 465–481.

McGahan, P. (1972) 'The neighbour role and neighbouring in a highly urban area', *Sociological Quarterly*, Vol. 13, Summer, pp. 397–408.

Shulman, N. (1967) 'Mutual aid and neighbouring patterns: the lower town study', *Anthropologica*, Vol. 9, pp. 51–60.

Snaith, R. (forthcoming) 'Informal care and state intervention: choice in social policy' (Newcastle Upon Tyne: unpublished paper).

Walker, A. (ed.) (1982) *Community Care*, Blackwell/Martin Robertson, Oxford.

7

Neighbours

SUZY CROFT and PETER BERESFORD

Lil Curtis was in the community care system for quite a short time. It was just over three years from her GP arranging for her to have a home help and her dying, aged 80, in a psychiatric hospital.

We knew Lil for about 13 years. She was a warm and friendly woman. We lived in the same private rented block of flats in Battersea. She lived alone after her husband died when he was 40. They couldn't have children.

For a long time our relationship with her stayed the same. A wave or a nod when she was climbing the stairs to her flat or an occasional chat. Then things started to change. We saw her driven to distraction as she became increasingly confused. She sat rubbing her hands, crying, and said: 'What have I done to deserve this? What would my mother say if she could see me like this?'

It started with things getting on top of her. Mrs Curtis came to us in confusion and tears about her gas bill. She'd had a final demand after she'd paid. Though she had been to the Gas Board to sort it out, it still worried her. 'Oh no, not Lil again!' they said when we went. She'd wanted a slot meter but they wouldn't fit one, and she kept getting estimated accounts because the meter reader didn't wait long enough for her to get down her stairs.

Other problems sapped her confidence and unsettled her more. Her pension book was stolen. 'A really nice smartly dressed young woman helped me carry my shopping home. She took the bag up the stairs and then asked for a glass of water. While I was in the kitchen, I heard the front door bang.' Later that afternoon Mrs Curtis found her pension book was gone, together with the £40 she'd just taken out. She cried and cried. Her sister told her she was a fool. 'That'll teach you a lesson.' She felt humiliated.

A week after she got her new pension book, Lil lost it. We looked everywhere. This was the first time we'd seen all over her flat. It was beautifully clean and tidy. There were ornaments everywhere going back years: brasses, pots, small plaster dogs and little framed pictures of flowers and cottage gardens. In the living-room, where she had her meals and watched TV, was the large old cabinet radio her huband had bought and colour photos of her great-nephews and nieces. 'He did all this,' she told us, about the brickwork surround of her fireplace behind her heater. This time we had to write a letter of explanation to get a new pension book.

Water kept coming in through her living-room ceiling. She had an outside lavatory and no bathroom. We've got a bad landlord. We had to phone the agent three times and go to the Citizens Advice Bureau before anything was done. Then it was no good and she had to keep a bucket and newspaper out to catch the water running down the wall.

Next we noticed that her train of thought was often interrupted. She'd lose her thread halfway through a sentence. At first she would see a funny side. Then she started to lose things, and finding them didn't help. She was frightened more and more of the time. She'd wander to the shops. She stopped cooking and washing herself regularly. Her nephew, Dave, and Cath, his wife, took on an increasing responsibility, coming to visit, arranging payment of her bills, taking her to lunch with her sister every other Sunday. People began to avoid her. She became more and more lonely. She came to see us at all hours.

One Saturday afternoon we found her shaking and crying. She didn't know why she was so upset. Making her a snack helped to calm her. She hadn't been eating. But, as we were sitting down for Sunday dinner with Gran and the children, Mrs Curtis knocked and came in distraught again. We spent two hours talking to her, trying to sort out what was wrong and to calm her down.

At this point we really began to worry. The children had gone to bed late and we hadn't been able to take Gran home when she wanted. We were spending more and more time with Mrs Curtis while trying to bring up three small daughters on a low income. Our growing fears were confirmed when Mrs Curtis knocked on the door early next morning before we were up.

We decided we'd have to set limits. We would have to explain to Mrs Curtis if we had to do something else when she was with us. We told each other this was only realistic and we shouldn't feel guilty. But, of course, we still did. We were getting just a taste of the sometimes insuperable conflicts full-time carers know only too well. If you try to restrict your responsibilities, you feel mean and selfish; if you don't, you sacrifice yourself or someone else.

But our friendship with Lil wasn't all problems. We'd got to know her better. It was still a two-way relationship. She'd give pocket money and Christmas presents to the children. She played with them, singing 'Knees up Mother Brown' with Rebecca. We had shared interests. We talked about Latchmere Baths, where she had worked, and about how the area was changing. Where we live, gentrification meant there were fewer and fewer neighbours Lil could turn to for help.

Mrs Curtis's GP arranged a psycho-geriatric assessment after we phoned him. Then the community psychiatric nurse (CPN), Liz, started to call. The home help came twice a week. Meals on wheels were organised, but shortly afterwards Lil cancelled them. She didn't want to go to a day centre. Social services installed a telephone and intercom, but these only seemed to confuse Lil more.

We've been impressed by the professionals working with Lil. The psychiatrist took the trouble to phone us after making his assessment and spent time explaining the situation properly. Liz has kept in close touch. So has Annie, the home help. She's been a real support to Lil.

On New Year's Day we saw Lil on her doorstep in a terrible state. She said she hadn't been to bed the night before. There was no food in the fridge. She said she felt better after we made her some tea and toast. After the holiday, we phoned Liz. She feels that Lil is coping well generally, although she sometimes gets confused and depressed over a minor crisis like a light bulb going. She'll try and get meals on wheels again, but she'll only be able to have a home help a maximum of three times a week.

A few days later we saw Lil outside her front door again. We took her back upstairs. She was incoherent. She said: 'The water just came down my legs.' She's going to her next-door neighbour's more and more. She just can't bear to be on her own.

The CPN was on leave. We spoke to the team leader. We tried to convey how lonely and desperate Lil was, without making it seem that she couldn't cope. She said, 'It sounds like she needs to be in a secure place.' We repeated how much Lil clung to her home. She said she'd get on to social services straightaway.

A note was pushed through our door. Mrs Curtis was in hospital. Dave found her. She'd had a minor fall in her bedroom. She was in casualty all day. It was agreed she could stay for one to two weeks to get her walking and stronger again.

When we visited, she was sitting in a chair next to her bed, munching some chocolates that Dave had brought. Her face was content. She seemed happy. Her hair was clean and combed. But she also seemed confused. We weren't sure if she knew who we were.

All along, what Lil most wanted was to stay in her own home. She also wanted company. From the start, Liz seemed to understand this. She had appreciated that the stairs were difficult but said that if the time came when Lil couldn't manage, then she would press for more support so that she could still cope indoors. She had explained that no certain prognosis could be offered. Mrs Curtis wouldn't get any better, but she might be able to carry on in her home for years. Seeing our relief, she'd said: 'Oh I'm glad you feel like that. Lots of neighbours go, "Oh no!" when they hear that.'

Liz thinks that Lil still wants to be in her own home. The problem lies in the level of support she could have. Her chances of getting domiciliary support are 'very slim' – almost non-existent. Lil is 'too well' for that. There is a waiting list and this level of help is only offered to people who would otherwise definitely go into a home. It's also clear she won't get occupational therapy. She 'might possibly' get a home help up to four times a week. When Lil went home initially she'd see Liz two or three times a week, but then Liz's visits would have to drop back to once a month 'as I've got 30 Mrs Curtises'.

Dave phoned. He wants our support to get Lil into the old people's home just round the corner. He's been told there's a waiting list. He's been to see her every day in hospital. Sometimes she's happy, other times she cries and is confused. He seems worried that Lil will go home and he and Cath will end up having to do everything for her like before. He's frightened of being left with all the responsibility. They already have to look after his mother who is confused.

It was at this point that things really changed. Before, we'd been worried about how much responsibility we might have to take on for Lil. Now we realised more and more how little say Lil, her family and friends would have in what happened to her. Cath told us the news. Lil isn't coming home any more. She was taken to her flat for a home visit as planned. She went with the CPN, a nurse and a social worker. The visit was a failure. Mrs Curtis collapsed in tears. She said she did not want to be in her flat. She was unable to do anything like make a cup of tea. According to Cath, she now seems to be unable to do quite a lot of things for herself. Often she can't remember how to dress and she has started to be incontinent at times. Cath says she can no longer cope with going to see Lil. 'Anyway, she doesn't know who I am.' Dave goes every evening and she sometimes knows him. 'She knows he is *someone*. Sometimes she knows he is Dave. Other times she thinks he is her husband or her brother.'

She's going to Greenways, a home for 'confused elderly persons', 'for assessment'. She's staying there a fortnight, 'to see if she is suitable for a home'. We went to see Lil. The assistant officer-in-charge told us that it had been decided that Lil would stay there for six more weeks, then: 'if she wants to, she can stay here. . . . She's been fully assessed here.'

Lil was standing in the middle of a large lounge. Old women were sitting in chairs against the walls. Most were asleep. In one corner the television was on very loudly, showing children's programmes. Two old men were watching it. It was on all the time we were there. We went and sat in a corner of the lounge with Lil, next to a cage with two budgies in it. She looked very pleased to see us. She clearly recognised us, although we had to remind her of our names.

We asked Lil how she was. She shook her head and cried. She told us she didn't like Greenways. She didn't know how long she had been there. She wasn't sure who had been to see her. 'I know them when they're here, but I can't remember who they've been after,' she said. She thought the food was good and she said she did talk to people, but she didn't feel she had made any friends. She has to share a room. She thought she wasn't supposed to go out of the home. She told us it wouldn't 'be allowed'. She didn't know where the local shops were. We offered to take her out but she felt she wouldn't be up to it. She spoke to a woman with a walking frame who was just coming into the lounge, but they couldn't hear each other because of the television.

When we visit Lil and ask her how she is, she starts to cry almost at once. 'It's terrible, terrible.' She's been frightened to go to bed because the woman she shares with bullies her. She does less and less and cries more and more, in spite of medication. She told us: 'Sometimes I don't know what I'm doing. Sometimes everything can be so clear and then I don't know what I'm doing at all.' She's not allowed to make herself a cup of tea because 'someone might break a cup'. She showed us both her blue lacy long johns, something she'd never have done when she'd been our neighbour.

In the dining-room there's a large noticeboard which says 'Today is Tuesday. The month is April. The weather outside is dry. The next meal is supper.' All the workers, except the officer-in-charge, are black. All the residents are white.

We went to see Lil again with a picture we bought her on holiday. She was sitting in the same chair as last time. Her face lit up and she smiled when she saw us, although she didn't remember our names. She was very pleased to see Rebecca, our youngest daughter. She couldn't remember her name, but said she knew she wasn't 'one of Dave's children'. She was very pleased with the picture. She held it up and said how beautiful it was. Another woman sitting nearby said, 'How lovely.' We said we'd put it up for her. We'd brought a hammer and nails. She was pleased, but anxious that we check with the staff that it was alright to put it up.

She explained to Suzy that she wets herself now and has to wear a pad, 'like for a period'. It obviously upsets her a great deal. It took a long time to understand what she was saying. She cannot speak very clearly and seems to find it harder than ever to put sentences together. We wonder if she gets much chance to practice.

We asked the officer-in-charge how Lil seemed to be settling in. 'Well, very well at first but we had a lot of trouble with her a few weeks ago.

She was very, very depressed, crying all the time.' Lil has been wandering out of the home. Apparently she is now on anti-depressants. 'Before, she was crying for days. She was unmanageable.'

We haven't seen Lil for about a month. We called in. She was asleep in a chair. She woke up when we spoke to her and recognised us. She seemed far worse than we'd ever seen her. She looked crushed and was tearful almost as soon as we spoke to her. Then we noticed her legs. They were very swollen and the skin was red raw and peeling. We asked her what was wrong. A care assistant sitting nearby said that Lil had got water on her legs, caused by sitting down too much and not moving around. The care assistant said, 'Of course, it is difficult to get them to do anything here. They go from their rooms into the sitting-room here and then from here into the dining-room and that's it.' We asked her what they could do. She said, 'Well, there isn't much they can do if they can't go out'.

Lil now goes to a day centre three times a week. 'She goes out in tears and she comes back in tears.' We asked Lil about it. She pulled a face but couldn't tell us what she did there. She didn't know where it was or how she got there. The care assistant said, 'At least it gets her our. It's better than sitting here all day.'

Lil can hardly walk now. We tried to help her to her room, but after a few steps she said that she would have to go back to her chair. She clearly didn't have the confidence. She also didn't feel up to going in the wheelchair. She has her own room now. The picture we bought her isn't there any more. Lil has deteriorated very rapidly in the last few weeks. She finds it even more difficult to talk than before.

We called in at Greenways today as we had heard that Lil is in the large local psychiatric hospital, Wellheath. She's been there a month now, in Victoria ward. She was at Greenways for nine months. A care assistant tells us there's a panel/case conference this week to decide whether she goes back. 'I hope she does as she is nice to have around. Not incontinent, can feed herself and all that. She's been on a diuretic to get rid of the water on her legs and a sedative to help her sleep'.

We visited Lil in Wellheath. She was sitting, asleep in a chair, in the ward. It took her quite a while to wake up. At first she didn't seem certain who we were. But after a few minutes she seemed to remember. She was slumped down low in her chair and looked uncomfortable. We asked if she would like to sit up and she said yes. She gets very distressed when she is moved. One of her legs is bandaged and the other looks red and painful. She said she doesn't walk around by herself. She cried out in little whimpers as we and a nurse helped her up.

She seems to be more herself in little flashes. When I said, 'It's Suzy. I used to live next door to you in Winders Road,' she said, 'No, not next door, down the road.' We share an orange. She is sitting next to a table with a plateful on it and she asked if we'd like one. We peel it and she did seem to enjoy it. Otherwise we didn't really understand what she was saying. This hasn't happened before.

While we sat there another old woman came and sat opposite. She said, 'Please help me. Can you help me?' We asked what was wrong, but she didn't answer. Later on she said, 'Oh, God help me.' We again said 'What's the matter?' But she didn't answer. She sat repeating 'Please help me' in a desperate tone of voice. Another old woman came to sit next to her and after a bit said fiercely, 'Shut up can't you.' She repeated this three times, but it had no effect. Then she said, 'Someone will come and help you in a bit. Try not to go on.' The woman continued to cry out until a nurse took her into lunch.

Before we left we spoke to the charge nurse about Lil. The panel/case conference was held yesterday. No one came from Greenways because of staff shortages, Mrs Curtis won't be going back. According to the charge nurse, she was admitted to Wellheath because of her demented behaviour. We said that we thought Greenways was for confused elderly people. She said yes but that her 'behaviour had deteriorated'. She was continually distressed, not eating or sleeping. She cried and wailed. We asked what treatment she has been receiving. 'Oh well, it was also thought that she might have been hearing voices' so she was put on a 'mild tranquilliser' and 'that has helped calm her down'. But she has a recurring urinary infection and we were told that increases her dementia. Lil will be admitted to a long-stay ward.

Today we phoned Greenways to ask if they knew which ward Mrs Curtis was in now. A man said he would check for us. After a few minutes he came back and said, 'I'm afraid I've got some bad news for you. We heard this afternoon apparently that Mrs Curtis is dead. She was buried last Friday.' He didn't know any more details.

We spoke to Cath on the phone. She said that Lil died of a urinary tract infection. Cath sounded bitter. Dave had not been at all happy for Mrs Curtis to be in Wellheath. 'They told us she was going in for two weeks for tests and then Greenways wouldn't have her back.' They both feel that Greenways 'slung' Mrs Curtis out. 'They pushed her out of there.'

Lil was cremated and her ashes will be buried with her husband. Dave went to see her body. 'Her eyes were all sunken in like hollows and her temples had fallen in.' We wish we had been able to see her once more. We wish we'd known about the funeral so we could have gone.

After Dave closed up Mrs Curtis's flat, the builder who works for the landlord did it up. The roof was at last repaired. He showed us around. He'd put in wall-to-wall carpet throughout – 'People like that.' The fireplace Mrs Curtis's husband made for her and of which she was so proud has gone. The builder has knocked out the outside lavatory and extended the kitchen. The boxroom has been converted into a bath-room. The walls have all been painted white.

A month before she died we saw a 'Sold' sign on the flat and a hired van parked outside. A young man called Charles and his parents were carrying furniture in. Now Lil's flat is his. The only sign of her is the metal hand-rail social services fixed on the outside stairs. It's still there as we write.

8

Two Views of Community Service

(a) Reflections of a Voluntary Worker*

MARGARET SIMEY

Everybody was taken by surprise by the sudden huge increase in the demands for the relief of families following the call-up of so many of the bread-winners [during the First World War]. No machinery existed which could cope with such a situation, apart from a fading organisation set up to deal with the relief of soldiers' and sailors' families during the Boer War. Sympathy ran away with sense and what had been a chaotic situation before became much worse. In despair, the Lord Mayor turned to his cousin, Eleanor Rathbone, who had for some years been training women for voluntary work under the auspices of the Victoria Settlement. Mary Stocks describes in her biography of Eleanor (Eleanor Rathbone, 1949) the astonishing speed and efficiency with which these cohorts of women rose to an opportunity such as they had never dreamed of. By the end of the war, two lessons had been learned. Firstly, a great increase in state intervention had to be accepted. Secondly, women, especially from the middle classes, must be allowed to play a far larger part in the world at large than ever before.

But what of voluntary work? Where did the social conscience of the individual come in? Burdened though they were, Eleanor and her colleagues on the working party never gave up their search for an answer. Many of the dreamers had been killed in the war, but the dream lived on. An increase in state benefits would have to be accepted, but they were wholly convinced that material relief was not the whole story. The more benefits the state provided for people's needs, the more complicated the machinery required for their administration. Such pub-

---

*This is an abridged extract from *Active Citizens: new voices and values*, Fielding, N., Reeve, G., and Simey, M., Bedford Square Press, London, 1991, pp. 5–11.

lic assistance as was available was hedged about with a labyrinth of rules and regulations which defeated many of those who applied. 'The poor' needed someone to be on their side, to advise them in their dealings with those in authority and, more subtly but none the less importantly, to care about their distress. Moreover, it was in meeting that need and maintaining a personal relationship between the community and those in need that all those who hungered to give service to others and to be of value to society would themselves find fulfilment.

The outcome was the setting up of a Personal Service Society (PSS), effectively a splinter group of members of the LCVA [Liverpool Council of Voluntary Aid] who banded together to defend the principle and practice of personal voluntary service. Their purpose was to provide the machinery whereby each and every citizen could voluntarily give and receive service, according to their capacity and their need. Out of that modest attempt to provide a counter-weight to what was one day to become the welfare state developed the nationwide service provided today by the Citizens Advice Bureaux.

The instant demand which deluged the little agency brought major difficulties. When Dorothy Keeling, who was appointed as organiser, wrote her autobiography, she called it *The Crowded Stair* because of the queues of applicants who chronically blocked the passage up to her office. The sheer bulk of poverty had always been a particular problem in Liverpool, but the aftermath of the First World War multiplied to unmanageable proportions. The agency had to face the fact that volunteers simply could not deal with such a volume of demand and that a nucleus of paid staff would have to be employed. Moreover, the complexity of the problems brought by the clients demanded a response that was plainly beyond the capacity or the good-will of the average volunteer. Every worker would have to be trained and supervised. Casework, as it came to be called, could no longer be a matter for spontaneous charity; it must become a recognised profession. [. . .]

Eleanor Rathbone and her colleagues, who fought so hard for education and opportunities for women, can have had no idea of the far-reaching consequences of that apparently minor decision by a small voluntary society to pay women to do what they had previously done voluntarily, and to train them for it. As it turned out, opportunities for employment such as were offered by agencies like the PSS came as a heaven-sent chance for the regiment of 'superfluous women' left high and dry after the First World War ended. Their wartime service had enabled women to escape from domesticity. They had tasted independence. They had undertaken all kinds of jobs and knew that they could do them. But once the war had ended, they found themselves unwanted. There was no room for them. Men back from the forces inevitably claimed priority for such work as was available; the Great

Depression was already casting its dark gloom over the economic scene. At the same time, there was no hope of retreating into marriage because of the slaughter of young men in the war. The option of staying at home as an unmarried daughter was no longer available in the changed economic climate.

[. . .] I had been reared in the tradition of the unpaid voluntary worker, my mother being an active member of the church women's section and I myself a Sunday School teacher. What more natural than that when I went to University, the first woman in the family to do so, I should be attracted to the prospect of earning my living as a social worker. [. . .]

Little did I foresee what a threat I and others like me were to become to the established order. I blush to remember with what condescension we regarded volunteers. We were professionals. We knew. Volunteers were of a lesser species, only to be tolerated as handmaidens, hopefully to be phased out as amateur dabblers who might well do more harm than good. Inevitably, the paid workers rose to the top, meekly though they might address the members of their Committees. The high-handed way Dorothy Keeling treated her voluntary chauffeur, the daughter of an important local family, became part of the folklore of students in training. As in the PSS so elsewhere, women flooded into this new and expanding job market. As fast as a new social need was uncovered, and a new specialism was devised to meet it, women swept in and took over. It could almost be said that women invented social work as a career in order to meet their own desperate need. There was little room here for amateurs.

It had been expected of me as a degree student that I would pioneer the entry of women into the expanding civil service brought into being by the increase in state welfare provision. What was, at the time, a high ambition held little attraction for me. I was even less tempted by the prospect of a career as a case worker: the closed-shop attitude of the professionals who dealt with the relief of the miseries of the poor repelled me. I was an out-going type, an enthusiastic folk-dancer who was essentially sociable. I had myself belonged to a curious little girls' club attached to a church, called the Camp Fire Girls. Without hesitation, I headed for what was called group work.

[. . .] The girls' club movement depended almost entirely on voluntary effort, although it had begun to attract a certain degree of official approval as a response to the 'youth problem' of the war years. [. . .]

It was on the back of the youth movement that voluntary work by local people for the benefit of the community as a whole began to develop. In particular, those men and women returning from the forces to the new housing estates found much to be desired in the land fit for heroes which they had been promised. These were people with no experience of voluntary work in the middle-class tradition of charitable effort, but quite spontaneously they began to come together in little local groups to struggle to improve conditions. Unhappily, the pressure of problems on big new estates deflected the energies of such groups into arguments with their landlord, the corporation of 'corpy', and this earned the community movement, as a whole, opposition from councillors and officials alike. [. . .]

To be fair, the official lack of appreciation has to be seen in the context of the Great Depression of the 1930s. Houses and jobs were not just a top priority; they were the only things that mattered. Demands for social facilities such as community centres or shops, or even churches, simply could not compete with that fearful urgency. Only public houses were available on the new estates and, in those days, women were not welcome in them. As official schemes for tackling the continuing distress multiplied, the drift to central control over their administration increased. There was little scope in those days of universal stress for the amateur endeavours of voluntary citizens, however active.

It was a drift which received a fresh impetus as a result of the evacuation of children from the inner cities on the outbreak of the Second World War in 1939. People living in the suburbs and affluent country dwellers were scandalised by the way of life of 'the poor' who invaded their orderly homes. The evacuees for their part, as in the case of the little family who arrived on my own doorstep, were equally dismayed by the lack of warmth or communal feeling in the welcome they received from the local community and quickly returned to wherever they had come from. I doubt if any increase of compassion or mutual understanding resulted from that entire exercise, but there was at least a fixed determination that 'something must be done' to improve conditions in the inner cities. So urgent was the need for action seen to be, that the Beveridge Plan for the setting up of the welfare state was actually published before the end of the war, in 1943. From then on, every energy was devoted to the preparation of the intricate legislation required to implement Beveridge's proposals and the setting up of the machinery necessary for their administration. Once again, as so often before, voluntary workers were left standing on the side-lines, bewildered and uncertain as to what to do next.

(b) Community as Service*

EILEEN and STEPHEN YEO

Local Liberal leaders first created this meaning [community as service] in response to the socialist practice of community. But it also featured in twentieth-century Labour Party politics and can be identified with politicians like Clement Attlee, Hugh Gaitskell, and with many would-be progressives in modern Britain. Community as service was important to professional men like doctors and lawyers, who grew rapidly in numbers from the mid-nineteenth century onwards, and who tried to establish their legitimacy by stressing their competence to treat social disease and their service to individual clients and to the community. Middle-class women, trying to move out of the home into public work, presented themselves as social mothers doing self-sacrifical service to the poor and to the community. These men and women also co-operated to reinforce each other's service role, especially in the area of public health, where women supposedly sweetened medical inspection, while doctors upgraded traditional philanthropic visiting into scientific activity. [. . .]

Mid-nineteenth-century civic leaders tried to transcend conflict and create community by making the municipality (as a city-state) into an object of service. Through service in local government and voluntary associations, public life was to bring 'the community', in the sense of everybody within the local state, into 'community' in the sense of a new kind of caring union. In the words of the Reverend Dale of Birmingham, where the 'civic gospel' received its clearest formulation in the 1860s, 'new ideas about municipal life and duty were pressed on the whole community'. The Reverend Dawson spoke of the Birmingham Public Library movement as

> capable of bringing about a better union of classes . . . There could not be anything more valuable than men [sic] finding rallying points at which they might forget sectarianism and political economy, which they did not half understand, and find a brotherhood removed from the endless grovellings, and the bickerings . . . This then was the new corporation, the new church, in which they might meet until they came into union again.[1] [. . .]

Community was to be created by public facilities notionally available to all classes. These would displace or absorb similar facilities supplied

---

*This is an abridged extract from *New Views of Co-operation*, Yeo, S. (ed.), Routledge, 1988, pp. 234–257.

by working people for themselves. Bought for a song from the socialists, the Manchester Hall of Science became the first free Public Library in Britain and was hailed as the product of a 'common effort for a common purpose . . . that public domain for mental culture which is the joint heritage and ought to be the common enjoyment of rich and poor'.[2] These fine words must not obscure the fact that this idea of 'common' was displacing mutuality with hierarchy. [. . .] It is safe to say that in bringing the public facilities into being and then in running them, bourgeois men had decisive power. The Public Subscription Committee which often raised the funds was multi-class, but it was divided into a complement of wealthy donors, a large body of affluent subscribers and a separate 'Working Men's Committee'. The resulting hospitals, libraries, town halls, and parks were turned over to local government to be made into state 'services'. They were never controlled, or actively produced, by the users. This was very much a version of community provided through the service of middle-class governors and philanthropists for the people, however much energetic participation in it was urged and however much it was recommended with the rhetoric of mutuality.

Indeed a key feature of community as service and a clear contrast to working-class mutuality has been the continuing middle-class attempt to harmonise social relations without disturbing inequalities of class or gender power. A characteristic project of middle-class groups has been to marry the two oldest definitions of 'community' and to conceal, or, as they would see it, transcend, social antagonism. They have tried to force a union between the community as supplied from above with its basically unequal social structures and community created from inside with its supportive and more ethical human relations. The transforming agency was to be their own *voluntas* expressed in service to a formal entity (e.g. the municipality or a Community Association) together with equivalent though unequal working-class participation. This strand of community thinking has remained strongly committed to locality (the city rather than the nation) and to voluntary effort. But the emphasis has been on co-ordinating voluntary and state activity so that, despite the presence of democratic and visionary anti-state rhetoric, the state has been left in place and in control. Ernest Barker, a member of the National Council for Social Service and the chief ideologue of the Community Association movement, drew upon the whole radical rhetoric of essential Englishness (including the Saxon precedent and the Norman Yoke) to celebrate 'Voluntary Community and a New Democracy', even calling the Community Centre 'a "moot-stow" for their deliberations'. But however representative, Barker argued that a Community Association was 'not a unit of local government, and does not attempt to replace the Local Authority' (which usually, he noted, filled people with massive apathy).[3] This view differed from working-class anti-statism which sought to constitute a (new) state (of affairs) through its own associational activity. [. . .]

People seeing community as service have often been preoccupied with formal institutions and with constructions in the literal sense – buildings as the symbol and the location of community life. We have noted the mid-nineteenth-century bourgeois concern with public buildings. Community Associations put a lot of energy into fund-raising and into lobbying local Councils for a Community Centre or Community Hall. Not least, this building was necessary to provide a venue for middle-class service. [. . .]

The idea of community as service was usually located away from economic production, in leisure life after work. As Park of Chicago, an advocate of Community Centres, put it, 'politics, religion, and community welfare, like golf, bridge and other forms of recreation, are leisure-time activities and it is the leisure time of the community that we are seeking to organise'.[4] This was another contrast with the socialist vision, where production of every kind, including economic production and production of family life, was to be reorganised in order to embody community. [. . .]

Although situated where people had their homes, the middle-class view of community with its stress on service within formal organisations tended to restrict working-class women and to displace their communities. Women's informal networks of relatives and neighbours were a continuing experience of mutual aid. But Community Associations, while purporting to answer the sexism of Working Men's Clubs, had few women officers in their committee structures and few women writers for the CA newspaper. It is true that groups like the Women's Co-operative Guild and the Townswomen's Guild did affiliate, for example, to the Norris Green Community Association in Liverpool and that this Association started a benevolent fund to give members 'a little immediate help'. But the Community Associations never seemed to relate to the neighbourhood networks among women which provided economic and emotional support so important for survival.[5]

Sometimes middle-class women tried to absorb poor women's networks into a notion of community in which social workers and their service was indispensable. Helen Bosanquet was an activist in the Charity Organisation Society and, together with the Women's University Settlement, a pioneer proponent of training for social workers in Schools of Sociology and Social Economics. She argued that social workers would haves to coerce into being the very family and neighbourhood networks which were already there and on which the poor had always relied. She inflated the service of social workers at the expense of poor people's sacrifice:

the unceasing sacrifice of patiently unintelligent women and selfishly unintelligent men is of little use to the community. It does not rise to the level of self-
sacrifice, for there is seldom anything voluntary about it; it is submission to
the brute forces round them.[6]

Only much later, in the 1950s, did the pendulum swing the other way.
Just when social services, public housing and private materialism
seemed to be undermining the informal networks in fact, groups like the
Institute of Community Studies resurrected these neighbourhood networks in theory as the 'traditional' (and desirable) working-class
community.[7]

The example of Bosanquet and other women social workers illustrates
a key feature of most of the middle-class practice of community. This
was the inability to leave independent working-class mutuality alone
and the recurrent attempt to absorb it or replace it with a practice
designed to make middle-class service indispensable. This was the case
even where the mutual aid was informed, as in the case of women's
networks, and perhaps even more the case when mutuality was organised into formal and sometimes militant associations. Community as
service has been continually invoked in and against situations of
working-class militancy. [. . .]

Notes

1. Dawson quoted in E. P. Hennock, *Fit and Proper Persons: Ideal and Reality in
   Nineteenth Century Urban Government*, Edward Arnold, London, 1973, p. 75.
2. Quoted in A. Briggs, *Victorian Cities*, Odhams, London, 1963, pp. 199–200.
3. *Norris Green Life*, June 1937, pp. 14–15, reprinting his address to the 8th
   Annual New Estates Conference in London.
4. R. E. Park, E. W. Burgess and R. D. Mackenzie, *The City*, University of
   Chicago Press, 1925, p. 117.
5. *Norris Green Life*, January 1937, p. 7. *The Wilbraham World: The Official Organ of
   the Wilbraham Association*, Vol. 1, No. 1, December 1932 – Vol. 2, No. 12, April
   1935, in the Manchester Central Reference Library, is a rich source for the
   aspirations of a high-minded Community Association on a Manchester
   estate. From 1929 to 1935 their secretary was Emily J. Jenkinson; see her
   Utopian dream of what the Wilbraham estate could be like in 1999 in *The
   Wilbraham World*, Vol. 1, No. 3, p. 29, and her disappointed departing letter in
   WW, December 1934. 'A change of heart in their neighbours' seemed to be
   what the Wilbraham Association was trying to achieve, although there is also
   evidence, for example from Wythenshawe (*WW*, June 1934), of tenants'
   union/area impulses at work.
6. H. Bosanquet, *Rich and Poor*, Macmillan, London, 1899, p. 103; *Social Work in
   London, 1869–1912*, London, 1914, reprinted Harvester Press, Brighton, 1973,
   pp. 403–4.

7. E.g., P. Willmott, *The Evolution of a Community: a Study of Dagenham after Forty Years*, Routledge and Kegan Paul, London, 1963, p. 109, the follow-up study to Willmott and M. Young, *Family and Kinship in East London*, Routledge and Kegan Paul, London, 1957. S. Laing, *Representations of Working-Class Life, 1957–1964*, Macmillan, London, 1986, pp. 37ff., for genres of community study in the 1950s.

Part II

CARE

9

Introduction

This section begins with an anthology of care. The extracts in this anthology are drawn from fiction, research, autobiography, diary, oral history, newspaper articles and taped interview. They focus mainly on the personal and experiential dimensions of care, and cover a range of different groups who provide and receive care and support. From a different angle, the anthology also attempts to place 'care' in a historical and international context and to see it operating over a wide range of relations.

The first two chapters in this section open with a detailed look at caring processes. The first, an extract from Janet Finch and Jennifer Mason's work, explores the nature of obligation and responsibility to care within kin groups and looks at how far principles of obligation shape the care and support offered by daughters and sons to their elderly parents. The second is drawn from Jane Hubert's searching, candid and closely observed research study of 20 families with young adults who have severe or profound learning difficulties or display challenging behaviour. She pieces together the complexity of reasons why parents in this situation find it difficult to let go of their adult children into care outside the home.

This is followed by work that in different ways opens up the field of research on caring. The first, by Yasmin Gunaratnam, fills an important gap. It looks at the experiences of Asian carers, drawing on both her own research and her experiences as an Asian carer. She argues for the necessity to understand the needs of Asian carers and the people for whom they care in a context wider than just 'care'. Many of the people she interviewed experienced poverty, poor housing conditions and racial harassment along with inappropriate and inaccessible service provision.

Hilary Graham continues with this theme of widening the context of care. She suggests that studies of caring need to account for the experiences of those who *receive* as well as those who *provide* care and to bring out more of the class and race differences in women's experiences of caring. The extract from Sarah Arber and Nigel Gilbert's work also represents an important refinement to research work on carers. Using data from the 1980 General Household Survey they map the significance of *male* carers, particularly men who care for their wives.

Clare Ungerson's article looks at care in the yet wider context of social rights. The notion of *citizenship* has enjoyed a resurgence in the 1990s, but how far is it applicable to the needs and lives of carers?

In 1988 the publication of Gillian Dalley's book *Ideologies of Caring*: *Rethinking Community and Collectivism* represented a consolidation of feminist research and writing on care. We reproduce here a short extract on the principles of collective care. The final extract represents a further significant development in work on caring. In this Jenny Morris, a disabled feminist, provides a critique of research on care which, she explains, has rendered invisible the experiences, perspectives and demands of those who receive care and support.

10

Anthology: Care

Compiled by FIONA WILLIAMS

These extracts have been grouped under five headings. The *process* of care focuses on the day-to-day experiences of those involved in caring for an older person. The *context* of care demonstrates the variety of historical, cultural and social sites and relations of care through extracts drawn from domestic service, institutional care, mothering, neighbouring and caring for a gay partner. In *struggles* of care both the carer and the person cared for describe the particular problems and difficulties that their situation gives rise to. Similarly, *dilemmas* of care illustrates the conflicts and constraints placed upon those committed to providing the best possible care. Under the heading of *rights* those who use care and support services give a powerful voice to the right to determine the kind of care and support they want. Overall, the anthology helps us to see care not only in terms of different contexts and relationships, but as a manifestation of different feelings and motivations: control, responsibility, obligation, altruism, love and solidarity.

10.1 The process

*An abridged extract from **Have the Men had Enough?**, a novel by Margaret Forster, Penguin, Harmondsworth, 1989, pp. 94–8.*

Adrian and I take Grandma to the chiropodist at the clinic. She, the chiropodist, would come to Grandma's home but it makes an outing for Grandma so we keep taking her. And it is what Mum calls a nice little job for Adrian. He does the driving. (Adrian is *very* proud of having passed his driving test first time last year.) He does the driving but for reasons unknown to me he cannot do the taking-into-the-clinic-and-divesting-of-stockings. Mum says Grandma would be embarrassed if Adrian took her stockings off. It would mean fiddling with suspenders – Grandma cannot be parted from her suspenders – and Mum says that is too much to expect. I can't see why but Mum also keeps saying

81

Grandma would mind. How this could be proved I don't know. But I go as well, to be the stocking-taker-offer. Women's work, again.

Adrian has no idea how to get Grandma into the car. He just stands there, helpless, saying why can't she sit down and Grandma stands, equally helpless, and they stare at each other and Grandma asks Adrian if his name is Duncan. He says no, of course, and she says that's a pity because she knows a poem about Duncan Davidson that puts her in mind of him and it goes etc. etc. I say if we stand here any longer, we'll miss the appointment. Then I show off. I point to the floor of the car and tell Grandma to pick that sweetie up, it's going to waste. She bends slowly and, when she's nearly there, reaching into the front of the car, I put my hand on her head to protect it from getting knocked and I push her bottom sideways and she half-falls into the car and I lift her legs to join the rest of her. Mission accomplished. Adrian is aghast. He says I'm cruel. I tell him to shut up. He hasn't the faintest idea of how to manage Grandma. He drives slowly, as though he had a cargo of porcelain.

I sit outside. I suppose the chiropodist wouldn't mind if I stayed but when she asks would I like to wait outside, I always obey.

I go back in to put the stockings on. The chiropodist explains to me what she has done and what she will do next time. She refers to Grandma as 'she' and 'her', as though she was an idiot. When it comes to putting Grandma's shoes on, I have difficulty. They're very old shoes. They're made of brown leather, the sort that are laced and have good strong soles. The leather is very worn. In fact, there's a small hole, rapidly widening into a tear, where Grandma's largest bunion is pushing through. The chiropodist watches. She says maybe 'she' needs some new shoes. Grandma flares up. She says these are good shoes they cost a fortune, there is nothing the matter with them. I'm sweating. Grandma is not helping. She holds her foot rigid, won't even attempt to bend her toes. One shoe is on and laced but I can't get her left foot into the other. All this pushing and shoving is useless. Grandma is getting angry. She starts kicking her foot deliberately so that the shoe flies across the room.

> One, two, buckle my shoe.
> Grandma, behave.
> You mind yourself.
> You mind yourself, keep your foot still.
> I like a wee jig now and again.
> Not when you're putting your shoes on.

The chiropodist has retrieved the other shoe and comments sympathetically that she does feel sorry for me. Now I am angry. I snap at the chiropodist. Then I hand Grandma her shoe and I stand up and I tell her that if she doesn't hurry up, the men will be in for their tea and nothing ready. She proceeds to put her own shoe on, stumbling only over the tying of the laces which I bend and do quickly.

When we get home, I say to Mum straight away that Grandma must have new shoes, that her shoes are in a terrible state, that it's no wonder her walking is deteriorating. I put Grandma's slippers on her feet and then I flourish the offending shoes under Mum's nose. Mum says I'm not telling her anything she doesn't know. She has taken Grandma to a shoe shop and there is no such thing as a shoe which will fit her appalling misshapen feet. But she will mention to it Bridget and see if she has any ideas. Adrian chips in. He says how about men's trainers? I scoff but Mum nods. Adrian brings his new trainers and tries them on Grandma. They appear to go on quite easily. She looks so funny, sitting on the sofa with Adrian's white trainers plonked on the end of her lisle-stockinged legs. We're still laughing when Bridget arrives. Grandma is laughing too, she knows she's a good turn. She has taken the tea cosy off the tea pot – the tea cosy she crocheted herself years ago and loves to see on the tea pot, so Mum tries to remember to put it on – and she has put it on her head because she says she can feel a bloomin' draught. She has one ear poking out of the hole for the spout and the other out of the hole for the handle. The vivid reds, blues, greens and yellows of the tea cosy stripes straddle her large head. Adrian is crying with laughing and I am almost as bad. Then Bridget arrives. She snatches the tea cosy off Grandma's head. Grandma yelps and tells her to get lost. Bridget's face is red and angry. She *hates* Grandma to be a laughing stock even though Grandma loves to be the cause of mirth. Bridget says, 'Mother!' furiously and also yanks off Adrian's trainers. Now Grandma starts moaning her feet and head are both cold. Bridget grabs the tartan shawl from a chair and ties it round Grandma's head. She looks around and finds Grandma's shoes and forces them on. Mum looks annoyed. She says to Bridget it was only a joke. Bridget says some jokes go too far. Mum makes an exclamation of irritation and goes into the kitchen. I start to speak but Mum motions that I should say nothing. Really, Bridget is very odd.

10.2   The context

*A home help talking about her job. An extract from an interview with Muriel Arncliffe, from the Open University course P654 **Working with Older People**.*

I used to enjoy me Fridays, that were a little old lady I had down there. She were great. She were crippled with arthritis but she was always right cheerful, you know, and she used to love me to go. [. . .] There is the type of people that appreciate whatever you do. I could have gone in there and just sat and she'd have never been bothered. [. . .] It's knowing you've achieved something isn't it? You've done that for them but they wouldn't be able to do it if you hadn't had time. [. . .] I mean it's alright sitting and talking but when you've gone they're still sit in a mucky house aren't they?

Mrs—, she was nasty. She couldn't understand why she had to have home help that's what it was. But she couldn't do it, you see, she'd got rheumatics, you know, arthritis. [. . .] You'd tell her why and then she'd forget and then she'd say well why are you here? And you'd tell her again and then ten minutes later she'd say but why are you here? And that's how it was all the time. [. . .] It gets you down. You know, I used to go back and say I think I need four hours there, it's driving me mad.

You panic when you go to the door and they don't answer . . . you look through t' letter box and if they're there on t' floor and they're not moving you do panic. You think, my God she's died, you know. Part of the job, isn't it?

Kevin Brompton, on caring for his lover, Alan. An abridged extract from **Who Cares? Looking after People at Home**, *by Cherrill Hicks, Virago, London, 1988, pp. 186–8.*

I suppose, looking at it now, all of last year on and off he was ill: there were lots of silly little things. If you're gay it's always at the back of your mind – every time you sneeze. He had had psoriasis, it got very bad; he had had problems with his bowels, as well as shingles and gout. He'd always been quite healthy before; he was the sort of person that everyone said: it will never happen to Alan.

I suppose, at first, we both sort of hoped we'd got a couple of years. We thought we had plenty of time for them to get a cure: in that situation, you grasp at any straw.

[Alan's parents, who live in a different part of the country, do not know that he is dead: there had been no contact between him and his family for years.]

There was a big bust up several years ago; they [Alan's parents] weren't happy because he was gay. At a later stage they said maybe they'd been a bit hasty, but it was too late for Alan. He got rid of everything to do with them: in all his belongings there was nothing, no papers or anything, not one reference to them. He didn't want them to know that he'd got AIDS, and he said they weren't to know about his death.

My own family have been as supportive as they could be. My father and stepmother: we're quite close, although we never openly discussed the fact that we were gay. It was referred to obliquely though. Just before Alan died, they guessed what was wrong.

We've got lots of very good friends, mostly gay, but some straight: they've been absolutely marvellous, and they still are. I don't think I could have done it otherwise, to be quite honest. In the last few months there were not enough hours in the day; I was working, but we had a rota of friends with keys who would all pop in.

Alan was always OK to be left. I used to give him his breakfast and leave a meal out, and a friend would drop by to see if he was OK; then he would snooze until I got home. I'd see to all the lotions and potions and ointments for his skin; he needed special cream for his fingers and feet. When he was in hospital I used to bath him.

When Alan first went into hospital, there was no proper AIDS ward. It was a fairly old ward and fairly crowded: not a very wonderful place. But later, when he went back, there was a new ward: they'd obviously spent a lot of money. Most of the time he had his own room with a shower, his own TV. The attention and love they got from the staff – it was quite exceptional. Especially the nurses. The doctors were good as well; but then, doctors have to be doctors, don't they?

I think it's affected all of us really. I can't speak for the whole of the gay community, of course; I can only speak for my circle. We all think we've got to live very much for today, but then most gay people have always felt like that.

He knew I'd look after him and I did, as best I could. That's all there is to it, really.

---

*From **A Woman's Place: An Oral History of Working-Class Women, 1890– 1940**, by Elizabeth Roberts, Blackwell, Oxford, 1984, pp. 189–91.*

The neighbours were far better than they are today. They were not as clannish. If the next door neighbour was poorly we would go in and help. We'd do her washing, do her ironing, and we'd take them back and if they wanted any messages going we used to do it. They were always willing to help you. Now today, they're more clannish, they seem as if they want to be on their own.

When they were ill they used to get a sheep's head and a marrow bone and then twopennyworth of pot herbs and make a good pan of soup, and some split peas and barley and take them a good bowl of soup in at night. We perhaps used to take them their dinners. [. . .] Really they were better friends than what they are. They're good friends today but they're more for themselves. In the olden days it was sisterly love and more motherly love. I used to be knocked up time out of time when anybody died. They used to come and knock at the door at midnight and say, 'Will you come and lay the baby out? Will you come and lay so-and-so out?' I used to go and lay them out.

An abridged extract from **Life As We Have Known It**, *edited by Margaret Llewellyn Davies, 1931; reprinted by Virago, London, 1977, pp. 20–5. The narrator, Mrs Layton, was born in Bethnal Green in 1855.*

Ten years of domestic service

When I was ten years old I began to earn my own living. I went to mind the baby of a person who kept a small general shop. My wages were 1/6 a week and my tea, and 2d. a week for myself. I got to work at eight in the morning and left at eight at night, with the exception of two nights a week when I left at seven o'clock to attend a night school, one of a number started by Lord Shaftesbury, called Ragged Schools. I was very happy in my place and was very fond of the baby, who grew so fond of me that by the time he was twelve months old he would cry after me when I went home to my dinner and when I went away to school before he was in bed. I felt very proud of my influence over my baby, and got into the habit of taking him home with me rather than let him cry.

When I was thirteen years old I went into service at Hampstead where I stayed twelve months. I had a very kind mistress and plenty of good food. I was fairly happy, but had to sleep in a basement kitchen which swarmed with black-beetles, and this made me very wretched at nights. I was only allowed out on Sundays to go to church. Sometimes I got a change by going on to the heath with the three children.

At the age of fifteen I had my first experience of maternity nursing. I went to service at Kentish Town, where there were four children, and in a few months another baby was born. A few days after the birth of the child the mother died of puerperal fever. [. . .] From that time till I left, two and a half years later, I had the principal care of the baby. I loved it as I love my life.

'Bloodmothers, othermothers, and women-centered networks,' an abridged extract from Patricia Hill Collins, **Black Feminist Thought**, *Unwin Hyman, London, 1990, pp. 119–20.*

In African-American communities, fluid and changing boundaries often distinguish biological mothers from other women who care for children. Biological mothers, or bloodmothers, are expected to care for their children. But African and African-American communities have also recognised that vesting one person with full responsibility for mothering a child may not be wise or possible. As a result, othermothers – women who assist bloodmothers by sharing mothering responsibilities – traditionally have been central to the institution of Black motherhood.

The centrality of women in African-American extended families reflects both a continuation of West African cultural values and functional adaptations to race and gender oppression. This centrality is not characterised by the absence of husbands and fathers. Men may be physically present and/or have well-defined and culturally significant roles in the extended family and the kin unit may be woman-centered.

Organised, resilient, women-centered networks of bloodmothers and othermothers are key in understanding this centrality. Grandmothers, sisters, aunts, or cousins act as othermothers by taking on child-care responsibilities for one another's children. When needed, temporary child-care arrangements can turn into long-term care or informal adoption. Despite strong cultural norms encouraging women to become biological mothers, women who choose not to do so often receive recognition and status from othermother relationships that they establish with Black children.

In African-American communities these women-centered networks of community-based child care often extend beyond the boundaries of biologically related individuals and include 'fictive kin'. Civil rights activist Ella Baker describes how informal adoption by othermothers functioned in the rural southern community of her childhood:

> My aunt who had thirteen children of her own raised three more. She had become a midwife, and a child was born who was covered with sores. Nobody was particularly wanting the child, so she took the child and raised him . . . and another mother decided she didn't want to be bothered with two children. So my aunt took one and raised him . . . they were part of the family.

Even when relationships are not between kin or fictive kin, African-American community norms traditionally were such that neighbours cared for one another's children. Sara Brooks, a southern domestic worker, describes the importance that the community-based child care a neighbour offered her daughter had for her:

> She kept Vivian and she didn't charge me nothin either. You see, people used to look after each other, but now it's not that way. I reckon it's because we all was poor, and I guess they put theirself in the place of the person that they was helpin.

Brooks's experiences demonstrate how the African-American cultural value placed on cooperative child care traditionally found institutional support in the adverse conditions under which so many Black women mothered.

An abridged extract from **A Price to be Born**, *New Directions, Colchester, 1981, pp. 91–3, the autobiography of David Barron, who spent many years in institutions. He was born in Leeds in 1925 in Street Lane Orphanage. At the age of 5 he went to a foster-mother who ill-treated him. He describes how at 14 he was removed.*

One evening, just as I was ready to go to bed, there came a knock on the front door and Miss Bellamy answered it to admit a lady and two gentlemen, one of whom asked my foster mother if they could see my bedroom.

The man turned to me, 'Come on David, you are to come with us.'

It might not have been so bad if they had let me get dressed again but before I knew what was happening they had taken me, still in pyjamas, to their care. I was never to see my foster mother again.

I was immediately placed in a home with children of my own age where I stayed for the next two days, but the worst was yet to come. From this short stay home I was taken to an institution which was to be very much my long stay home, and a very big home at that. The name of the Institution was the Mid-Yorkshire Institution, Wixley, near York. The reader might care to note that I was a mere fourteen years of age when I was taken to what was a mental institution, but in those days these places had to take in all kinds of homeless persons who were in no way mentally ailing. The Institution was to be my home for the next eighteen years, beginning as a so-called patient and finishing as a supervisor. It is now run by the Clifton Mental Hospital, York.

How my life proceeded from the formative years of early adolescence into adulthood is another story which may or may not be written, but the reader will appreciate that fate had decreed that the price to be born in my case was to go on being paid for right up to the present day.

10.3   Struggles

'Carers may be angels but does that make their dependants devils?', an abridged extract from the **Guardian**, *2 January 1991, by Kate Cooney.*

Maria's pale green eyes sparkle in the candlelight, ablaze with wine and desire. Slowly, carefully, she unzips the front of her dress. The black silk slips from her shoulders, caressing the lengths of her naked body as it rustles to the floor. Dropping to the bed, she slithers out of her shiny, thigh-high boots as a snake sheds its skin. She leans back, beckons to him and he obeys, stumbling and with shaking hands. At last, he is beside her, paralysed with anticipation. Turning boldly towards him, she whispers, 'Will you take my socks off, please?'

There is something terminally unsexy about not being able to take your own socks off – even if they're clean, without holes and have never belonged to your dad. It's been some years since I have been able to do it, yet it still rankles to see my partner peeling back those little black ones from M&S for me after a particularly sweaty day. It also peeves me that I need him to insert a suppository for me every night, that I've stopped wearing earrings because I don't want to bother him to put them in for me, that the air does not always smell of lavender when he has to help me off the loo.

I am 31 and have had rheumatoid arthritis since the age of 18. Like most people, I once plucked my eyebrows, made a cup of coffee when I felt like it, shaved my own legs. Slowly, the ability to do these things has been taken away from me.

Allowing someone else into the yuckier side of your life is hard. Even the most intimate of relationships do not contain the grossly earthy things that are par for the course in ours. I have next to no privacy. My partner knows my every nook and cranny, and I am left without a millimetre's worth of mystery.

No, it's *not* easy, being 'cared for'. It's not just the messy bits. It's no longer being able to nick a chocolate biscuit out of the fridge, or experiment with make-up, or grab just the right scarf to set off your jumper as you rush out of the door. Always, *always*, you have to ask.

These things may seem insignificant nit-pickings compared with the more obviously dramatic changes wrought by disability, but taken together they are as momentous as the arrival of the wheelchair or the loss of your job. As they are given up, a little bit of what outwardly makes you an individual is eroded.

Your carer has to run part of your body for you. If you insist it is run exactly the way you would have run it, you will be ridiculously demanding. But it still hurts to let go and it's still hard, getting used to the new, circumscribed you – should I ask for that or shouldn't I?

No one would deny that looking after another person can be tough. The current rash of articles written by and about carers bears witness to this. It is also often a job reluctantly undertaken. Knowing all this, reading all the accounts of ruined lives, it can be just as tough finding yourself in the position of having to receive all this 'care' – your self-esteem can easily be drowned out by guilt and gratefulness. If carers are way down the ladder, then those they care for are at the bottom, popularly seen as exacting tyrants, as indifferent to their helpers' feelings as pampered pet poodles.

Caring isn't just about changing incontinence pads and wheeling inert lumps of flesh, draped in tartan blankets, around the shops on Saturday mornings. Give the carers the recognition they deserve. Give them the money. But don't reduce those who depend on them to dehumanised burdens, don't let their handicaps cancel out their identities. After all, you are only one visit to the doctor, one dash across the road, one hair's breadth away from being one too.

———————

From **Carers at Work**, *based on the National Carers' Survey, carried out by Opportunities for Women, London, 1990, p. 5.*

Carers in general face tremendous problems, fears. I mean just look at the financial worry, constantly trying to make sure bills are paid, trying to juggle the different incomes, make them stretch far enough.

And then there's the isolation. A lot of carers get sucked into isolation. It depends on the relationship they have with the person they are caring for. I mean I am very very lucky, I have a good relationship with my mother-in-law and she is very easy to care for considering her disability. Other people get bogged down, and people stop calling and they can't go out. You don't have much of a social life. You can't really roll home at two o'clock in the morning and then get up at 7 or 8 o'clock to breakfast people and things like that . . . there's lots of problems.

It would be good from the psychological point of view for carers to be able to go out to work, but they would need to have some very secure support system. Because you don't actually know from one day to the next what's going to happen or what's going to meet you when you get up in the morning, or if the person's going to be more ill than usual. Or if you're going to be up during the night. If you are, you're not going to be bright-eyed and bushy-tailed first thing in the morning. So halfway through the next day you would be very very tired. Then it would be difficult to work because your concentration would go. Carers in the main, the ones who work and who I have contact with, are generally in low-paid menial jobs, just very part-time hours and very very low wages, which is very unfortunate.

The support system and the benefits for carers at the moment are by no means adequate. I mean they just don't cover anything. There's nothing out there comparable to what it would cost to keep a person in a nursing home or in a long-stay hospital or whatever.

10.4 Dilemmas

An abridged extract from A. Richardson and J. Ritchie, **Making the Break: Parents' Views about Adults with Mental Handicap Leaving the Parental Home**, *London, King's Fund, 1986, pp. xx.*

Matthew is 36 and mildly handicapped as the result of an accident at birth. He can read, write, has an excellent memory and is a keen musician. According to his parents, 'he's definitely a character. He's an extrovert in every sense of the word, with a tremendous sense of humour.'

Matthew's parents are in their 70s and his father, after a major operation, is now in very poor health. They have a very close relationship with Matthew and both are quite devoted to him. They feel they are over-protective with Matthew, but there is clearly a real dilemma. 'Being a parent you automatically do for them – you can't help it. Partly you want them to look good all the time and partly it's because you just want to keep on doing things for them.' Again they are aware that they could have done more to encourage Matthew to be independent. 'You want him to be independent but at the same time it's difficult to put over this independence, and you are forced to do things that *they* want you to do although you know you shouldn't do it. For example, he won't tie his shoe laces so in the end we finally buy shoes for him that have *no* laces – slip-on shoes and that gets over the problem. Well it's wrong.'

Matthew's mother admits to it having been a wrench when her three older sons left home but saw it as a natural progression. With Matthew it's different. 'I always thought I'd look after him as long as I could. [. . .] I'd keep myself in good health and look after him, and I have done.' But at the same time, both parents are aware that it's not necessarily the best thing for Matthew. 'I mean, that's obvious . . . you think you're doing the best for them but deep down you know damn well he'd been better off in a place where they'd have given him a thorough education – but would they have looked after him? Would they have given him a home life?'

Because of his father's illness, Matthew's parents have begun very reluctantly to consider the issue of his move from home. They have written for information about village communities and asked around about the local hostels. They feel that life in the 'village system' would be best for him because of the small, family type living arrangements. But if a place became available, 'a lot's dependent on Matthew – if he puts his foot down and doesn't want to go – I can't go against that, can I?'

Matthew's parents think it is most likely that he will eventually go to live in one of the local hostels. Deep down, his father knows that they should be taking some steps to effect a move in the very near future. 'We're not youngsters any more . . . [if he agreed to try to live elsewhere] I would be happy; it would be so terribly important for him.' But his mother is less sure that she could ever part with Matthew. 'He's part and parcel of my life . . . my life is Matthew. It has been for such a long time that I can't visualise it any other way. And I don't think I would want to.'

An extract from Frank Thomas's diary in **The Politics of Mental Handicap**, *by Joanna Ryan and Frank Thomas, Free Association Books, London, 1987, pp. 36–7.*

Helping at meal times on my first day nearly drove me into getting my coat and heading for home. Standing at the patients' meal trolley, wearing my crisp white clinical uniform, hearing the high-pitched abuse, the constant shouting at the patients to sit down and shut up, was enough to make me jack it all in on the spot.

There was perhaps one staff, Bruce, who treated the patients as humans, as individuals. In the following days I jolted him out of the apathy and despair he was experiencing with the situation. He at the same time convinced me that if we worked together we might get a few things done. The potentialities of the situation could be exploited only if I chose to stay.

Could I help the lads get through the day without feeling too bad, soften the blows they constantly received, give a more humane aspect to their nursing care? With Bruce's help this seemed possible. The snag was of course that there were the other staff to contend with. What was needed was an attempt to break down the rigid staff/patient dichotomy, to be a friend of the lads, with all that entails. Completely reject the authoritarian side of my role as staff.

All the bizarre happenings on the ward would still go on, but at least I could define a purpose in being there. To stay meant to a certain extent accepting the situation, but at the same time not being part of it – an insider and an outsider simultaneously.

You change. Whether you change the system or the system changes you, you change. Circumstances change to change you. People hit other people. Horrific. A daily occurrence. A norm. You want to vomit at the ever present reek of urine. You get used to it. People swear, defile, bite themselves, scream incessantly, say nothing, do less, go beserk at you, dribble for ever, have dried food all over their clothes, look a terrible grey mess. A superficial overview. You get to know the lads, it doesn't take too long. Each lad is a highly individual person in his own right. Such relationships can be very satisfying, rewarding and enjoyable experiences.

As far as I could, every time I saw a patient being harassed or bullied or abused, I would attempt to relieve the suffering, for suffering it was. And with those lads who were up to it, we discussed their situation freely – the hospital, the staff, the food, what it was all about. It was an opportunity to take a look at their situation for themselves without the other staff interfering, an experience they had not had before. If this smacks of anarchy, well – maybe what these hospitals need is a revolution to sort them out.

10.5 Rights

*Mukti Jain Campion defends the right of women with disabilities to be parents. An abridged extract from the **Observer**, 14 July 1991.*

'It's obscene, people like you shouldn't be allowed to have children.' These were the words of a complete stranger thrust at a young pregnant woman out shopping one day in her wheel-chair.

The assailant knew nothing about her disability, her domestic situation or about her preparations to become a parent. Like many people, she had made a lot of assumptions:

- Disabled women shouldn't have sex (young people with disabilities don't need sex education or family planning advice).
- Disabled women are ill (so the child will be too).
- Disabled women cannot be adequate mothers (so it's selfish).

They are prejudices which are no more true of most disabled women than they are of the able-bodied. What is worrying is that these misconceptions are so prevalent that even professionals, such as teachers, doctors and social workers, are often infected by them.

The result is that thousands of healthy, fertile women are put off having children or pressured into abortions. And if they decide to have children, they have to negotiate a painful series of obstacle courses. Few hospitals have staff trained in disability awareness or in signing for the deaf. Childbirth itself can be made more frightening because of the lack of accurate information and optimistic support.

Then when the child is born the mother is often labelled as either a pathetic victim in need of pity, or a courageous heroine with no need of help. Both labels deny the woman's right to be treated as normal. The threat of children being taken into care also looms when fitness to parent is questioned.

So are disabled women fit to be mothers? The question suggests there is a norm, established by able-bodied parents, that disabled parents have to match. This is ludicrous.

All the research shows that, as far as the welfare of the child is concerned, disability is not a bar to being a competent, caring parent. Disability takes so many different forms that no outsider can generalise on whether it might prevent mothers from being fit to look after their own children. Thousands of women – with arthritis, multiple sclerosis, spina bifida, women who are blind or deaf, disabled since birth or in later life – have successfully borne and brought up children. Each has contributed her own version of normality and in the process enriched our society.

Some women with disabilities may need additional medical help in pregnancy or practical help with childcare, but then so do many able-bodied mothers. If disadvantages arise, they are often due to social repercussions of disability, such as poverty, poorly-adapted housing, isolation and, above all, public attitudes. These are society's failings, yet it is disabled mothers and their families who are penalised.

Things are changing slowly. Peer networks such as the one run by ParentAbility are springing up all over the country. These enable prospective mothers to tap into the wealth of advice and experience of others with similar disabilities.

Professionals, too, are putting disability and parenthood on their agenda.

It is often argued that not everyone has a right to be a parent. But if that is the case, selection criteria should be agreed and applied to everyone, not just to those who appear different.

In a historic case in the US, a judge returned a child to the care of a disabled mother whose fitness to be a parent had been questioned. He suggested that other people, as well as parents, could help with the physical aspects of childcare, but said the essence of parenting 'lies in the ethical, emotional and intellectual guidance the parent gives to the child throughout the formative years and beyond'. In this, he judged, the mother was thoroughly able.

Mike Lawson, from Survivors Speak Out, an organisation for people who use psychiatric services, and Jane Campbell, from the British Council of Disabled People, discuss the meaning of care to them as users of services. Extract from an interview for the Open University course K259 **Community Care***.*

Mike:
I want the choice when I want to be cared for and when I want to be left alone like any other human being would and I don't want a special set of circumstances to be considered simply because I've been labelled as psychiatrically ill or whatever and I assume that this is a mutual sort of feeling.

Jane:
I'd say we don't want to be cared for at all. I would say that we want to be facilitated, supported and empowered. Care to me has connotations of custody and of lack of control and of looking after somebody who is sick and getting worse basically. Several people have actually become more and more to actually loathe the term care because it is being used

in such a way to fudge the issue. You know, we have care and repair for all these wheel-chair companies; now we have the caring government that really is going to look after us and make sure that care in the community really works well. Nothing could be more far from the truth. Then there's the carers – you know these paragons – these people who who care at the expense of their own lives, the burden of the disabled person who they look after. I'm just quoting some of the tabloids. This has actually made disabled people become very touchy around the whole notion of care because it's not what they want. What they want or what we want or what I want is to have control over my life, but at the times when it's difficult to do that then I want the support to actually get through that particular time. I would say caring and care in the community is about control – maintaining us in a certain position – and it's about seeing disabled people as people with individual problems. It's not empowering at all.

11

Filial Obligations and Kin Support for Elderly People*

JANET FINCH and JENNIFER MASON

11.1 Introduction

Research on the family care of elderly people has been a major growth area in recent years, in Britain as elsewhere. Underlying much of it – but often not addressed directly – are questions about the nature of obligation and responsibility within families, and how far these underscore the support which may be offered to elderly people who can no longer fully care for themselves. Research which has attempted to encompass these issues has tended to be conducted on a fairly small scale.[1]

This chapter is based on a large research project, which includes qualitative and quantitative data on kin obligations and support. We are confining ourselves to discussing data upon the care of elderly people and upon the obligations of children in particular. The central focus of our research is support which passes between kin and adult life, and how far this is underpinned by concepts of obligation, responsibility and duty. We are therefore concerned with issues about norms and morality in family life, and how far these constitute explanations of what people do, or do not do, for their relatives. Other explanations of what people do are possible, of course: personal preference or liking, pragmatic considerations or patterns of exchange built upon reciprocity over a lifetime. We are not excluding any of these – indeed we are very interested in trying to understand how they mesh together – but our central concern is the issue of normative obligations and how they

---

*This is an abridged version of a paper that was first published in *Ageing and Society*, Vol. 10, 1990, pp. 151–73.

operate. To put it very simply, in what sense do people support their kin because they see it as 'the proper thing to do'?

Our discussion locates these issues in the context of contemporary Britain, because the study upon which we draw was based in the north-west of England. However, the issues which we raise are fundamental to understanding the nature of final obligations in any society. Existing literature on kinship in Britain would suggest that if we are going to find a strong sense of duty or obligation anywhere, we will find it in parent–child relationships. It is variously described in this literature as the central kinship bond, the least ambiguous of adult kin relationships and the relationship most clearly founded upon a sense of obligation.[2]

The classic kinship literature indicates that it is widely seen as legitimate for parents who are elderly to make demands on their adult children, but that literature also suggests that it is possible for parents to overstep the mark by demanding *too much* and also by making demands in the *wrong way*. Alongside this we also have to place the substantial evidence that a situation of total dependence of elderly people on their children seems to be widely regarded as undesirable. Townsend's classic study of the family life of old people[3] popularised the phrase 'intimacy at a distance' to describe the desired relationships between elderly people and their children, and later studies do seem to keep confirming that.[4]

There are also predictable sources of variation in the support which passes between elderly people and their children, most obviously related to gender and ethnicity. The classic kinship literature documents the central role which women play in the maintenance of family relationships ('kin keeping'), and there is also ample evidence that when it comes to the more arduous of the practical tasks, these are usually performed by daughters, or indeed daughters-in-law, rather than sons.[5] Clearly that reflects the gender division of responsibility and labour in the performance of domestic tasks more generally, a division which itself varies in different ethnic groups. There is a separate, but linked, question about whether women and men display a different sense of obligation and duty towards their parents, or their relatives more generally. Some feminist writers have argued persuasively that 'a sense of responsibility' permeates women's approach to family relationships in a way which is not replicated for men.[6]

These then, are the kinds of issue which form the background to our study. The questions which we are raising are:

(1) Do people in contemporary Britain clearly acknowledge that parent–child relations are founded upon norms of obligation (rather than personal preference, pragmatic considerations, etc.)?
(2) What is the substance of these norms? Is there anything

approaching a consensus about what parents can expect from their children?

(3) How do norms operate in practice?

11.2   Public norms about filial obligations

We begin with some of the data from the Family Obligations survey. This was conducted in the Great Manchester area in late 1985 and involved interviews with 978 adults of all ages.

The purpose of the survey was to investigate how far it is true to say there is a public normative consensus about obligations between adult kin. We wanted to see if there is any level of agreement among a random sample of the population about what counts as 'the proper thing to do' for relatives in specified circumstances. We were not trying to use the survey to generate data about what people *actually* do for their own relatives – that came at the second stage of the study, which was based on in-depth interviews with some of the people who had been in the survey, and some of their relatives. Nor were we wishing to make any prior assumptions about the relationship between beliefs and values expressed in our survey and the ways in which people arrive at commitments to their own relatives. Again, it is in the second stage of the study that we have tried to explore the extent to which people are guided by a sense of 'the proper thing to do' in relationships with their own relatives.[7] In the survey, our method was to assess whether there is agreement about proper forms of obligation between kin, mainly by using questions about hypothetical situations concerning third parties, in which people were invited to indicate what the participants 'should' do.

11.2.1   Do people give assent to the idea of filial obligations?

At the most general level, our survey data suggest that most people do give assent at this normative level to the idea of filial obligations (i.e. that adult children are obligated to their parents), but that this assent is neither universal nor unconditional. When presented with a bald attitude statement: 'Children have no obligation to look after their parents when they are old', 57 per cent of our sample disagreed and 39 per cent agreed. Disagreement with this statement indicates assent to the idea of filial obligations, and we can see that although a majority fall into this category, a sizeable minority do not.[8]

In various other more specific questions concerned with examples of middle-aged or elderly people needing assistance, again a majority seemed to give approval to the idea of filial obligations. We had a whole series of questions in which we spelled out a situation, asked respondents to presume that some relative was going to provide assistance and invited them to say *which* relative this should be. Respondents were not presented with a list of options so that, in effect, they could propose any permutation of relatives they wished. In all circumstances where a child could be presumed to exist, children were the clearest targets. Tables 11.1–11.4 give some examples from these questions, which are concerned both with financial and practical assistance.

A number of points could be explored in relation to these tables – for example, the variations in people's responses according to the type of assistance needed. However, we use them here for a fairly limited purpose: to focus upon what is being said about *who* should offer help. Although there is some variation in the preferences expressed, it is noticeable that they remain concentrated in a very narrow genealogical range. Of course there is nothing startling about this pattern, but it does confirm empirically that, at the level of publicly expressed norms, most people do see children as the people who should step in first and offer assistance even when other relatives are presumed to be available. A few people did mention siblings, grandchildren or more distant relatives, but they were in a very small minority.

Thus the data contained in these tables suggest fairly strong support for the idea of filial obligations specifically – the special responsibilities of children over other relatives. This seems to hold for all the questions where we asked our respondents to assume that *some* relative was going to provide assistance for an elderly person. These answers have to be understood in the light of knowing that a sizeable minority of our survey population would not necessarily have wanted care to come from relatives at all – or at least did not regard this as the optimum solution. That is illustrated in Table 11.4, for example, where 35 per cent thought that relatives definitely should not offer money to pay for decorating. In relation to the situations posed in Tables 11.1–11.3, earlier in the interview between 56 per cent and 70 per cent of our respondents had opted for some solution other than family care, when they were given the choice of state care, privately paid for care, care by relatives or care by friends. Presumably what these respondents were telling us is: I would prefer the responsibility not to fall on the family, if it *has* to be relatives, then it should be children.

However, although our data suggest that people generally see it as appropriate that adult children should do *something* to support their parents, there is less broad agreement as to exactly what children should do. In fact, our data often point to different ways of fulfilling obligations legitimately. One of our questions which illustrates this particularly well is concerned with a middle-aged couple facing the dilemma of what to do about the husband's parents who live several hundred miles away,

TABLE 11.1   Caring for an elderly woman: which relatives should offer assistance?

Introductory statement to tables 11.1 to 11.3

I would like to ask you about some situations in which people might need personal care. This time, let's suppose that the help is going to come from a relative.* In each case, the person has a lot of relatives living nearby who could help.

An elderly woman who can manage well living alone but who needs help getting up and going to bed. Which relative should be the first to offer help?

	Number of respondents	%
Daughter	663	67.8
Children	102	10.4
Son	43	4.3
Sister	42	4.2
Brother/sister	10	1.0
Other named relative	18	1.8
Whole family/all equally	33	3.3
Immediate/closest	9	0.9
Who is available/can cope	8	0.8
Other	16	1.6
Don't know/not applicable	34	3.4
Total	**978**	**100.0**

* Respondents had been asked to consider these same situations earlier in the interview, but had been asked different questions about them.

TABLE 11.2   Caring for a woman recovering from a hip operation: which relatives should offer assistance?

An elderly woman who lives alone and who has to stay in bed all day for the next few months following a hip operation. Which relative should be the first to offer help?

	Number of respondents	%
Daughter	646	66.0
Children	94	9.6
Son	33	3.3
Sister	59	6.0
Brother/sister	9	0.9
Other named relative	12	1.2
Whole family/all equally	53	5.4
Immediate/closest	12	1.2
Who is available/can cope	4	0.4
Other	13	1.3
Don't know/not applicable	43	4.3
Total	**978**	**100.0**

TABLE 11.3   Caring for an elderly and confused man: which relatives should offer assistance?

An elderly man who can move about well, and who lives alone, but who gets confused and who needs someone to go in regularly several times a week to check that everything is safe. Which relative should be the first to offer help?

	Number of respondents	%
Son	382	39.0
Daughter	299	30.6
Children	90	9.2
Brother	46	4.7
Sister	28	2.8
Brother/sister	7	0.7
Other named relative	19	1.9
Whole family/all equally	43	4.3
Immediate/closest	9	0.9
Who is available/can cope	7	0.7
Other	15	1.5
Don't know/not applicable	33	3.3
Total	**978**	**100.0**

TABLE 11.4   Decorating an elderly couple's house: should relatives help to pay?

(*a*) Suppose an elderly couple need money to redecorate their home. Do you think that relatives should offer to pay to have the work done?

	Number of respondents	%
Yes	538	55.0
No	342	35.0
Depends	98	10.0
Total	**978**	**100.0**

(*b*) Respondents who said 'yes' or 'depends' – up to three answers post-coded. Assuming that they could all afford to help which relatives, if any, should be the first to offer money?

	Number of respondents	%
Son	247	38.8
Children	138	21.7
Daughter	27	4.2
Other named relatives	24	3.8
All equally/whole family	113	17.7
Whoever can afford it	32	5.0
Immediate/closest family	11	1.7
Don't know/not applicable/other answer	44	6.9
Total	**636**	**100.0**

and who have been seriously injured in a car accident. Proportions of our sample choosing the various options were as follows: move to live near the husband's parents 33 per cent; have the parents move to live with them 24 per cent; give the parents money to help them pay for daily care 25 per cent; let the parents make their own arrangements 9 per cent. Only the last option suggests that the couple have no filial responsibility, and even there people may well have expected that they would, in fact, provide some kind of support. Viewed in this way, we can say that 82 per cent of our sample were assenting to the notion of filial responsibility, but were acknowledging different ways of fulfilling it.

11.2.2   Do people distinguish between children in relation to their filial obligations?

We did not have any questions in the survey which explored in detail whether people distinguish between different children when allocating responsibility for parents, but our data do give us some clues here.

First, there does not seem to be any significant inclination to distinguish children by birth order. We had expected that people might see the obligations of an eldest son or daughter as 'stronger' than the rest, but very few specified this on those open-ended questions where we invited them to name a relative (as above).

Second, there is a clear sense in the data of people wanting to follow an 'equal shares' principle if at all possible. Tables 11.1–11.4 all have substantial proportions of respondents who say that the 'children' should assist the elderly people in question, without making any further distinction, or who specify that it should be 'the whole family' or 'all equally'. This occurs in questions where people were asked to say who should offer *first*, directing them to name a single individual, so we take this to be quite a strong response.

Third, there is clearly some tendency to distinguish between sons and daughters in the allocation of responsibilities, although this is not as straightforward as stereotypes would predict. The equal shares principle suggests that many people see both sons and daughters as targets for providing assistance to parents, although in the case of providing money (Table 11.4) a substantial proportion of our respondents specify that it should be a son. When it comes to providing care (Tables 11.1–11.3), the question of where the responsibility should fall apparently depends upon the gender of the person needing care, at least for some of our respondents. Where an elderly woman needs care (Tables 11.1 and 11.2), a daughter is the clear preference of two-thirds of our respondents. For an elderly man both daughters and sons are regarded as appropriate to take prime responsibility. (What 'taking responsibility' means could, of course, be different for daughters and sons, but we cannot explore that on the basis of these data.) This pattern is repeated elsewhere in all these questions is quite complex, and certainly does not just follow gender stereotypes, there are some situations in which gender does seem to have a clear impact upon people's normative judgements: daughters are rarely chosen as the appropriate people to provide money, and sons are rarely chosen as the people who should provide care for an elderly woman.

11.2.3   Do filial obligations have limits?

One important way to test out the significance of publicly expressed norms about filial obligations is to consider whether they have limits and, if so, of what kind. Our data enable us to make two points about this.

First, the quality of the relationship between a parent and adult child does not seem to have much impact upon the way responsibilities are allocated – at least not at this level of publicly acknowledged norms. We asked one question about whether a person should be prepared to make daily visits to look after his or her elderly father, even if they have never got on well together (Table 11.5); 72 per cent of people said 'yes'. Neither respondents' gender nor their social class was apparently related to the answers they gave, although there was a small tendency for people over the age of 65 to answer 'yes' more frequently than younger people. Table 11.5 also shows that, for about half of the respondents who thought that a child should visit despite a poor relationship, a key consideration was the fact that the relative in question was a *father* since, when we substituted 'uncle' for 'father', the proportion saying 'yes' dropped to 40 per cent.

This 'strong' view of filial obligations is supported elsewhere in our survey data. For example, one of our examples concerned an elderly woman and her daughter, who had never got along well. They had quarrelled, and the older woman had cut the daughter out of her will. Yet in this case, 37 per cent of people still thought that the daughter should offer her mother a home when she needed it – a proportion very similar to answers given in other questions about children giving a home to elderly parents, where the circumstances were less contentious. So it appears that the particular circumstances in this question, including a very poor relationship between mother and daughter, have little effect on the number of people prepared to endorse the principle of filial obligations. In general, people do not seem to 'count' the quality of the relationship as a factor which legitimately puts limits upon the obligations of children to their elderly parents.

Second, the fact that the quality of the relationship does not set limits does not mean that there are no limits at all to filial obligations. In

TABLE 11.5   Obligation to visit and 'getting on'

(*a*) Should a person be prepared to make daily visits to look after his or her elderly father, even if they have not got on well together?

	Number of respondents	%
Yes	704	72.0
No	220	22.5
Depends	49	5.0
Not applicable	5	0.5
Total	978	100.0

(*b*) And should a person be prepared to make daily visits to look after his or her uncle, even if they have never got on well together?

	Number of respondents	%
Yes	390	39.9
No	486	49.7
Depends	90	9.2
Don't know/not applicable	12	1.2
Total	978	100.0

another of our examples, we set up a situation where a middle-aged couple would be torn in two directions – between moving several hundred miles away to care for the husband's parents, or staying put because their own children were at a crucial stage in their education (coming up to O-levels). Here there was much clearer agreement about the proper thing to do: 78 per cent said that they should stay put, and 20 per cent that they should move, which we interpret to mean that four out of five of our respondents thought that the needs of the younger generation should take precedence over the older. Thus there *are* normative limits upon filial obligations and, in this instance, these are set by the need to fulfil other responsibilities which are seen as taking precedence.

In summary, our findings do seem to confirm the normative strength and importance of filial ties, but also underline that they do not entail unconditional responsibilities. It seems then that there is a degree of public normative consensus (although by no means universal) that children should do *something* to assist their parents in these types of circumstances, but it is not always clear what that should be, who should do it, or what limits might apply to filial obligations.

If various different courses of action *could* constitute the 'proper thing to do', then two consequences follow. First, on an individual level, each person necessarily has to engage in a task of 'working out' what to do for his or her own parents in a given set of circumstances. The appropriate course of action does not present itself as obvious, as if it were a well-defined rule where the only choice left to the individual is to obey it or break it. Second, there is the task of presenting one's actions publicly and getting other people to accept that they lie within the legitimate range of filial obligations. These two processes might be consecutive (you decide what you are going to do first then you sell it to other people), but equally they might operate in parallel (your assessment of what other people will accept as legitimate may well influence precisely what you decide to do for your parents).[9] On the basis of our survey findings, it seems likely that both processes have to be worked at actively, but clearly we need quite different kinds of data to get further with understanding that.

We can say that relationships between parents and children *are* importantly founded on a sense of obligation, but one which recognises definite limits. There is not a clear consensus about what it is reasonable to expect. However, there are well understood principles which can be mobilised when you are working out 'the proper thing to do' in practice. People do have an understanding of what would be generally accepted as proper, but they use it as a resource with which to negotiate rather than as a rule to follow.

Notes

1. For example, Ungerson, C., *Policy is Personal*, Tavistock, London, 1987; Lewis, J. and Meredith, B., *Daughters Who Care*, Routledge, London, 1988.
2. Morgan, D. H. J., *Social Theory and the Family*, Routledge and Kegan Paul, London, 1975.
3. Townsend, P. *The Family Life of Old People*, Routledge and Kegan Paul, London, 1957.
4. Firth, R., Hubert, J. and Forge, A., *Families and their Relatives*, Routledge and Kegan Paul, London, 1969; Allan, G., 'Kinship, responsibility and care for elderly people', *Ageing and Society*, Vol. 8 (1988), pp. 249–68.
5. Firth *et al. op. cit.*; Wenger, G. C., *The Supportive Network*, Allen and Unwin, London, 1984; Qureshi, H. and Simons, K., 'Resources within families: caring for elderly people', in Brannen, J. and Wilson, G. (eds) *Give and Take in Families*, Allen and Unwin, London, 1987.
6. Graham, H., 'Caring: a labour of love', in Finch, J. and Groves, D. (eds) *A Labour of Love: Women, Work and Caring*, Routledge and Kegan Paul, London, 1983; Cornwell, J., *Hard-Earned Lives*, Tavistock, London, 1984; Ungerson *op. cit.*
7. The findings from this aspect of the study have not been included in this extract.

8. This and other attitude statements in our survey were taken from another study, in Scotland in 1982, directed by Patrick West. Patterns of response to this question were similar on both surveys. (See West, P., 'The family, the welfare state and community care: political rhetoric and public attitudes', *Journal of Social Policy*, Vol. 13, No. 4, (1984), pp. 417–46). There were some differences among our survey population in answering the attitude statement about filial obligations. Notably, older people were more divided in their views than younger people. In the 18–29 age group, 65 per cent supported the principle of filial obligations.
9. Finch, J., *Family Obligations and Social Change*, Polity, Cambridge, 1989.

Acknowledgement

The project discussed in this paper was funded by the Economic and Social Research Council 1985–89 (Grant number GOO 23 2197).

12

At Home and Alone: Families and Young Adults with Challenging Behaviour*

JANE HUBERT

This chapter is based on an intensive study of 20 families with teenagers or young adults who have severe or profound learning difficulties and challenging behaviour living in one county of southern England. . . . The 20 young people are between the ages of 14 and 22 years old, have or no speech and have few basic skills. Some are very physically disabled, and spend much of the time in wheelchairs, whereas others are highly mobile. Most are subject to epilepsy, and the majority are incontinent. Their challenging behaviour, where it exists, ranges from aggression and self-injury to destructiveness and non-compliance.

[. . .] Since the birth of their children, the parents had been waging an almost continuous battle to keep going, with help and support from the local health and social services often proving unreliable and inadequate. Many of them, determined to keep their child at home in spite of the enormous problems this often caused to themselves and to their families, found that other people, including professionals, often responded to their crises and their cries for help with defeatism, suggesting that permanent care away from home would 'solve' the problem. To parents who are asking for help to do just the opposite this response is unhelpful, and indicates a lack of understanding of what they actually want and feel. It also tends to add to their sense of frustration, since it appears to them that they are fighting a battle which the professionals already consider to be a losing one. [. . .]

---

*This is an abridged extract from a chapter in *Better Lives: Changing Services for People with Learning Difficulties*, Booth, T. (ed), Social Services Monograph, (1990), pp. 105–114.

Almost all the mothers find it difficult to manage if their young adult child is at home all day every day – which often happens during holidays or bouts of illness. The daily routine is already extremely demanding. In addition to all the usual day-to-day tasks involved in family life, they must attend to the almost continuous basic needs of a young adult – washing, dressing, toileting and changing incontinence pads, feeding, carrying and in most cases having to be in the same room for almost every minute of the day. For many the task continues at intervals throughout the night – in response to cries of discomfort, to change wet bedclothes, or to hold and comfort their child through each epileptic fit.

Families such as these walk a narrow tightrope, and any upheaval or crisis within the family – not necessarily related to the disabled young adult – can upset a delicate balance between managing or not managing to get through each day. Most of the mothers work to a precise and precarious schedule, easily thrown out of gear by any lack of response by professionals to relatively simple requests for such things as more incontinence pads, wheelchair repairs, dressings or even a lift to the hospital, let alone requests for more major help, such as the provision of a downstairs toilet or bedroom, a stairlift or the widening of a bathroom door.

The most essential service, according to most parents, is access to short-term residential care, which allows them at least an occasional night without their disabled child at home. Many say it is these breaks that make it possible to keep going, although two families have found their experience of the units so unpleasant, for them and for their children, that they no longer make use of the service. In the county under study, short-term residential care is available in long-term National Health Service residential units, run by senior, qualified nurses, with a staff of trained and untrained care assistants. In most cases the young adults spend a weekend away at regular intervals, with perhaps a week or two in the summer holidays.

Many parents spoke of the children's residential units as sympathetic and friendly places, but at the age of 16 their children have to leave these, and the transition to adult units is often abrupt and distressing for both parents and children.

Apart from this unwelcome change from children's to adult services, parents are often, at this stage, facing all kinds of other changes and crises: for example, other children in the family having adolescent problems or leaving home, mothers facing hysterectomies, grandparents slipping from potentially useful roles into increasing dependence. Altogether, it is often a trying time during which parents feel they need greater support than ever before. Instead, many of them find there is less support, less interest in their children and a correspondingly greater battle to get an acceptable level of care for them.

The transition from children's to adult units is considered by most parents to be too early, and in most cases far too abrupt. Ideally there would be no administrative switch, but if there must be one then it should happen a few years later. Such a move should also be made gradually – preferably with others of the same age group to reduce any sense of isolation – so that the young people can grow accustomed to the new environment before being finally cut off from the children's unit. Few parents feel their 16-year-olds are ready to be plunged into an adult environment. Not only are adult residential units very different from the children's unit, but they are also full of many older people who may have been institutionalised for most of their lives. Parents would prefer small, home-like units which cater for short-term residents only.

Although almost all of the parents in this study do make use of short-term care facilities, many still feel guilty about letting their children go away even for one night, mainly because they feel that the level of care is inadequate. In spite of this dissatisfaction with the quality of the care, they know that they need occasional breaks even though for many of them these few days are spent worrying about what might be happening to their child, rather than enjoying a recuperative and stress-free period of rest.

In fact the demands that parents make of the short-term residential care services are very basic, and all are aspects of the same thing – quality of care. This is the fundamental issue, and one that is determined by a wide range of policies and people from national policy-makers and health authority administrators to the care staff working in the units.

An important part of this care is basic physical care: the provision of adequate and appropriate food, warmth and rest. It also includes the right to cleanliness and comfort, which may involve constant vigilance and work with those young people who are incontinent or who are unable to move or who dribble continuously. It is the inadequacy of this physical care that angers and saddens many of the parents, especially those whose sons and daughters cannot walk and are sometimes left sitting in their urine, even in faeces, their tee-shirts stiff with dried dribble. Parents believe that attention to such basic needs is an essential right of their young adult children, and that they are only treated in this way because they are unable to protest or to express their discomfort.

Another aspect of care that concerns parents is the protection of their children from harm of any kind. Few of these young people are able to protect themselves from the actions of others, whether these are direct acts of aggression or merely mistakes made by the staff responsible for their well-being. Mistakes of this kind do occur – in such things as the preparation of food for those who cannot chew, or in the administration of drugs. Often it is the latter – the prescription and administration of drugs – that causes the most acute concern to parents.

Almost all the young people concerned are on regular medication of one or more kinds. Three-quarters are on anti-convulsants to control their epilepsy, the majority on more than one. Other drugs include anti-psychotics, anti-depressants and hypnotics. Apart from general anxiety about the number and levels of regular drugs, parents are particularly worried, when their children are in short-term care, by the possibility of unacceptably high dosages of drugs being given, either deliberately – to suppress violent behaviour or to deal with sleep problems – or by mistake. Such overdosages have occurred, and tend not to be adequately explained or excused.

Parents are well aware that mistakes are easily made in a situation where there are few staff and many people to be cared for, each with specific individual needs. However, when such accidents happen, they are justifiably angry and become even more unwilling to let their children out of their sight. They may not blame the members of staff involved, but this does not affect their basic complaint that their adult children are receiving inadequate care.

As their children grow older and become adult, parents know there will be even fewer people who will want to look after them and who will be concerned with their individual needs. To them it is a labour of love, but they have few illusions about the nature of the task. Moreover, parents sometimes feel that because their physical needs are so time-consuming care staff only respond to the young people at this basic level and seldom pay attention to their emotional or intellectual needs. The young people are often left to sit alone, or to wander around the building for most of the day, receiving very little affection or understanding, and with few opportunities to try to communicate in whatever way they can.

Many parents feel that care staff do not respond to the changes that are taking place in their children, and that they often disregard their intellectual, perceptual and emotional development – including sexual awareness. They consider that carers should take account of this as they attend to the personal needs of these young people. Allowances should be made for feelings of embarrassment and pride, even if they cannot be expressed. Carers should act on the assumption, for example, that those they care for would prefer their incontinence to be treated as a private matter, and would rather not be seen to be sitting in wet clothes, or be changed in front of other people.

At the same time, one of the criticisms parents level at the adult residential units is the apparent assumption that those who are transferred to them for short-term care at 19 suddenly cease to be children altogether, and become fully-fledged adults. Often they are deprived of the physical and emotional comforts that they are used to at home and used to have at the children's unit, but which are no longer considered 'age-appropriate' – a concept which, in this context, seems to override individual needs and desires.

Through their intimate experience with their children since birth, parents are aware of the infinite complexity of their abilites and disabilities, of their likes and dislikes, and recognise the many different 'ages' they may be at any one time. The fact that someone enjoys sensations such as chewing, squeezing and banging does not mean that this source of enjoyment is the sum total of their intellectual and physical needs.

Because of their disquiet about the quality of care for their young adult children, the parents in this study are faced with a very real dilemma. Two families resolved this by refusing to allow their children to go into short-term residential care at all, whatever the cost to the main carer and the other members of the family. For the other 18 families, the choice has been to make use of the service, however distressing this may sometimes be. In fact, most feel they must have these breaks to survive, and as a result consider it essential that they should be able to count on a reliable short-term care service. The survival of these families has often relied upon a fragile balance between the various needs of different members of the family, including agreements – whether explicit or not – between husband and wife. For this balance to be maintained it is essential that there is a reliable agreement with the service agencies. Any unexpected gaps in availability of short-term care, or changes in frequency of breaks, or in agreed dates, may threaten the stability of the families concerned.

One of the major penalties paid by many families, especially the mothers, of keeping a highly dependent child at home is the loss of any social or community life, and a gradual erosion of relationships with friends and kin outside the household. This is especially true when there is also very challenging behaviour to contend with. The problems involved in maintaining relationships are less acute when the children are small. They are more portable, more easily contained by car seats and pushchairs. As they grow older, behaviour that is tolerated in a young child may, in an adult, be seen by other people as threatening or even dangerous. Even trips to local shops or to a neighbour's house may be too daunting to contemplate with a teenager who is likely to start shrieking, 'throw a wobbly', or kick and grab at people and objects within reach.

Apart from the problems involved in taking their young adults out, it is also difficult to leave them at home. Few of them can be left at home with a 'sitter'. Thus any outing has to be planned far in advance and often depends on the availability of a short-term bed for the night. Ordinary social relationships, based on mutual visits and joint outings, often lapse to the point that mothers, at least, sometimes cease to have any social life whatsoever. In many cases fathers, or partners, may well continue to have an outside life, at least during the day.

Thus, ironically, by keeping their children at home 'in the community', the families as a whole and the mothers as individuals may, in effect, cut themselves off from the community. This is not only the result of practical problems and lack of mobility. Relationships may well be affected by infrequency of contact, but many mothers in the study also feel their isolation is greater because, as the years pass, they have less and less in common with their kin and friends who have children of the same age. It is when other people's children are beginning to live adult lives – getting jobs, going to college, leaving home and getting married – that these parents feel particularly excluded. The things that happen to them in their daily lives, and the successes and failures that they experience in connection with their children, have no counterpart in the lives of their relatives and friends.

In spite of such social isolation, and the awareness of a potentially very different life, these parents continue to resist pressure to put their adult children into permanent care. Most of them are used to this sort of pressure, whether it be from kin or friends or professionals, but as their children become adults there is often a new wave to overcome. Professionals tell them it is normal for teenagers to leave home, to become independent of their parents, and abnormal for a mother to devote her life to an adult child. But these parents know their children will never have any real independence and will remain totally dependent on other people for their most basic needs. In fact, if they left home, they would move into an environment in which they would be even less autonomous than they are now, since their needs and wishes would be less understood by those around them, and in most cases there would be no one prepared to try to interpret the often minute signs that parents have learnt to understand. Thus many would probably live the rest of their lives without ever having another close and reciprocally satisfying relationship.

Many of these parents would be pleased to let their children live away from home, at least for longer periods of time, if they knew there was any *viable* alternative for them somewhere else. So far, all their experiences have proved to them that there is no acceptable alternative to keeping them at home. In particular, their wide and varied experience of short-term, respite care has convinced many of them that, judged by the low standards and level of neglect suffered in a week away, the prospect of a life in residential care is intolerable.

This chapter has only covered a small part of the results of the research carried out with these families but it will, perhaps, have given some idea of the sorts of problems faced by parents who want to keep their adult children at home. Because they see no acceptable alternative they are determined to continue, whatever happens, to have their children living at home. Three-quarters of them say they would rather their children should actually die than go into permanent care away from home.

There are many conclusions to be drawn. Among the most obvious is that services to families should be better co-ordinated, and so arranged as to make it possible for them to keep a young adult at home for as long as they choose. This calls for simple and quick ways of getting help when necessary both at the basic level (of having incontinence pads delivered, wheelchairs mended, support at home in crises and so on) and also at the level of providing alternative care of an acceptable quality away from home as regularly and as frequently as individual parents required.

Increased funding and adequate staffing (in terms of numbers, training and quality) would go a long way towards achieving this goal, but this is only part of the answer. This study has revealed that it is not only adequate staff and funding that is lacking. Most parents feel that once their children are adult no one – except their families – really cares about them or what happens to them. As they become adult, it is as though their learning difficulties and challenging behaviour are all that most people see and react to. They often cease to be treated as fellow human beings, with the same needs, preferences and dislikes as other people. Even more disturbing is the lack of understanding of these young people's doubts, confusions and fears.

The professionals may consider parents' 'overprotective' of their young adult children, but such protectiveness generally arises from an intimate knowledge and understanding of them as whole people, who lack only the ability to care for themselves and to communicate their own needs and fears to others.

Until there is a major change in attitudes towards adults with severe and profound learning difficulties, these families will continue to watch and worry, and will be forced to continue to fight their own individual battles for the basic rights of their adult children.

13

Breaking the Silence: Asian Carers in Britain

YASMIN GUNARATNAM

This chapter focuses on Asian people's experiences of caring. It is drawn from research as well as from my own experiences as an Asian woman carer. The chapter therefore reflects a particular perspective and overview. Above all it represents the recognition that while mainstream research into carers' lives has provided us with useful and valuable information it has often not enabled us to 'see it like it really is': to explore the depth and intricacies of issues in some carers' lives and to reach beyond the generalisations.

Within this context, and by enabling carers to speak for themselves through case studies and quotes, this chapter attempts to address some of the experiences of Asian carers in Britain. It is by no means a comprehensive account. As well as using existing research sources, it will also refer to my own research for the King's Fund Carers' Unit on a project to produce information for Asian carers of elderly people (Gunaratnam, 1991). During the course of the project, which began in September 1989, 33 Asian carers were interviewed, mainly in London, Birmingham, Bradford and Derbyshire. The largest representation of carers in the sample were from the Bengali-speaking community (11); the remaining language representation of the sample was Punjabi (7); Hindi (2); Sindhi (1); Gujerati (8) and Urdu (4). The experiences and views of the carers involved with the project will be referred to throughout. The names of carers quoted in all the case studies have been changed to respect their privacy.

It is also important, at this stage, to begin by addressing the analytical clumsiness of conceptualising 'Asian carers' as a unified, homogenous group. Asian peoples come from a variety of countries and cultures, representing different dialects, languages, religions, histories and customs. These differences have meant that not all Asian carers in this country have the same experiences or needs. For example, in my own research I was able to identify patterns of social and economic relations that were related to the sex, age and country of origin of the carer, which directly affected their caring experiences. These patterns will be referred to later in this chapter.

13.1   Myths and stereotypes

For a Black family (irrespective of 'ethnicity') the popular image is one of an extended family network, 'families within families', providers of care and social and psychological support.

(Patel, 1990, p. 30)

To the 'outsider' English neighbour in the same area the apparent segregation of the population is perceived as a deliberate statement of not wanting to mix or adapt.

(Khan, 1979, p. 8)

Before we can begin seriously to examine some of the different experiences of Asian carers in Britain, it is important also to address some of the 'popular' myths and stereotypes about Asian communities generally, and Asian carers in particular. This is not just a theoretical exercise. In many instances ill-formed assumptions about different minority communities have practically influenced policies and service provision.

Perhaps the most significant stereotype about Asian carers is that all Asian families live within an extended family, where roles and responsibilities are clearly defined and caring for ill or disabled family members is a 'natural' function. While research clearly indicates a high proportion of Asian extended family households (18 per cent: Brown, 1984; 21 per cent: Westwood and Bachau, 1988), information on household size and structure does not actually tell us anything about patterns of caring or about the impact of immigration controls and housing and welfare provisions on family structures. For example, the 'no recourse to public funds' clauses in immigration legislation, has restricted the right of some people from black and minority communities to apply for public housing or to claim welfare benefits.

While there is inadequate data to enable us to cut through the stereotypes about Asian extended families and patterns of care, it is clear that much more subtle and complex relations exist. For example, a study by Bhalla and Blakemore (1981) of 400 European, Afro-Caribbean and Asian elders in Birmingham found that although 95 per cent of Asian elders (compared to 59 per cent of Afro-Caribbean and 11 per cent of European elders) said that they were looked after by relatives when discharged from hospital, one-quarter of the Asian sample had no close relatives in Britain.

My own research showed a variety of relationships and patterns of care that included elderly couples living alone who were 'mutual' carers; elaborate systems of shared secondary care by relatives and friends living separately from the person requiring care and single isolated carers whose relatives either did not live in the country or who lived some distance away. In fact only 8 out of the 33 carers interviewed lived in an extended family network.

However, perhaps the most interesting factors were not just kinship networks and living arrangements but also the identities and perceptions of the carers themselves. The carer's identity and perceptions were in many cases of central significance in determining the distinction between the simple presence of family networks and the actual practical help available and how it was received. For example, in the following quotes from carers it is useful to consider, in the first case, the carer's reluctance to 'trouble' her son for help and the second carer's feelings of isolation and frustration with the lack of support from the wider family. The first case is that of Pritam Kaur, an elderly Punjabi woman of 65 years of age, and the second case reflects the feelings of Ishfaq Ahmed, a Pakistani woman of 34.

Pritam Kaur:

> We live in my son's house. The toilet and bathroom are upstairs and we live in the downstairs. So every time he wants to go to the toilet my son has to take him [husband] up and down. I can't do it. I'm too old and I haven't got my eyesight. I would like to live near to my son in another house. We are too much trouble to him and he has three small children to look after.

Ishfaq Ahmed:

> My brothers and sisters-in-law don't want to look after my mum because they think that she is too demanding on them. They can't take looking after her, it would take up too much of their time and energy. So they have left it all to me.
>
> I'd like to spend more time with my mother, looking after her, but it is difficult. I have so much pressure from my husband, my in-laws and the business. I don't know what to do. . . I'm the only daughter and I should be looking after my mother, and I want to, it is just all the circumstances that are making it difficult.
>
> I think it's probably easier for men. My brothers do not see my mother as their responsibility but I'm the only daughter, how can I turn my back on her?

A related myth about Asian communities is that the communities are insular and self-servicing and therefore do not 'need' mainstream service provision. It is certainly true that Asian communities' take-up of services is comparatively low; however, this appears to be directly related to lack of knowledge about service provision and inappropriate information-giving. The Birmingham study (Bhalla and Blakemore, 1981) found that out of the Asian sample, 64 per cent had not heard of any of the services mentioned in the study, such as home help, day centre or meals on wheels, as opposed to 35 per cent of the Afro-Caribbean sample and 2 per cent of the European sample.

It was significant that 10 out of the 33 carers I interviewed were illiterate in English and their own language. All of them were women who were over the age of 50; five were Bengali and five were Punjabi. For these carers even translated information in their first language was of limited value and information about service provisions was exclusively gained through word of mouth from relatives, friends and community groups. The need to address illiteracy among different sections of minority communities and to prioritise alternative forms of information-giving is being slowly recognised by service providers:

> Is written information the best way of getting your message across? Leaflets may not be the best way, as people may not be literate in their mother tongue. Many elderly Chinese women for example are most illiterate . . . as there was no free education in China until the 1950's and until 1971 in Hong Kong . . . Perhaps written material when appropriate could serve the purpose of being a handy reference guide rather than the primary source of information.
> (London Borough of Camden, 1990, p. 24)

Given the inaccessibility of information about services to some Asian people it is perhaps not surprising that the Birmingham Asian study found that Asian elders were 'pitifully lacking in knowledge about basic services and help available to them'. Similarly a recent study of 40 Asian, Afro-Caribbean and Vietnamese carers in a London borough (McCalman, 1990) found: 'In most cases carers were unable to say whether services were suitable to their needs because they did not know about them or use them' (p. 16). In the study only 21 per cent of the people requiring care used social services day centres, and meals on wheels was only used by approximately 3 per cent of the sample.

It was significant that only approximately half the carers I interviewed (17) had had contact with service providers, and very few of the carers had gone on to use services. It should be pointed out, however, that the lack of take-up of services by the carers was seen in terms of the inappropriate nature of the service provision:

> He used to have meals on wheels, but even though it was useful to have them delivered, because they were so appallingly bad . . . I don't think they had even heard of halal meat . . . it was just a waste of money.

I see some of the old people in this area, they just sit and look out of the window all day. They have no rights. No Asian people that I know go to day centres. People have nowhere to go. In the day centres there is no food for them, culture for them, music . . . nothing . . . so they just stay as they are – housebound.

There aren't many Asians working as home helps and my mum doesn't speak English. She doesn't want an English person who is a stranger to our ways in the house.

The low take-up of services by minority communities is now being recognised as the responsibility of service providers rather than the 'problem' of uncooperative communities. A recent report by the London Borough of Camden on 'The needs of women carers whose first language is not English' (1990) stated:

At present there seems to be scant understanding of dietary rules . . . and little provision of halal meat or vegetarian or vegan meals.
  Current home help and respite care provision caters poorly for minority ethnic communities and the take up of services is likely to be closely related to how sensitive and responsive the service is to those needing it.

(p. 20)

The following case study highlights the experiences of Joshim Miah, a 28-year-old Bengali man caring for his elderly father. In addition to drawing attention to the inappropriate nature of services it also indicates the significance of the wishes of the person cared for in determining the take-up of services and places such feelings firmly in the context of wider racism.

13.1.1 Case study: Joshim Miah

The only advice on looking after him I got from the hospital. My father doesn't like outside bodies. The only time he had help was when it was a friend of mine who was a social worker and a black woman and he trusted her . . . My dad gets very frustrated at people's lack of understanding of his English because his understanding is perfect and as far as his speaking is concerned he thinks that he can speak well. So he gets frustrated because people don't understand him and what's worse than that is that they pretend to understand him and he is not stupid so he gets more frustrated . . .
  It is difficult because even though I am articulate and educated I also have a distrust of agencies and a lack of knowledge of them. It is difficult because you do not know the right questions to ask and who you should ask, like 'This is my dad, this is his situation. What help can you give him?' . . .
  It is not something that is static, his needs change and develop. You can't say at one moment, 'What does he need?' At his age you can't suddenly

introduce people into his life . . . Because he has always managed on his own, you can't suddenly say, 'You can have a home help or district nurse.' Just because they are there doesn't mean that they are available to him . . . He doesn't like to ask. Why should he? He also has a real attitude about not wanting to scrounge, which is something that gets instilled in you. This country doesn't encourage you to get your entitlements. It is not just a case of knowing what is available.

It should also be pointed out that the provision of accessible and appropriate services that benefit residents irrespective of their ethnic origin is not simply a matter of good practice but is also a question of legality. Section 20 of the Race Relations Act 1976, which covers the provision of goods, facilities or services, makes it unlawful for service providers to discriminate directly (through less-favourable treatment) or indirectly (through applying a requirement or condition that has a disproportionately adverse effect on a particular racial group and which cannot be justified). Unfortunately for some Asian carers, racism from service providers is a day-to-day reality:

When he first got the stroke, I didn't know what to do. My GP said we should go back to India.

One of the after-effects of a stroke is an intense headache. They would give him painkillers but they didn't do much. One of the things we do when we are in pain is to give massages. It might not take the pain away, but it helps you to relax. He used to like having his head massaged at that time. The Sister [nurse] used to get really annoyed. She said 'Why are you touching him? All you Asian women mollycoddle your men' . . . My mother had become frightened to sit with him or even hold his hand.

13.2   Caring in focus

13.2.1   Case study: Abdul Azizz and Moyna Khanum (not their real names)

Abdul Azizz is approximately 70 years of age, his wife, Moyna Khanum, is approximately 65 years of age (the couple do not know their exact birth dates). Mr Azziz is partially sighted and asthmatic; Moyna Khanum is also in poor health and has high blood pressure and 'heart problems'. The couple help to look after each other and do not use any service provision. The couple are originally from Bangladesh; they speak no English and are illiterate in Bengali.

Mr Azziz and his wife live alone in a small, run-down council flat in a London borough. When I visited them, the house was in a state of obvious disrepair, there was visible damp on the walls and the toilet was cracked, with water leaking from it down to the internal stairway. At the time of my visit there was no central heating or hot water. The flat was also infested with cockroaches.

The following quotes are extracts from a longer interview with the couple:

> The thing that I most want to talk about is the house. There are a lot of problems with the house. We moved in here eight years ago, but I've got nobody to help look after it or decorate it . . . The toilet doesn't work and the floor of the toilet is broken and dangerous. For over a year we have had no heating in the bedroom. The hot water is not steady and we have to go to the station to have a shower . . . we have been to social services and housing people.

> Mr Azziz:
> My wife does everything, housework, cooking, cleaning, washing – she struggles herself to do it, she has no other choice . . . We need most help to sort out the house. When you are ill and the house is also in a state it makes you feel much worse.

What is significant about the case of Abdul Azziz and Moyna Khanum is that caring issues and their caring relationship were not identified as a central concern in their lives. The couple clearly and repeatedly identified their housing conditions as a priority. Similarly McCalman's research (1990) found that in the Asian sample of carers where housing conditions were bad, 'this seemed to take precedence over their caring' (p. 47).

In talking to a variety of different Asian carers, I found that caring issues were rarely identified in isolation and for some carers were not even a priority. Issues raised by carers included poverty, poor working conditions and racial harassment, which directly related to the wider social and economic position of black and minority communities in this country.

For many of the carers it was a cause of concern that service providers had failed to recognise and respond to the interrelationship and cumulative effects on caring of such issues as racial harassment. Carers spoke of the frustrations of being 'shunted' back and forth between different departments, and could not understand why social services dealt only with their 'caring' issues and the housing department dealt with racial harassment.

The most responsive and helpful agencies repeatedly cited by carers were community organisations, although it should also be recognised that only just over one-half of my sample of carers (17) had had contact with such organisations. In fact the most effective organisations I consulted with during the research were community groups who had recognised and responded to the interrelatedness of issues in black carers' lives. For example, an Asian carers' and users' lunch club in a Tower Hamlets community centre had provided much effective support for the Bengali carers attending the club. It was significant that the club had started out in 1987 as a club for Bengali disabled elders. However, due to a lack of resources and help carers started attending the club primarily to provide support for the elders. The carers, mainly women, then began meeting together and their presence slowly transformed the club. Today the two stated objectives of the club are:

> 1. To provide a day-care facility for older disabled members of the Bengali community and through this create respite for their carers, as well as carrying our direct support through home visits.
> 2. To actively involve carers in activities, providing a forum for them to voice concerns, exchange mutual support and receive information.

In the club regular verbal information-giving is supported by an advice facility, which has taken up a variety of issues, from home helps and poor housing conditions to racial harassment. The support the club provides is vital to the area, where there are no day centres for Bengali elders or specific support for Bengali carers. Significantly, the club has yet to receive funding from its local social services office.

While I met with a number of community organisations who were concerned with black and minority carers, there is no national information on the scale and scope of community provisions for black carers. It is also true that a network of services, not specifically targeted at carers, for example day and advice centres, may indirectly meet some of the needs of black carers. There is further evidence of 'informal' support for black people generally from a variety of community groups and resources. For example, Norman's (1986) research on black elders found that in the absence of agencies providing specialised advice and counselling services, various religious and cultural organisations as well as individuals provided levels of support. Far from being 'helpless victims', Asian communities, like other black and minority communities, have been resourceful in establishing a range of support services when faced by a lack of appropriate and responsive 'mainstream' provision.

13.3   Community care: opportunities or threats?

The National Health Service and Community Care Act (1990) was hailed as involving a major shake-up in the way services are provided to people requiring care in their daily lives. Whatever the actual effects of the legislation are, the fact that the government had put off the full introduction of the proposed new community care arrangements until 1993 meant that all carers and service users had been left in the middle of the administrative hiatus to 'wait and see'. So what does this all mean for black and minority carers?

The government's White Paper on community care addressed 'people from ethnic minorities' in 57 words, culminating in a catch-all statement that: 'Good community care will take account of the circumstances of minority communities and will be planned in consultation with them' (Department of Health, 1989, p. 11). Unfortunately in addressing the existing information that we have about Asian carers in particular, the immediate picture is quite grim. First, in terms of carers, lack of accessible information about services and inappropriate provision has meant that the proposed move to care in the community is at some levels quite meaningless. Asian carers have always provided not only care *in* the community but also care *by* the community in the face of inaccessible services. Second, the very resources valued by carers and service users in community organisations are threatened in the 'contracting out' of services by social services departments. Although there was an assumption in the White Paper that achieving the most cost-effective services and stimulating 'independent' provision were compatible, it has been pointed out that: 'pressure on local authorities to achieve low unit costs, will push them into block contracts with large scale providers, which will disadvantage small black groups or users with unusual [*sic*] patterns of need' (Local Government Information Unit, 1990).

Clearly, at the time of writing there is still a lot that we don't know about the exact impact of changes in the organisation of community care on the lives of all black and minority communities. However, for Asian carers existing research has shown that radical and imaginative changes are needed to enable services to meet the wide-ranging and specific needs of carers: changes that will entail a whole new approach to the interrelationships of issues in the lives of Asian carers and that will empower self-determined choices.

References

Bhalla, A. and Blakemore, K. (1981) *Elders of the Ethnic Minority Groups*, All Faiths For One Race, Birmingham.

Brown, C. (1984) *Black and White Britain: the Third PSI Survey*, Heinemann, London.

Department of Health (1989) *Caring for People: Community Care in the Next Decade and Beyond*, Cm 849, HMSO, London.

Gunaratnam, Y. (1991) *Call for Care*, Health Education Authority, London.

Khan, V. (ed.) (1979) *Minority Families in Britain: Support and Stress*, Macmillan, London.

Local Government Information Unit (1990) 'Caring for people – the government's plans for care in the community', special briefing.

London Borough of Camden (1990) 'The needs of women carers whose first language is not English' [Report of the Director of Law and Administration (Women's Unit)] (unpublished).

McCalman, J. A. (1990) *The Forgotten People: Carers in Three Ethnic Minority Communities in Southwark*, King's Fund Centre, London.

Norman, A. (1986) *Triple Jeopardy: Growing Old in a Second Homeland*, Centre for Policy on Ageing, Policy Studies on Ageing, No. 5.

Patel, N. A. (1990) *'Race' Against Time: Social Services Provision to Black Elders*, Runnymede Trust, London.

Westwood, S. and Bachau, P. (1988) 'Images and realities', *New Society*, 6 May.

14

Feminist Perspectives on Caring

HILARY GRAHAM

14.1 Introduction

Since the late 1970s, feminist researchers have been engaged in a sustained critique of government policies on community care, speaking out against the orthodoxy that communities should be the major source of care for people with long-term needs for support. While questioning the orthodoxy, feminist perspectives have themselves been subject to little by way of development or critique. Instead, the perspectives appear to have become fixed in the form in which they developed in the early 1980s. They have remained largely untouched by recent debates within and beyond feminism, debates that challenge many of the assumptions on which feminist approaches to care have been based.

The chapter reviews the British feminist literature on caring, focusing on some of the complex issues raised and obscured by this important body of research. It begins by outlining what feminists have added to the debate about community care before exploring dimensions of care neglected in feminist accounts. The chapter moves on to highlight how, along with gender, other social divisions are also built in to the exchange of care within communities. It pays particular attention to class and 'race' as axes of difference among women which are reflected in their experiences of giving and receiving care.

14.2 Challenging the orthodoxy: feminist perspectives on caring

Care by families and within communities has long provided the corner-stone of Britain's welfare system. The centrality of such care has been highlighted in recent debates about the support of those who need help with day-to-day living. Here, the 'community' figures prominently, linked to 'care' in ways that convey the sense that they go naturally together. In this linking of community and care, communities are seen as both the major and the best source of care for people with physical disabilities, with physical and mental illnesses and with learning difficulties. As the Griffiths report on community care put it, 'families friends, neighbours and other local people provide the majority of care . . . this is as it should be' (Griffiths, 1988, p. 5).

The assumption that communities are the major and best source of care has informed, in increasingly explicit ways, welfare policy since the 1970s. Both Labour and Conservative governments have seen community care as self-evidently the right way to support individuals who find it difficult to live independent lives. While a question mark has hung over its resourcing, few have spoken out against the principle of care within communities. One of the most sustained and systematic critiques has come from feminist researchers, in a steady stream of studies over the last decade. Their critiques were developed in a series of empirical studies that described the experience of looking after people with long-term health and mobility problems. Alongside these empirical studies were theoretical papers, which tracked the impact of caring on women's lives. This seam of empirical and theoretical research has continued into the 1990s, with the result that there is now a sizeable feminist literature 'on caring'.

This literature has pointed to ways in which community care is resourced by women's unpaid labour. It notes how care within communities is largely care by families, which, in turn, is largely care by female kin. Using a definition of care that may well underestimate the extent of care by women, the recent national study of informal carers none the less reminds us that women make up the majority (two in every three) of those caring for at least 20 hours a week. Underlining the kinship-base of community care, the survey suggests that the majority of female carers (over 70 per cent) are caring for relatives (Green, 1988).

In explaining these patterns, feminists have pointed to the way in which gender divisions take shape within families. They have pointed, in particular, to the fact that family life is sustained by the responsibility that women assume for the health and care of children and for the welfare of male partners. Women's care of those with long-term needs, they suggest, builds on and extends these private caring responsibilities. Low-waged and part-time work limit the opportunities most women have to pay for high-quality and reliable care from others, while their caring role restricts their employment opportunities. Presented by policy-makers as a way of supporting the social independence of those receiving care, community care is re-cast by feminists as a policy that reinforces the economic dependence of women.

This critique of community care developed in the late 1970s and early 1980s. Since then the frameworks that informed the critique have themselves become the focus of intense debate within feminism. It is to these debates that the chapter now turns.

14.3   Feminist perspectives on caring: recent critiques

Feminist research on caring is marked out by a uniformity of perspective. Instead of the sharp lines of theoretical division that characterise other fields of feminist enquiry, it is consensus that is the hallmark of feminist studies of caring. This consensus can be traced back to a series of articles published in the early 1980s, which opened up women's experiences of caring to feminist analysis (for example: Finch and Groves, 1980; Stacey, 1981; Graham, 1983). These articles articulated a common perspective, one that defined caring in terms of the unpaid responsibility that women have for the welfare of their families. As the previous section suggested, such an approach identifies gender divisions as determining the organisation and the experience of care within families.

The perspectives developed over a decade ago have continued to inform feminist studies, both empirical and theoretical (see, for example, Dalley, 1988; Lewis and Meredith, 1988). The enduring influence of the early critiques gives this literature a somewhat dated feel, speaking to past rather than present currents in feminism. Recent debates appear to have largely passed it by. As a result, feminist research on caring has become distanced from the arguments that made the 1980s such a difficult but productive period for feminism as an intellectual and political movement. It has yet to engage in a systematic way with the debates about differences and divisions among women, with the critiques that accuse academic feminism of masking 'race' and class, sexuality and disability as crucial dimensions of women's lives. Yet many of these arguments – which were emerging at around the time when feminist research on caring was developing its frameworks – apply directly to the organisation of care within families (see, for example, Carby, 1982; hooks, 1982; Mama, 1984). They suggest that, while couched in terms of women in general, feminist research on caring has a more exclusive focus. An inclusive language that speaks of 'women's lives' and 'women's experiences' hides the fact that perspectives are grounded in the lives and experiences of some, rather than all, women. Specifically perspectives are grounded in studies where most (if not all) of the respondents are white, heterosexual women whose lives are structured by the giving of care within their families. As a result, some relationships and experiences find a secure place within feminist

research, while others are left on the margins of analysis. Three examples may help to illustrate what has been eclipsed in feminist perspectives on caring.

First, the emphasis in most feminist studies of caring is on the
experience of providing care. Like the orthodox perspectives on community care that they critique, feminist studies tend to see 'care' and
'caring' services as that carers give rather than others receive. When
studies talk about 'the meaning of caring' and 'the cost of caring', when
they describe 'caring relationships' and 'the experience of care', the
frame of reference is typically that of care-providers. It has been left to
women excluded from this frame of reference to point to the tacit
alignment of feminist and carers' perspectives. This exclusion is powerfully conveyed in the juxtaposition of 'feminists' and 'women with
disabilities' in Nasa Begum's account of women receiving personal care.
She notes that:

> *To feminists* community care is a means of reinforcing women's oppression. It
> traps women within the private domain of the family home and leaves the
> carers struggling with the emotions of love and duty.
> *To women with disabilities* community care is a policy which can perpetuate
> oppression and/or promote their right to independence. It is the mechanism
> which enables them to receive personal care outside institutional settings; yet
> it is also the tool that can leave them dependent for intimate personal care at
> the mercy of others.
>
> (Begum, 1990, p. 18; italics added)

Recognising the contradictory position that women with disabilities
occupy in caring relationships, other studies have also argued for
perspectives that reflect the experiences of those receiving as well as
giving care (Campling, 1981). They have argued, too, for a recognition
that 'receivers' and 'givers' are not rigid, mutually-exclusive groups.
Many women with disabilities are heavily involved in both self-care and
in servicing other family members. For women who were carers prior to
the onset of their disability, this involvement can have a deep psychological significance. As Morris notes, many women who experience
disability in their adult lives measure their progress towards independent living 'in terms of whether or not they are still able to look after
their families' (Morris, 1989, p. 48, see also Morris in this volume).

Secondly, in exploring the lives of those who give intimate personal
care, feminist studies are populated primarily by white, heterosexual
women in established family networks. On the basis of their experiences, researchers in the UK have identified a 'hierarchy of caring',
which runs from spouse (first choice) through daughters (second choice)
to other close relatives (Qureshi and Walker, 1988). The importance of

marriage and the nuclear family is borne out in the national survey of informal carers, which confirms that these social relationships provide the setting for most caring relationships. However, while feminist studies of caring have explored the consequences of having family ties, they have paid less attention to the experiences of lesbians seeking and providing care for women outside the nuclear family. These studies have paid little attention, too, to how 'race' structures the hierarchy of caring. Yet Black feminists have argued that it is the absence rather than the presence of family networks that has shaped the domestic lives and health experiences of many Black women in Britain. The struggle was, and is, to build families and to care for, and be cared for by, one's kin. Thus, while caring can be a negative and oppressive experience, it can also be experienced as a way of resisting the divisions of class, 'race' and sexuality, which have worked to separate women from those they care about.

Third, like policy-makers, feminist studies typically define 'care' and 'caring' in terms of the unpaid health-related activities that go on at home and between relatives (and, more rarely, friends). Caring is seen primarily as being about the unpaid work of those who are related to each other through birth or marriage. This kind of definition makes it hard to see forms of home-based care that are not shaped by marriage and kinship obligations. One major example is domestic service, a relationship that constrained the lives of many white and Black working-class women in eighteenth- and nineteenth-century Britain. Its influence continues today in the divisions within women's paid work, which mark out 'caring' work, like nursing and social work, from 'service' work, like laundry, catering and domestic work.

These three examples suggest that gender alone can not explain the patterns of care within families and communities. Women occupy different positions, both in terms of their access to and responsibilities for care, with these positions linked to their experiences of disability and their place in the hierarchies of 'race', class and sexuality. The next section looks in more detail at two of these dimensions, focusing on how the social divisions of 'race' and class are reflected in women's needs to receive and opportunities to give care within their families.

14.4   Social divisions and the patterns of care within families

The social divisions of class, 'race' and gender are etched into the patterns of care within families and communities in ways that, as yet, are only partially understood. While research remains limited, the available studies highlight three important aspects of the relationship between these social divisions and family care. The aspects relate to the distribution of illness and disability, the patterns of access to informal networks and the forms of care within families.

First, social divisions are reflected in people's exposure to illness and disability, with prevalence linked to gender and socio-economic status and rising sharply with age. Thus, the proportion of adults reporting a long-standing illness or disability that limits their activities ranges from 10 per cent among men aged 16 to 44 years in non-manual households to 51 per cent among women aged 65 and over living in manual households (Office of Population Censuses and Surveys, 1990). While national surveys, like the General Household Survey and the OPCS surveys of disability, do not address 'race' as a dimension of disadvantage, small-scale studies have begun to compare the experiences of white and Black ethnic minority populations. These studies remind us that 'white' and 'Black' are not homogeneous groups – the patterns of health and illness vary both within and between ethnic groups. However, they do point to a high incidence of chronic ill-health and physical and sensory disability among Afro-Caribbean and Asian elders (Glendinning and Pearson, 1988).

Second, the social divisions reflected in the distribution of illness and disability emerge again in the family networks that govern access to care within the community. These networks have long been recognised by governments as the 'irreplaceable' and 'principal source of support and care' in old age (Department of Health and Social Security, 1981, p. 37). As the Griffiths report put it, they are 'the primary means by which people are enabled to live normal lives in community settings' (Griffiths, 1988, p. 5). Yet the evidence suggests that this primary and irreplaceable resource is unequally distributed. Resources in 'the community' are not universally available. Like access to health, access to communities of carers appears to be linked in systematic ways to racial and class divisions. Studies have highlighted how poor employment prospects have combined with the progressive tightening of controls on immigration to leave many Black elders without access to kin. In one study of 400 older people, one-third of the Asian respondents and one-half of the Afro-Caribbean respondents had no family in the neighbourhood. One-quarter of the Asian respondents had no family in Britain (Bhalla and Blakemore, 1981). Other studies, too, have described the isolation experienced by those who have no family here and for whom family reunification is no longer seen as a real possibility (Fenton, 1985 and Gunaratnam in this volume).

It is not only Black elders who find themselves denied access to the family networks that government policies have defined as irreplaceable. White people, too, can find themselves without informal sources of support for the tasks they find it difficult to perform alone. The OPCS survey of disability, for example, found that four in ten (44 per cent) of disabled adults were not receiving informal support with the everyday tasks where help was needed (Martin *et al.*, 1989). As the studies of Black elders suggest, low social class, and poverty in particular, is associated with restricted access to informal sources of help. In one recent study of working-class older people living alone, four out of five were women and the majority lived on social security benefits. A large proportion of the respondents (over 50 per cent) were housebound. Yet despite their location 'in the community', 45 per cent had no living children. Only one in three had a relative living in the neighbourhood (Sinclair *et al.*, 1988, p. 25).

The social divisions of class, gender and 'race' are reproduced in the patterns of family care in a third way. As a number of feminist historians have noted, the lives of many women have been shaped by colonial labour patterns in which women's care of other families took precedence over the needs of their own families. 'The family' was the setting for domestic service as well as the care of kin.

In the seventeenth and eighteenth centuries, Black slaves were brought to Britain from Africa and the West Indies to work as personal and household servants: as cooks, maids and valets (Fryer, 1984, p. 72). Through the nineteenth century, Afro-Caribbean women in Britain continued to be employed as servants, while colonial expansion beyond Britain established domestic service as a major source of employment for Black women in India and the Caribbean.

For white English working-class women, and for Irish and other ethnic minority groups, the maintenance of white middle-class families has also been a major source of paid employment. In the 1880s, it is estimated that one in three women aged 15 to 20 had entered domestic service (Lewis, 1984, p. 56). In London in 1861, 55 per cent of women in employment were engaged in personal service (Stedman Jones, 1984).

Residential domestic service remained the largest single occupation for women well into the twentieth century, with over 1,000,000 women 'in service' in the 1930s. Today domestic work continues to characterise the labour market position of many Black and white working-class women engaged in low-paid, low-status work that services the needs of those working in more privileged positions in the household/ organisation. Within the health service, an organisation centrally concerned with meeting daily needs for care, racial hierarchies are in evidence in the organisation of women's care and service. For example, the evidence suggests that Afro-Caribbean women are disproportionately placed in posts where the emphasis is on domestic and personal service rather than on nursing care (London Association of Community Relations Councils, 1985).

In looking at the building of families and kinship networks, it appears that white middle-class women have had greater access to a family life sustained by their care. Many white working-class women and Black and ethnic minority women have found their care arrangements structured by employment opportunities and immigration restrictions in ways that restrict their opportunity to receive and give care within their families. While not underestimating the difficulties, women have emphasised their resistance to the restrictions placed on them by racism and poverty. In their accounts of their lives, many women have described the strategies they use to protect their own health and the health of those they care about. They emerge not as the passive recipients of oppression, but as agents struggling actively to get help and to achieve change for their families (Fenton, 1985; Lewis and Meredith, 1988; Eyles and Donovan, 1990; Phoenix, 1991). They are, in Linda Gordon's evocative phrase, 'heroes of their own lives' (Gordon, 1988).

14.5   Concluding remarks

The chapter has been concerned with a seam of British feminist research on caring that has emerged over the last decade. This research provides a critical commentary on community care, highlighting the way in which both the ideology and the practice of community care rests on, and reinforces, gender divisions. While offering a critical review of policy, feminist perspectives on caring have become strangely insulated from recent critiques of feminism. These critiques challenge the assumption that gender divisions provide a catch-all explanation of care within families. They suggest that other social divisions are also deeply embedded in the past and present organisation of family care.

What are the implications of recognising that the day-to-day care for people in families is structured by many, rather than one, social division?

First, it suggests the need for a broader understanding of 'care' and 'caring'. This understanding should take account of women's experiences of receiving care within families, as well as their experiences of giving it. A more inclusive concept of care needs to confront, too, women's differential need for and access to the communities of kin who provide day-to-day support.

A feminist concept of care should recognise, also, that unpaid care between relatives and friends is not the only kind of home-based care that has defined women's place in British society. Other forms of care have played a crucial part in the reproduction of gender as an identity that has class and racial divisions embedded within it. A focus on care and service within the home provides one way of recognising that the everyday reproduction of families is linked to the reproduction of class and racial differences among women.

Broadening the concept of care highlights a second issue for future analysis. It suggests the need to approach the concept of women critically. Feminists should be wary of treating 'women' as a homogeneous group, with identical interests born of their common experience of gender oppression. Black feminist and lesbian researchers, together with those describing the lives of women with disabilities, have pointed to the profound differences between women. These differences affect, in direct and powerful ways, the kinds of caring relationships that women experience.

Differences and conflicts are part of the reality of many women's lives. As the Black feminist researcher bell hooks has put it, 'none of us experience ourselves solely as gendered subjects. We experience ourselves everyday as subjects of race, class and gender' (Childers and hooks, 1990). Her comments suggests that a woman's experience of caring is mediated through her multiple (and potentially conflicting) identities. She is a carer, but she is also middle class, she is Black, she is a mother, she is disabled, she is heterosexual, she is in paid employment. These different dimensions of her life are likely to shape, in complex ways, the choices she can make about how she cares for her family.

Third, and finally, the arguments of the chapter suggest that the development of one all-embracing feminist perspective is an inappropriate as well as an unachievable aim for those concerned with community care policies. Instead it suggests that the strength of future feminist analyses of caring is likely to lie in their tolerance of the uncertain and unfinished business of understanding women's lives. I anticipate – and hope – that these analyses will more explicitly recognise that feminism is a changing landscape of ideas, with feminist perspectives on caring representing not a fixed intellectual position but a provisional body of knowledge under continual review. With these more fluid and open-ended frameworks, feminist research on caring may be better able to take up its rightful place, at the centre rather than on the margins of contemporary feminist thought.

References

Begum, N. (1990) *Burden of Gratitude: Women with Disabilities Receiving Personal Care*, University of Warwick, Social Care Practice Centre/Department of Applied Social Studies.

Bhalla, A. and Blakemore, K. (1981) *Elders of the Ethnic Minority Groups*, All Faiths for One Race, Birmingham.

Campling, J. (ed.) (1981) *Women with Disabilities Talking: Images of Ourselves*, Routledge, London.

Carby, H. (1982) 'White women listen! Black feminism and the boundaries of sisterhood', in Centre for Contemporary Cultural Studies, *The Empire Strikes Back: Race and Racism in 70s Britain*, Hutchinson, London.

Childers, M. and hooks, b. (1990) 'A conversation about race and class', in Hirsch, M. and Fox Keller, E. (eds) *Conflicts in Feminism*, Routledge, London.

Dalley, G. (1988) *Ideologies of Caring*, Macmillan, London.

Department of Health and Social Security (1981) *Growing Older*, HMSO, London.

Eyles, J. and Donovan, J. (1990) *The Social Effects of Health Policy*, Avebury, Aldershot.

Fenton, S. (1985) *Race, Health and Welfare: Afro-Caribbean and South Asian People in Central Bristol*, University of Bristol.

Finch, J. and Groves, D. (1980) 'Community care and the family: a case for equal opportunities?' *Journal of Social Policy*, Vol. 9, pp. 487–511.

Fryer, P. (1984) *Staying Power: the History of Black People in Britain*, Pluto Press, London.

Glendenning, F. and Pearson, M. (1988) *The Black and Ethnic Minority Elders in Britain: Health Needs and Access to Services*, Health Education Authority, London, in association with the Centre for Social Gerontology, University of Keele.

Gordon, L. (1988) *Heroes of Their Own Lives*, Virago, London.

Graham, H. (1983) 'Caring: a labour of love', in Finch, J. and Groves, D. (eds) *A Labour of Love: Women, Work and Caring*, Routledge and Kegan Paul, London.

Green, H. (1988) *Informal Carers: General Household Survey 1985*, HMSO, London.

Griffiths, R. (1988) *Community Care: Agenda for Action*, HMSO, London.

hooks, b. (1982) *Ain't I a Woman: Black Women and Feminism*, Pluto Press, London.

Lewis, J. (1984) *Women in England 1870–1950*, Wheatsheaf, Brighton.

Lewis, J. and Meredith, B. (1988) *Daughters Who Care: Daughters Caring for their Mothers at Home*, Routledge, London.

London Association of Community Relations Councils (1985) *In a Critical Condition: a Survey of Equal Opportunities in Employment in London's Health Authorities*, LACRC, London.

Mama, A. (1984) 'Black women, the economic crisis and the British state', *Feminist Review*, Vol. 17, pp. 21–35.

Martin, J., White, A. and Meltzer, H. (1989) *Disabled Adults: Services, Transport and Employment*, OPCS Surveys of Disability in Great Britain, Report 4, HMSO, London.

Morris, J. (ed.) (1989) *Able Lives: Women's Experience of Paralysis*, Women's Press, London.

Office of Population Censuses and Surveys (1990) *The General Household Survey 1988*, HMSO, London.

Phoenix, A. (1991) *Young Mothers?*, Polity Press, London.

Qureshi, H. and Walker, A. (1988) *The Caring Relationship*, Routledge and Kegan Paul, London.

Sinclair, I., Crosbie, D., O'Connor, P., Stanforth, L. and Vickery, A. (1988) *Bridging Two Worlds: Social Work and the Elderly Living Alone*, Gower, Aldershot.

Stacey, M. (1981) 'The division of labour revisited or overcoming the two Adams', in Abrams, P., Deem, R., Finch, J. and Rock, P. (eds) *Practice and Progress: British Sociology 1950–1980*, George Allen and Unwin, London.

Stedman Jones, G. (1984) *Outcast London: a Study in the Relationship between Classes in Victorian Society*, Penguin, Harmondsworth.

15

Men: The Forgotten Carers*

SARA ARBER and NIGEL GILBERT

The financial, psychological and social burdens of caring for the infirm elderly have been widely explored. However, many studies, such as Nissel and Bonnerjea's pioneering work (1982) have focused specifically on married daughters as carers, leaving the impression that it is they who are most likely to take on caring responsibilities. For example Allan's recent textbook on the family comments:

> Just as the bulk of housework and childcare is undertaken by mothers, so too by far the largest portion of routine tending for the elderly is provided by daughters . . . The support at a daily level is almost wholly given by women and is defined as an extension of their routine domestic role.
>
> (Allan, 1985, p. 130)

Who cares for the infirm elderly is of increasing importance. The number of people aged 75–84 has risen by 38 per cent over the last fifteen years and the number of very old elderly people, aged over 85, has risen by 46 per cent (Office of Population Censuses and Surveys, 1987, Table 7). These major changes, together with government policies to shift care into the community, have well-recognised implications for those who provide care for the elderly living at home. From the 1980 General Household Survey (Office of Population Censuses and Surveys, 1982), we estimate that 10.7 per cent of elderly people living at home find it difficult or impossible to manage basic daily activities such as walking outside or bathing and washing all over. In varying degrees they need help from others, and in practice, this usually means help from their family. The proportion needing help with these basic activities is 6 per cent of those aged 65 to 74, 15 per cent of those aged 75 to 84, and 41 per cent of those aged 85 and over.

---

*This paper was first published in *Sociology*, Vol. 23, No. 1, 1989, pp. 111–18.

The idea that the burden of caring falls mainly on daughters coupled with the belief that men are unable to care for themselves is widespread and deeply rooted in social policy on community care (Land, 1978). The result is that it is commonly assumed as almost self-evident that

- men are very unlikely to be the primary carers of infirm elderly people;
- elderly men receive much more support from statutory and voluntary services than equally disabled elderly women; and
- when men do perform a caring role, they are more likely to obtain support than women carers.

In fact, our research on a nationally representative sample of elderly people living at home shows that each of these assumptions is far from the truth.

15.1   Men and caring

The few studies which have systematically examined the gender balance of carers have shown that between one-quarter and two-fifths of carers are men (Briggs, 1983; Equal Opportunities Commission, 1980; Charlesworth *et al.*, 1984; Levin *et al.*, 1983). However, these studies used small samples, often from specific localities, that may have been unrepresentative of the wider population.

More reliable data can be obtained from the replies to a section of the 1980 GHS which asked people aged over 65 living in private households about their ability to carry out various domestic and self-care tasks and about their receipt of statutory health and welfare services. The extent of help needed by the 4,533 elderly people in the sample was measured using a series of questions about their ability to perform daily tasks. Six tasks formed a linear scale of increasing difficulty for most people: cutting one's toenails; getting up or down stairs; walking outside; bathing or washing all over; getting around the house; and getting in and out of bed. Elderly people who said they could do a task easily were given a score of zero for that task, those who could do it only with difficulty were given a score of one, and those who could not manage the task at all except with help scored two. Of people aged 65 and over 10.7 per cent had a total score of six or more on this scale and were defined as 'severely disabled'. They were unable to walk outside without help and most could not manage a bath or wash all over unaided (Arber *et al.*, 1988).

Table 15.1 shows that 38 per cent of 'severely disabled' elderly people live alone. The 1980 GHS only provides a broad indication of who helps

TABLE 15.1   Living arrangements of severely disabled elderly people and proportions living with male carers

Type of household	% of all severely disabled elderly	% with male co-resident carers	N for whom information on disability is available
Elderly disabled living alone	38.3	—	1,483
with Spouse			
Couple only	31.3	51	1,998
Couple and adult children	5.8	28–84	260
with Siblings or other elderly	7.3	9–33	178
with Unmarried child	9.0	38–45	277
with Married child	8.1	*	178
(and some lone parents)			
	100 (467)	35–44	4,374

*The wife is assumed to be the carer in all households including an elderly infirm person and a younger married couple.
Source: Derived from the General Household Survey, 1980.

such elderly people and does not distinguish their gender. For example, 'sons and/or daughters' are the main source of informal support for elderly people living alone (Evandrou *et al.*, 1986). Because of this lack of information on carers' gender, this note focuses on the two-thirds of frail elderly who share their home with others.

We have assumed that in these households, the primary carer of the elderly person is another member of the same household. Although this assumption is not always valid, earlier analyses of the 1980 GHS (Evandrou *et al.*, 1986) show that it is generally the case. For example, over 90 per cent of married persons were helped with domestic and personal self-care tasks by their spouse and, where an unmarried elderly person was living with younger household members, under 5 per cent received any help with activities of daily living from people living outside the household.

Table 15.1 shows that 31 per cent of 'severely disabled' elderly people live in households as couples with just their spouse. These couples are almost exactly equally divided between those in which the wife is caring for the husband and those in which the husband is caring for the wife. Another 6 per cent have a spouse and one or more younger unmarried adults, usually their children, living with them. It is difficult to identify from the GHS the gender of the carer among these latter families, because it is not clear whether it is the spouse of the infirm person or the younger person who is the main carer. However, it is possible to define a range: the proportion of male carers lies between 28 per cent (if a woman is assumed to be the carer in all the uncertain cases) and 84 per cent (if a man is always assumed to be the carer).

Seven per cent of severely disabled elderly people are living with other elderly people who are, in most cases, their brothers or sisters. Only from 9 per cent to 33 per cent of carers in these households are men.

A minority (17 per cent) of severely disabled elderly people live only with members of the younger generation, generally their adult children. In just over half these households, the younger people are unmarried and amongst these, there are nearly as many men as women carers, a fact which has often been overlooked.

Only 8 per cent of the elderly in need of daily support are living with a younger married couple, generally their married daughter and her husband. We assume that in these households very few, if any, of the husbands are the primary carers for the disabled elderly person. Thus, the gender balance of co-resident caring for the elderly differs according to four types of kin relationship: (a) caring as part of a marital relationship – men and women are equally likely to care for an elderly spouse; (b) a filial relationship involving an unmarried carer – slightly fewer unmarried sons than unmarried daughters care for an elderly parent; (c) a sibling relationship – elderly sisters are much more likely to be carers than brothers; and (d) a filial relationship involving a married carer – we assume that men are unlikely to be carers.

15.2 The contribution of men carers

Overall, therefore, although a majority of the carers of severely disabled elderly people are women, over one third of co-resident carers are men. Why, then, is there an overwhelming impression that carers are female and silence about the contribution of male carers? An explanation can be found in the life histories of the relationship between the carers and the cared for.

Three-quarters of the men are caring for spouses with whom they have probably lived for most of their lives. Love may be the major motivating factor, as suggested by three out of the four men caring for their wives in Ungerson's study (1987). The majority of the other male carers are unmarried men caring for an elderly parent and are most likely never to have moved out of the parental home since they were children or to have returned following a divorce. In all these households, there is likely to be a strong bond between the carer and the cared for.

The situation is very similar for women caring for their elderly spouse and for many of the unmarried women carers. There will have been a gradual transition from mutual support to a situation where the infirm person is very dependent and can provide little more than companionship. The relationship between the carer and the cared-for will have gradually changed from reciprocity to dependency. The carer has 'little choice' but to care and the transition to caring is often seen as 'natural' – it would be unthinkable to do otherwise than care for the spouse or parent with whom one has been living for many years. Lewis and Meredith (1988) describe unmarried daughters who have always lived with their mother as having 'drifted' into care; caring was seen as a 'natural' stage in their life course. We would expect this to be equally true for spouses and unmarried sons. There may be gender differences as to the primary motivation for caring. For example, Ungerson (1987) suggests that men are more likely to be motivated by 'love' and women by 'duty'. Nevertheless as Levin *et al.* (1983) found, carers of either gender who had lived with the elderly person for a long time were more likely to give love as a motivating factor.

In contrast, the married women who care for elderly parents in their own home are much less likely to have been living with their parents for most of their lives (Arber and Gilbert, forthcoming). The elderly person will often have 'moved in' to the household because of their infirmity and dependency. Caring will be motivated by kinship obligations, which in turn are influenced by norms about gender obligations and feelings of duty (Finch, 1987). This is the major source of gender inequalities in caring: married women are much more likely to be the carers when an elderly person moves into another household. The responsibility for caring is more likely to be the result of a conscious decision than the result of 'drifting into care'.

15.3 Help for elderly men

The second of the common assumptions about the disabled elderly which we suggest may be incorrect is that elderly disabled men obtain much more support from the statutory and voluntary services than women. This issue can be investigated using the 1980 GHS because the survey asked a number of questions about the receipt of community support services. We have chosen three as representative: home helps, where the provision is controlled by local authority social services departments, meals on wheels, primarily a voluntary service, and visits from a district nurse, a medical service. Because the amount of support someone receives depends greatly on how well they can manage for themselves, any useful analysis has first to control for the elderly person's degree of disability. This is particularly important if one is

TABLE 15.2   Receipt of services by the elderly living in different types of household

Type of household	Likelihood* of receipt of:		
	Home helps	Meals on wheels	District nursing
Elderly people living alone:			
man	5.66	15.27	1.91
woman	5.21	5.22	1.68
with Spouse			
Couple, both elderly	1.00	1.00	1.00
Couple, one elderly,			
one younger	0.24	0.00	0.56
Couple and adult children	0.00	0.00	0.90
with Siblings or other elderly	1.29	2.69	2.84
with Unmarried			
male adult child	0.74	1.48	1.43
female adult child	0.80	1.37	1.28
with Married child	0.30	0.36	0.72
(and some lone parents)			

*Odds ratio of receipt of the service within the last month, controlling for level of disability.
Source: Derived from the General Household Survey, 1980.

making gender comparisons, because it is known that a higher proportion of elderly women than men are severely disabled. It is also helpful to express the results in comparison to a common standard, which we have arbitrarily chosen to be the likelihood of one of an elderly married couple receiving the service. The likelihood of an elderly person in different types of household receiving home help, meals on wheels and community nursing services can then be compared to the likelihood of either partner of an elderly couple receiving each of these services (Arber *et al.*, 1988).[1]

Table 15.2 shows that after controlling for level of disability, elderly men and women who live alone are over five times more likely to receive home help support than elderly married couples. Comparing the figures in the top two rows of the table shows that men living alone are about 8 per cent more likely to have a home help than women on their own and about 14 per cent more likely to have been visited by a district nurse in the last month. However, an elderly man living alone is three times more likely to receive meals on wheels than an elderly woman with an equivalent level of disability. Thus there is a gender difference in the receipt of services by elderly men and women living alone, but it is to be found mainly in the voluntary sector, not in the public sector where, once disability has been controlled for, differences in likelihood of receipt are relatively small. The gender differences are much smaller than might have been expected from recent literature on gender and caring (e.g. Walker, 1981; Land, 1978; Ungerson, 1983).

15.4   Help for male carers

One reason which has been put forward to explain why men carers have been so 'invisible' to policy-makers and researchers is that it is presumed that men carers get much more support from the voluntary and statutory services and therefore do not suffer the burdens of caring in the same way as women. However, the evidence from the GHS does not bear this out. Table 15.2 shows that unmarried male carers living with an elderly severely disabled person (usually sons caring for an elderly parent) are marginally less likely to get home help support than unmarried women (usually daughters). Nor does the gender of a younger unmarried carer have any important influence on the elderly person's likelihood of getting meals on wheels or being visited by the district nurse in the last month.

Home helps are very infrequently provided for households in which an elderly infirm person is living with a younger married couple. An elderly person living alone is 18 times more likely to have a home help than an elderly person with an equivalent level of disability living with a younger married woman. The likelihood that these households will obtain meals on wheels is about one-quarter of the likelihood for households in which an unmarried person is the carer. The picture is similar for visits by the district nurse, where the likelihood is about half that for households with unmarried carers, suggesting that some of the tasks which are done by the district nurse where an unmarried adult is the carer are being left to the married daughter. Overall, it looks as though the variation in the provision of these services is not due to discrimination against women *per se*, but discrimination against households in which non-elderly married women predominate as carers.

It has been argued that men do not 'really' care for elderly people because they receive considerably more support from informal carers living outside the household. Data from the 1980 GHS show that men carers in most types of household receive somewhat more help than women (Arber and Gilbert, forthcoming). However, the difference is very small for elderly married couples. For example, 9 per cent of husbands receive help with bathing their wife from informal carers compared to 1 per cent where the wife is caring for her husband. Where a younger unmarried man is caring for an elderly parent, slightly more support is given by 'sons/daughters' living outside the household than where an unmarried daughter is the carer, but even unmarried sons provided nearly three-quarters of the shopping for their frail elderly parent. The least help from informal carers is provided where the elderly person lives with a younger married couple. Since men who care receive only slightly more help from informal carers than women, they cannot simply be dismissed as not being 'real' carers.

15.5 Conclusion

Once one has controlled for the level of disability, the major source of variation in the amount of support services received by elderly infirm men and women seems to be not the gender of the recipients or the gender of the carer, but the kind of household in which they live and, in particular, whether there are others in the household who could take on the burden of caring. Thus infirm elderly people living alone get much more support from formal services than those living with others. Elderly people living with their elderly spouse or with other elderly people get more support from formal services than those in households in which there are younger unmarried members. In all these households, the amount of support does not depend much on the gender of the carer.

Married daughers caring for elderly infirm parents receive considerably less support than unmarried carers, male or female. For these women, caring for an elderly person can conflict with the needs of their children as well as restricting their opportunities for employment and other activities. These burdens may be particularly onerous to married carers because of their relative lack of statutory and voluntary support, together with the fact that in most cases the elderly infirm person will have joined the household as someone needing care.

Note

1. A logit analysis was carried out using GLIM with receipt of services as the dependent variable and type of household and level of disability as the independent variables. The odds ratios in Table 2 are derived from the coefficients of a main effects logit model. There was no statistically significant interaction between disability and household type at the 5 per cent level.

References

Allan, G. (1985) *Family Life: Domestic Roles and Social Organisation*, Blackwell, Oxford.
Arber, S. and Gilbert, G. N. (forthcoming) 'Transitions in caring: gender, life

course and the care of the elderly', in Bytheway, W. (ed.) *Becoming and Being Old: Sociological Approaches to Later Life*, Sage, London.

Arber, S., Gilbert, G. N. and Evandrou, M. (1988) 'Gender, household composition and receipt of domiciliary services by elderly disabled people', *Journal of Social Policy*, Vol. 17, pp. 153–75.

Briggs, A. (1983) *Who Cares?* Association of Carers, Chatham, Kent.

Charlesworth, A., Wilkin, D. and Durie, A. (1984) *Carers and Services: a Comparison of Men and Women Caring for Dependent Elderly People*, Equal Opportunities Commission, Manchester.

Equal Opportunities Commission (1980) *The Experience of Caring for Elderly and Handicapped Dependents*, EOC, Manchester.

Evandrou, M., Arber, S., Dale, A. and Gilbert, G. N. (1986) 'Who cares for the elderly? Family care provision and receipt of statutory service', in Phillipson, C., Bernard, M. and Strang, P. (eds) *Dependency and Interdependency in Old Age*, Croom Helm, London.

Finch, J. (1987) 'Family obligations and the life course', in Bryman, A., Bytheway, B., Allatt, P. and Keil, T. (eds) *Rethinking the Life Cycle*, Macmillan, London.

Land, H. (1978) 'Who cares for the family?' *Journal of Social Policy*, Vol. 7, pp. 357–84.

Levin, E., Sinclair, I., Gorbach, P. (1983) *The Supporters of Confused Elderly Persons at Home*, National Institute of Social Work, London.

Lewis, J. and Meredith, B. (1988) *Daughters Who Care: Daughters Caring for Mothers at Home*, Routledge, London.

Nissel, M. and Bonnerjea, L. (1982) *Family Care of the Handicapped Elderly: Who Pays?* Policy Studies Institute, London.

Office of Population Censuses and Surveys (1987) *Population Trends*, HMSO, London.

Office of Population Censuses and Surveys (1982) *General Household Survey 1980*, HMSO, London.

Ungerson, C. (1983) 'Women and caring: skills, tasks and taboos', in Gamarnikow, E. *et al.* (eds) *The Public and the Private*, Heinemann, London.

Ungerson, C. (1987) *Policy is Personal: Sex, Gender and Informal Care*, Tavistock, London.

Walker, A. (1981) 'Community care and the elderly in Great Britain', *International Journal of Health Services*, Vol. 11, pp. 541–57.

Acknowledgements

The work reported in this article is based on research carried out under the ESRC Ageing Initiative under grant G01250003. We are grateful to Angela Dale, Maria Evandrou and other members of the Stratification and Employment Group for continued help and support.

16

Caring and Citizenship: A Complex Relationship

CLAIRE UNGERSON

16.1 Introduction

The idea of citizenship has a long and distinguished history; but like any idea with historical antecedents, it has, as a notion, become more and more complex, and therefore, eventually, vague. Different groups and political associations claim that they hold the true notion of citizenship, but all too often their definition turns out simply to be the one that suits their particular interests. But one thing about the idea is clear: it is always concerned with the relationship between the individual and the state. Of course, we can and we do argue about the nature of that relationship: whether, for example, it contains a notion of reciprocal rights and duties between state and citizen; whether citizens' rights are more important than citizens' obligations; whether there are different kinds of citizens' rights – such as legal, civil and social rights – and whether these can be placed in historical sequence, and/or normative hierarchies. We can also argue, as we shall see later, about whether the notion of citizenship is essentially masculine. But the one immovable feature of the idea of citizenship is that it is placed in the public domain: it is concerned with how the individual and the state relate to each other across public concerns, and how public institutions, such as the judiciary and the polity, mediate that relationship.

In this chapter, I will be using an idea of care to mean 'informal care', by which is usually meant the care, by relatives, neighbours and friends, of vulnerable people in their own homes, or in the homes of their carers (for a critique of this definition, see Graham in this volume). In Britain, over the last 15 years, an important movement of carers, often combined with feminists, has managed to make informal care a public and political issue (see, for example, Griffiths, 1988). But I will argue that even though caring has moved on to the public agenda, it nevertheless

143

remains difficult to put the public notion of citizenship together with the private notion of care.

16.2   Public and private rights

The fact that the notion of citizenship is essentially placed in the public domain, and that, in the twentieth century at least, it has come to contain within it a very strong emphasis on rights, particularly 'social rights' to personal security and welfare, poses two particular problems. The first problem is that carers are not in the public domain; they are physically located within the so-called 'private' world of hearth and home. Moreover, there is a panoply of ideology that reinforces this idea that caring is essentially a private activity, since – it is often and easily argued – the motivation to care commonly arises out of love, and, if not love, then obligations based on kinship and reciprocal biography. But love and kinship are particularistic, internal and domestic – unlike citizenship, which is most often taken to be general, external and public. Hence, logically, these essentially private constructs of love and kinship do not sit easily within the public construct of citizenship. This remains true at a logical level even though the state and its agencies may in actuality try, and often, in reality, succeed, in using assumptions about love and kinship as reasons (for excuses) for leaving people in need to their own and their family's private devices.

The second problem that arises when we try to link care with citizenship is that, particularly where we adopt a notion of citizenship that emphasises rights, we run into difficult water as soon as we try to *operate* a notion of rights within the domestic and private domain. It is notoriously difficult and controversial to operate and ultimately to enforce rights within the domestic domain, and if attempts are made to do so, these attempts are often sexist. For example: the question of rights to sexual intercourse is marriage and the related issue of married women's rights over their own bodies, and the question of women's rights to live free of the threat or actuality of their partner's violence, are both issues that demonstrate how generally complicated it is to translate the essentially public issue of rights into the domestic domain. It is particularly difficult because the state and its agencies, in the process both of defining and of enforcing rights, very frequently act in a patriarchal manner. One can immediately see similar difficulties when it comes to caring: do children have a right to their parents', or, more particularly, their mother's, continual attention? Do parents, once they have grown frail and elderly, have a right to be cared for by their children and a right to be financially maintained by their better-off kin? Do people deemed to be schizophrenic have a right to be looked after by their parents, or, conversely, a right not to be looked after by their parents? One can imagine deep controversies around these issues, and one can even imagine such 'rights' being placed on the statute book[1], but it is extremely difficult to understand how they would be enforced except within an exceptionally authoritarian state – which would in itself be in antithesis to the civil rights aspect of the idea of citizenship. Moreover, one can all too easily imagine how the operation of such 'rights' to be cared for would make those caring relationships fraught and even dangerous.

Another problem involved in trying to put the issue of rights into the domestic domain, is that, particularly within a caring context, people locked into caring relationships with each other may well have conflicts of interest, such that they want different rights. For example, it is arguable that it is in carers' interests, and that they should have the right, to be freed from caring, at least for, say, one week in six, by placing their dependent persons in respite care, or by having someone to replace them in their own homes while they go away. But it could equally well be argued that dependent people should not have to suffer the disruption of continuously changing where they live, or having strangers enter their homes in order to care for them in the most personal and intimate ways. In other words, carers and persons cared for may well have conflicts of interest, and want to claim rights to quite different types of resource and conditions for autonomy.

16.3   Citizenship and women

These problems of using an essentially public notion of citizenship to deal with the rights of people who spend most of their physical and psychological time in the private world of the home are not new. Such problems have been largely considered in relation to the question of how to integrate women as citizens. One aspect of this discussion has been a general feminist critique of the idea of citizenship within political theory, suggesting that it is essentially masculine – an analysis powerfully developed by the Australian political theorist Carole Pateman (see, for example, Pateman, 1988, 1989). Other feminist writers, such as Cass and Lister, have developed a feminist critique that contains suggestions as to how – in practical ways – women's social rights within a framework of citizenship might be underwritten. The basic question they have attempted to answer is how, given women's domestic roles and responsibilities, social policy can be used to guarantee women's autonomy so that women attain social rights quite independently of men (in particular, their husbands), and irrespective of their civil and legal status as wives, mothers or carers (see, for example, Cass, 1990; Lister, 1990). Clearly such critique and analysis is relevant when it comes to considering caring and citizenship, for at least two reasons. First, this feminist literature on citizenship is dealing with overlapping categories: most – although, as we shall see later, by no means all – carers are women. Second, this tradition of feminist commentary on social policy has critiqued the way in which the state has treated as natural and unproblematic the contribution that women make as unpaid reproducers at home, while, at the same time, it has had to use a variety of instruments, some of them quite draconian, in order to reinforce this unpaid contribution so that current social policy developments can be maintained (see, for example, Land, 1978). It is out of this 20 years or more general feminist critique that a considerable feminist literature focused particularly on caring has developed. In other words, much of the existing caring literature owes its origins to the general feminist claim that caring is a form of domestic labour.

Thus the feminist commentary on the issue of the integration of women as citizens is important for the purpose of putting caring and citizenship together, but, I am going to argue, it is not wholly adequate for our purposes. There are a number of reasons for this. For a start, the main focus of this literature has so far been concerned with finding ways of guaranteeing women's income in a way that loosens, if not banishes altogether, their dependency on men. This commentary stresses the way in which social policy can be used to underwrite women's full participation in the labour market. Second, the feminist critique talks about 'women' but usually, in the citizenship context, it talks most particularly about mothers. Often the feminist commentary on citizen- ship elides mothering with caring, and treats mother and carers as though they are in identical positions (see, for example, Cass, 1990). The difficulty is, however, that while mothers and carers may share a sex, they are also rather different, and they have different needs.

One of the important differences between mothers and carers is the question of age. Of course there are mothers who are carers too, and they have particular problems (see, for example, Ungerson, 1987), but it is interesting to note that most carers are beyond child-bearing age (if they are female), and that also, for many of them, the period of their lives devoted to child-caring is probably over. In 1985 a national sample survey found that of carers looking after someone dependent for at least 20 hours a week, 69 per cent were aged over 45; 26 per cent were aged over 65. Moreover, given the feminist literature on caring which claims that caring is very largely undertaken by women working on their own, a surprisingly high proportion of carers – 36 per cent – appear to be men (Green, 1988, Table 4.4). Thus the literature on women and citizenship, while claiming to be relevant to carers, has to be somewhat refined and qualified in order properly to take account of carers' needs. The first point is that if citizenship is to be operationalised to mean economic

independence underwritten by participation in the labour market supplemented by benefits, then, for many if not most carers, the labour
market, and participation within it, is no longer relevant since they are
largely beyond that point in their lives. It is possible, of course, to
envisage an insurance system, based on employment, which generates
rights for carers beyond employment – in much the same way as the
present National Insurance scheme generates pension and unemployment benefits (however inadequately). But such a route to 'carers'
citizenship' is a very long-term prospect, since the amount of contributions needed to generate the right to benefit would, no doubt, stretch
over the equivalent of a lifetime's employment. Second, while it is the
case that carers are often in desperate need of income, partially to cover
the additional costs of caring, but also simply to maintain themselves
while outside the labour market, it is also the case that most carers have
very pressing problems to do with the actual nature of caring – for which
income may be only a limited answer. Obviously money, particularly a
large amount of it, might help to alleviate some of these problems if the
money were used by carers to buy in support services, but such private
sector services might be difficult to find, unreliable, and create further
problems for the carer who would have to organise and manage them.
Thus an employment- and income-related discourse, which clearly is
salient to the general question of women and citizenship, and the more
particular question of mothers and citizenship, has to be qualified when
it comes to the issue of carers and citizenship.

Third, carers and mothers experience their caring in different ways
and have different needs for support. Mothers need help with the
socialisation of their children, their feeding, clothing and washing, their
education and recreation; but mothers can expect the state to take over
aspects of this socialisation – particularly education and some recreation
– at a particular point in their children's lives. In other words, the life
course of a normally developing child is relatively predictable, and
although the care of that child will demand a great deal in terms of time
and emotion from the mother, at least she can make plans for herself
within a fairly ordered universe, as can the state. Carers' needs for
support are ostensibly fairly similar to those of mothers. They too have
to feed, clothe and wash their cared-for persons, and provide for their
recreation, and, for younger people, their education. But one thing
about caring, particularly where elderly people are concerned, is that it
is unpredictable. A carer may expect to care for someone who appears to
be close to death for a brief period, only to find that their cared-for
person recovers to live for many more years but in a highly dependent
condition. Moreover, just as there is no predictability whatsoever about
when, if at all, the state will step in to take over some of these caring
functions, so there is no predictability for the state as to when, for

example, a previously employed carer might return to work. Hence the development of rights to, for example, carers' career breaks is much more problematic than the development of rights surrounding maternity.

If we are to operationalise rights in the context of informal care, then, in effect, we have to lay down standardised, minimum rights for carers and people cared for, irrespective of their circumstances. But it would be quite wrong to standardise rights to services across all dependencies: young disabled adults clearly have quite different needs from those of elderly mentally infirm people. Similarly, the needs of carers will vary. In part this will reflect the particular dependencies of the persons they care for, but carers themselves also vary widely in terms of, for example, age, length of time spent caring and the additional costs of caring that are incurred. Not surprisingly, in the field of community care we are constantly trying to find ways of dealing with variety of need: hence all the talk of flexibility of care, and packages of care tailored to the particular needs of individual independent people (Griffiths, 1988). I do not wish to rule out altogether the question of carers' rights; simply to recognise that there is bound to be a problem of matching highly various needs to standardised rights to services, and that there will always have to be a considerable place for the operation of discretion. Moreover, the operation of such rights – to respite care, for example – may, as has already been suggested, conflict with the needs and desires of the people that carers care for.

16.4   Rights for carers

So how might care and citizenship be put together, as far as carers are concerned? As I have argued, the situation is extremely complicated, and the concept of rights in this context is a slippery one. There are, however, a number of suggestions as to how to underwrite carers' citizenship, which are currently under discussion. There is too little space to consider them in any detail here; needless to say, each has its advantages and disadvantages. The first concerns the development of employment rights for carers (for example, so many days off in a year to care for someone; protection of pension rights; career-break rights) or social service rights (for example, rights to a certain number of hours, or weeks, of respite care; rights of access to a social worker or care manager; rights to a care allowance). While these may well be a step in the right direction, there is a danger that support services may be over-routinised, unreliable, and intrusive, and they may be services that suit the carer and not the person cared for, or vice versa. Another set of rather more radical proposals queries the direction of community care altogether, suggesting that residential care for dependent people remains the better alternative (Finch, 1984), or that forms of collective care, which might include high-quality residential care, should be developed (Dalley, 1988). The difficulty here is that institutional care is notoriously vulnerable to the risk of becoming authoritarian and even brutal. Within a citizenship framework, if institutional care is to avoid this danger, then the rights of residents and their families to high-quality and safe care has to be underwritten and enforced by widespread inspectorates, with teeth. Perhaps the best way of ensuring high-quality institutional care is to make it attractive to carers as well as the people they care for: Christmas for the family 'in the home', rather than 'at' home.

Other radical proposals accept that community care policies should continue, while at the same time acknowledging that the burden on carers is considerable, and that they should be compensated in some way. Two different kinds of proposal then emerge: the first is the 'basic income guarantee', which would be a benefit payable to all citizens, irrespective of their employment or marital status. Everyone over a certain age would receive the same amount, which they could then supplement by earnings, which, in turn, would be highly taxed. This is not specifically a carers' benefit, although those who support this proposal often argue that one of its main advantages is that it recognises the unpaid labour of housewives, mothers and carers, and provides them with an independent income (see, for example, Parker, 1991). Basic income has also been adopted by many commentators as a way of operationalising the concept of citizenship (see, for example, Jordan, 1989; Dahrendorf, 1990; Pateman, 1989). The difficulty here, as far as carers are concerned, is that if everyone gets the same, then the specific work of caring, in effect, remains unrecognised. There is also the more general problem that basic income proposals are extremely expensive, and not, in the current political climate, thought to be feasible. The second proposal along these lines is that carers should be paid for the work that they do. The feasibility of such a proposal is not so open to question since there are already systems of payment in place for, in particular, foster parents (Leat and Gay, 1987) and there are rapidly developing systems of payment for 'volunteers' (Qureshi, 1989; for a critique of these payments, see Baldock and Ungerson, 1991). Moreover, it is arguable that the present invalid care allowance, payable to all non-employed carers of working age in order to compensate them for not being in the labour market, is an embryonic form of payment for care. Of course, such a proposal commodifies care, and the effect is that it might alter – quite possibly for the worse just as much as for the better – the relationship between carer and person cared for. It is not that difficult, for example, to imagine a dependent person assuming that they have an infinite right to their carer's time and patience because their carer's time and patience is being paid for by the state.

16.5   Conclusion

This chapter has presented a somewhat sceptical view of the position of carers *vis-à-vis* citizenship in general and rights in particular. On the whole I have pinpointed the dilemmas and complexities that arise when we try to put caring and citizenship together, rather than the ways in which the idea of citizenship might lead to progress both for carers and the people they care for. But, more optimistically, it seems to me that it is also possible to argue that carers and the people they care for have interests in common and that these common interests can and should be underwritten by rights. The policies of community care are partially the result of a well-grounded critique of institutional care, and reflect the fact that as standards of living have generally risen, so elderly people have opted to stay in their own homes, forming their own separate households for as long as possible into their old age (Donnison and Ungerson, 1968). It is therefore in the interests of dependent people that they be enabled, through intensive and extensive support services, to continue to live in their own homes, and as independently of informal care as possible. The policies of community care do not and should not entail that dependent people wishing to remain 'in the community' should eventually have to move out of their own homes and into the homes of their kin, who then become their full-time informal carers, because the support services are non-existent or inappropriate. In this sense, then, carers and the people they care for have a joint project: to campaign for the development of support services that allow all of us who wish to remain in our own homes to do so. If such support services are of high enough quality and reliable enough, then the private aspects of care – the parts that contain the love and watchfulness – can flourish within a public framework, underwritten by the collectively guaranteed provision of caring services by the state.

Note

1. The German principle of 'subsidiarity', laid down in the German Social Assistance Act, states that before an individual can qualify for state social assistance they have to have tried – and demonstrate that they have failed – to change their own circumstances, and to get support from their immediate family, or from voluntary organisations (Jamieson, 1990).

References

Baldock, J. and Ungerson, C. (1991) ' "What d'ya want if you don' want money?" ' A feminist critique of "paid volunteering", in MacLean, M. and Groves, D. (eds) *Women's Issues in Social Policy*, Routledge, London.

Cass, B. (1990) 'Gender and social citizenship: the politics and economics of participation and exclusion', paper given at the Social Policy Association annual conference, University of Bath.

Dahrendorf, R. (1990) 'Decade of the citizen', interview with J. Keane, *Guardian*, 1 August.

Dalley, C. (1988) *Ideologies of Caring: Rethinking Community and Collectivism*, Macmillan, London.

Donnison, D. and Ungerson, C. (1968) 'Trends in residential care, 1911–1961', *Social and Economic Administration*, July.

Finch, J. (1984) 'Community care: developing non-sexist alternatives', *Critical Social Policy*, No. 9, pp. 6–18.

Green, H. (1988) *Informal Carers: a Study*, Office of Population Censuses and Surveys, HMSO, London.

Griffiths, R. (1988) *Community Care: Agenda for Action*, HMSO, London.

Jamieson, A. (1990) 'Informal care in Europe', in Jamieson, A. and Illsley, R. (eds) *Contrasting European Policies for the Care of Older People*, Gower, Aldershot.

Jordan, B. (1989) *The Common Good: Citizenship, Morality, and Self-Interest*, Blackwell, Oxford.

Land, H. (1978) 'Who cares for the family?', *Journal of Social Policy*, Vol. 7, No. 3, pp. 257–84.

Leat, D. and Gay, P. (1987) *Paying for Care: a Study of Policy and Practice in Paid Care Schemes*, Policy Studies Institute, Research Report No. 661, London.

Lister, R. (1990) 'Women, economic dependency and citizenship', *Journal of Social Policy*, Vol. 19, No. 4, pp. 445–67.

Parker, H. (1991) 'Terminology', *Basic Income Research Group Bulletin*, No. 12, February.

Pateman, C. (1988) *The Sexual Contract*, Polity Press, Cambridge.

Pateman, C. (1989) *The Disorder of Women: Democracy, Feminism and Political Theory*, Polity Press, Cambridge.

Qureshi, H. (1989) *Helpers in Case Managed Community Care*, Gower, Aldershot.

Ungerson, C. (1987) *Policy is Personal*, Tavistock, London.

17

*The Principles of Collective Care**

GILLIAN DALLEY

17.1 Essential principles of collective care

There are certain essential principles which must be observed in the development of any form of care. Responsiveness to individual need and inclination is clearly one. But perhaps overriding that and all others from the cared for person's perspective is the ability for that person to be responsible for his or her own life. This is a theme which emerges from many studies of disability and dependence (Blaxter, 1976; Shearer, 1982a), and it is precisely this quality which current provision denies. Disabled people recognise quite clearly that they are, to varying degrees, dependent on other people for the performing of certain basic tasks. They acknowledge that independence, in the sense that this might imply freedom from such dependence or reliance on other people, is not an option for them – however sophisticated mechanical aids and adaptations might become. What they are concerned with is to be able to control the way in which they manage that dependence and the degree to which they have options from which to choose. Dependence and interdependence are a part of ordinary life (Shearer, 1982b); a life of total *independence* would mean isolation and separation.

It is the recognition of dependence and interdependence as facets of all human relationships that validates the collectivist approach to the issue of caring. By the collectivity taking on responsibility for the provision of care, the tensions, burden and obligation inherent in the one-to-one caring relationship, which are the product of the family model of care, are overcome. Particular individuals are not forced into particular caring and cared for roles, dictated by their social and biological relatedness; for it is in those relationships that dependence becomes

---

*This is an abridged extract from *Ideologies of Caring*, Macmillan, London, 1988, pp. 114–18.

a warped and unhealthy pressure on the actors involved. In collectively shared relationships of caring, the burdens are dispersed and fewer pressures arise. The individuals who are being cared for are not forced into dependence on certain other individuals with whom they might have other kinds of relationships (of love, dislike, intellectual partnership, parenthood, siblingship, and so on).

Thus the first principle of collective care, which is also applicable to any form of care provision, must be for the disabled and dependent individual to be in a position to be responsible for his or her life choices – and they should not be once and for all choices. The possibility for change has to be incorporated. Equally, those who provide care should also be in a position to be responsible for decisions about their role in providing care. Women should not be forced into the position of having to care at the cost of other choices, and the status and economic rewards of caring should be comparable with alternative activities.

A second principle should be that the system of care should be responsive to the needs and inclinations of the individuals receiving care. This must mean that forms of care should be flexible in themselves – rigid routines and fixed expectations should play no part – and movement between different forms of care *when appropriate* should be possible. But this should not be mandatory; concepts such as the continuum of care which sees dependent people moving from one form of care into another as their dependency-related conditions improve or deteriorate often fail to recognise the regimentation that they may involve. Existing care should be responsive as far as possible to accommodate such changes, rather than the dependent person being expected to change location.

A third principle must be maximal opportunity to form as wide and varied a range of personal relationships as the individual might wish. This might be coupled with a fourth principle – an equally maximal opportunity to develop skills and talents in any way that the individual chooses. These two principles relate closely to concepts of integration, ordinary life and normalisation, although the normative and prescriptive implications of the latter concept may be inappropriate (Dalley, 1983) if one of the objects of this alternative approach to care is to open up new ways of being and doing. Dependent individuals should not be cut off from other areas of social life if they choose not to be; on the other hand, they should be free to develop their own social environment in the way they wish. An ordinary life means precisely that – that the lives of dependent people should be unremarkable, should not be *ab*normal.

A fifth principle should underwrite all the others – dependent people should be economically secure, to ensure that the other principles have real meaning. Shearer (1982a) and Blaxter (1976) describe vividly the effect that economic constraints have on disabled people endeavouring to live independently. Indeed, Williams (1983) notes that Shearer suggests direct monetary assistance is the most important resource permitting some people with disabilities to live independently. There can be no ordinary life and no control over choice or exercise of responsibility in conditions of poverty. Current levels of income maintenance for chronically disabled people are notoriously low; in Britain arbitrary limits are put on the levels of state support available for people in residential care, unrelated to the actual costs. Comparison of state pension levels between current and past provision, and between Britain and other countries, reveals how far Britain is from guaranteeing those who are not economically active a secure standard of living.

These then are basic principles for which collective systems of care must be tested. However, it is salient to note that the dependency groups are not homogeneous either in type and degree of dependency or, thus, in their need for care. The pertinence of the principles established may vary accordingly. The young physically disabled person is in a very different situation from a very elderly person suffering from senile dementia; likewise, a chronically mentally ill, middle-aged individual has different needs and wants from a child with a severe mental handicap. Young people at the beginning of their lives may be eager to develop social networks; old people facing the end of their lives may be more concerned with consolidating and maintaining existing social networks than seeking new ones. Physical disability requires physical care, especially related to problems of mobility; mental disability requires different forms of supportive care and chronic sickness may require constant nursing care. These differences have major consequences for the expectations which individuals themselves have of their own lives and for the varieties of care which should be available. Williams (1983) makes a pertinent comment on the heterogeneity of dependency in his critique of the independent living movement in the United States:

> The core constituency of the independent living movement is young, male and 'fit' as opposed to 'frail', whereas a major feature of the social reality of disablement is the elderly female, lacking in robustness and living far from the supportive confines of university campuses [where the ILM originated]. It may well be that the disadvantages and needs of an elderly arthritic in an urban slum have more similarity to the problems of her able-bodied neighbours than to the values of the movement for independent living.

There may be a danger, then, if the heterogeneity of dependency is ignored, that certain groups may be excluded from benefiting from developments in patterns of care. In policy and administrative terms, it is relatively straightforward to talk about dependency groups, priority groups or Cinderella groups as a whole, but the reality of the lives of the people who form those groups is far from straightforward. The flexibility and responsiveness to need, discussed above, has to include the policy and administrative levels, and from there permeate the whole system involving the people who are to be in receipt of care, or their advocates, from the outset. Indeed, some might argue that only those in receipt of care have any conclusive right to determine types and standards of care. If this is so, the right should also be extended to the other potential partner in the caring dyad – those who provide the care, both paid and unpaid, and who are predominantly women.

References

Blaxter, M. (1976) *The Meaning of Disability*, Heinemann, London.
Dalley, G. (1983) 'Ideologies of care: a feminist contribution to the debate' in *Critical Social Policy*, No. 8.
Shearer, A. (1982a) *Living Independently*, Centre for the Environment for the Handicapped and King Edward's Hospital Fund for London, London.
Shearer, A. (1982b) *An Ordinary Life: Issues and Strategies for Training Staff for Community Mental Handicap Services*, King's Fund Project Paper, No. 42, Kings Fund Centre, London.
Williams, G. H. (1983) 'The movement for independent living: an evaluation and critique', *Social Science and Medicine*, Vol. 17, No. 15.

18

'Us' and 'Them'? Feminist Research and Community Care*

JENNY MORRIS

Community care is a major area of concern for feminist academics yet the experiences of disabled and older women are missing from the debate, from the research and from the development of theory. This has meant that, in attempting to explore forms of care which do not depend on women's unpaid work within the family, non-disabled feminists have advocated residential care. Thus Janet Finch writes, 'On balance it seems to me that the residential route *is* the only one which ultimately will offer us a way out of the impasse of caring' (Finch, 1984, p. 16).

Disabled and older people experience daily the inadequacies of 'community care'. However, as individuals and through our organisations we have put our energies into achieving a better quality of life *within* the community. How has this conflict between non-disabled feminist academics and organisations of disabled people come about?

18.1 'Us' and 'Them'

For feminists writing and researching on carers, the category 'women' does not include those who need physical assistance. When Janet Finch asked 'Can we envisage any version of community care which is not sexist?' she went on, 'If we cannot, then we need to say something about how we imagine such people *can* be cared for in ways which we find acceptable' (1984, p. 7). In order to understand how she, and other feminists, answer this question we need to recognise who Janet Finch

*This article is an edited version of a chapter in *Pride Against Prejudice: Transforming Attitudes to Disability*, The Women's Press, 34 Great Sutton Street, London, 1991.

156

means when she says 'we' and whether 'we' are included in the term 'such people'.

The latter term refers to 'people . . . whose physical needs require fairly constant attendance' (p. 7). Throughout Finch's writing it is clear that the term 'we' does not include 'such people'. When Finch and others are assessing what policies would be acceptable to 'us' she means what policies would be acceptable to non-disabled feminists.

Feminist research on caring explicitly separates out non-disabled women from disabled women. This distinction has major implications for the issues which feminists consider important. Finch and Groves, for example, identified that the equal opportunity issues around community care concerned the sexual division of labour between men and women as carers (Finch and Groves, 1983). In none of the research is there any analysis of equal opportunity issues for disabled and older women.

This separating out of disabled and older women from the category of 'women' comes about because these feminist researchers fail to identify with the subjective experience of 'such people'. The principle of 'the personal is political' is applied to carers but not to the cared for. This is articulated by Clare Ungerson's account of why the issue of caring is of personal significance. She writes 'my interest in carers and the work that they do arises out of my own biography. The fact that my mother was a carer and looked after my grandmother in our home until my grandmother's death when I was 14 combines with the knowledge that, as an only daughter, my future contains the distinct possibility that I will sooner or later become a carer myself' (Ungerson, 1987, p. 2). Lois Keith, a disabled feminist, commented on Ungerson's inability to see *herself* as potentially a person who needs physical care, 'Most of us can imagine being responsible for someone weaker than ourselves, even if we hope this won't happen. It is certainly easier to see ourselves as being needed, than to imagine ourselves as dependent on our partner, parents or children for some of our most basic needs' (Keith, 1990).

Ungerson's failure to identify with those who need care is then carried over into her feminist analysis which must remain incomplete while she considers only one part of the caring relationship. Yet again disabled and older women are marginalised – but this time by those who proclaim their commitment to 'women-centred issues'.

18.2 Gillian Dalley's 'Collectivism'

Gillian Dalley presents the most fully developed feminist critique of community care, arguing for the development of social policy based on the principle of collectivism rather than that of familism and possessive individualism which she says motivates community care policies (see Chapter 17).

Most disabled people would thoroughly endorse Dalley's promotion of the principles of collectivism and mutual support. We would also welcome her insistence that disabled and older people should 'be in a position to be responsible for his or her life choices' (Dalley, 1988, p. 115). The problem is that she reaches a decision about which policies should be supported without allowing our voices to be heard.

One of Dalley's reasons for arguing against community care policies is that she believes that these policies are not necessarily supported by 'dependent people'. Unfortunately, the only evidence that she produces to back this up is from non-disabled people. The only time she cites the opinion of a disabled person, she quotes him out of context to support a position which he would never have agreed with. In advocating group living for disabled people, Dalley quotes Bernard Brett (whom she describes as 'heavily dependent') on the advantages of having more than one person providing personal care. 'Nothing is quite as corrupting for all concerned as being completely dependent on too few people' he says. 'I can promise you, there are few less pleasant things than to be cared for by somebody who is constantly tired and under too much strain. This makes life tense, unpleasant and unfulfilled' (quoted in Dalley, 1988, p. 120).

Far from advocating some kind of residential, group living situation (which is how Dalley uses this quote), Bernard Brett was describing a set-up where he had bought his own house, let rooms in it to non-disabled lodgers and employed a number of different carers. Like many disabled people, Bernard Brett described residential care as 'a form of living death' and like most non-disabled people he wanted a home of his own (see Shearer, 1982, pp. 37–48).

Bernard Brett was not, of course, receiving 'family care'. He was instead able to choose to pay (in cash and in kind) those who provided assistance to him. However, feminists such as Dalley and Finch have dismissed this as an option, arguing that even where assistance within the home is provided by a paid carer that carer is still likely to be a low-paid, low status woman and, although this is also true for care workers employed in residential establishments, residential workers are more likely to be able to campaign for better pay and conditions. They see the removal of caring for disabled and older people from a family setting as a crucial part of undermining women's dependency.

Dalley dismisses the demands that have been made by disabled people and their organisations for good quality services to enable them to live in their own homes, insisting that such demands are merely expressions of dominant ideology.

She argues, 'Propounders of the familist ideal favour it [a community care policy] because for them it embodies notions of the family as haven, as repository of warm, caring, human relationships based on mutual responsibility and affection and thus a private protection against a cold, hostile, outside world' (Dalley, 1988, p. 25). When disabled and older people express an aversion to residential care, according to Dalley, this must be set in the context of the strength of the ideology of the family.

There is no recognition here that disabled people are often denied the family relationships that she takes for granted. Insult is then added to injury by the assumption that for a disabled person to aspire to warm, caring human relationships within the setting where most non-disabled people looked to find them is a form of false consciousness.

Dalley also insists that disabled people's organisations are not representative. Anti-feminists often seek to undermine feminism by claiming that most feminists are white, young and middle-class. Dalley echoes this sort of divisiveness by quoting a critic of the Independent Living Movement (ILM). 'The core constituency of the independent living movement is young, male and "fit" as opposed to "frail", whereas a major feature of the social reality of disablement is the elderly female, lacking in robustness and living far from the supportive confines of university campuses [where the American ILM originated]' (G. H. Williams, quoted by Dalley, 1988, p. 117).

It is certainly true that the ILM is dominated by men. However, to use this to undermine the principles of the movement is to deny the basic human rights for which it stands. The aims of the ILM are not only relevant to young, middle-class, white men. Such men are merely demanding what young, middle-class, white, non-disabled men take for granted. The economic and social advantages of this latter group normally enable them to achieve such things – and this is why it is common for white, middle-class young men to react with such outrage when their social and economic privileges are suddenly threatened by disability. Why shouldn't those of us whose class, race, age, gender and disability mean that we are denied such advantages, insist on the same rights?

Given non-disabled feminists' inability to identify with our subjective experience, perhaps they should be wary of prescribing the kind of care that would be best for us. Dalley, however, is not inhibited by this. Dismissing the demands of the Independent Living Movement, she advocates new forms of residential provision on the grounds that it is only by removing caring and servicing functions from a family setting that the sexual division of labour (in both the private and public sphere) will be fundamentally undermined. A sceptical disabled feminist may comment that if communal living is such a liberating force for women, then perhaps non-disabled women should try it first.

Dalley argues that a group home would make it possible for a 'bed-bound' young mother to develop an 'ungendered' role. Such a woman, says Dalley, will not expect to 'take up a domestic role vis a vis housework and child-rearing as she would (because of normative attitudes at large) if she were able-bodied' (1988, p. 122). Others would perform this role for her and the advantage of a 'collective' setting, according to Dalley, is that her role would be performed by men or women, depending on who was employed.

Such a solution to accommodation and personal assistance needs would be firmly rejected by disabled mothers like Sheila Willis, whom I interviewed when writing *Pride against Prejudice: Transforming Attitudes to Disability* (Morris, 1991). Her aim after learning that she had multiple sclerosis was to remain living in her own home continuing her role of a mother caring for her daughter. Sheila rejected the term 'bed-bound' – 'What me? *Bound* to a bed?'. During the last years of her life, she spent most of the time on her bed, organising and taking responsibility for not only her own household but also setting up a voluntary organisation which would provide help to other disabled people. A feminist for 15 years, her role as a mother and her ability to run her own home were intensely important to her; to deny this would be a denial of her fundamental human rights – and those of her daughter.

18.3   Different questions, different answers

Feminists cannot claim to have developed a full analysis of and adequate strategies on community care until the experiences of disabled and older people are included within the research. Nasa Begum, a disabled feminist, recently carried out a piece of qualitative research into ten disabled women's experience of receiving personal care which illustrates some of the ways that this subjective experience can be incorporated into a feminist analysis of community care (Begum, 1990).

Disabled feminists (were they properly represented within the academic and research community) would raise new questions when carrying out research on community care and would not be faced with the stark choice which Finch has posed between community care or residential care.

Instead of focusing on the 'taking charge of' part of Hilary Graham's definition of 'caring about' (Graham, 1983, p. 13), such research would focus more clearly on the reciprocity involved in caring relationships and the threats to that reciprocity. Loss of reciprocity brings with it a vulnerability to abuse.

Little attention has been paid to disabled and older people's experience of physical and emotional abuse, which occurs within both residential and community care. Unfortunately feminism's concern with the various forms of abuse experienced by non-disabled women has generally failed to incorporate the experience of disabled women.

We should ask whether people want to receive physical care from someone they care about and who cares for them. For someone like Clare Robson, who has multiple sclerosis and lives with her lover and her children, the answer is clear 'I know that I am loved and that I love her. I feel very privileged and secure. I never, ever, anticipated a relationship that was so wonderful and loving. Obviously there are difficulties. There are, in effect, three of us – me, her and the MS – and we have to take account of the uninvited guest, the squatter' (Morris, 1991, p. 164).

On the other hand, Simon Brisenden identified that where there are no options than dependence on a relative or partner, then this can be 'the most exploitative of all forms of so-called care delivered in our society today for it exploits both the carer and the person receiving care. It ruins relationships between people and results in thwarted life opportunities on both sides of the caring equation' (Brisenden, 1989, pp. 9–10).

Research must examine what makes 'caring for' in a 'caring about' relationship possible in a way which meets the interests of both parties. Many disabled people have identified that 'caring for' in a 'caring about' relationship cannot work unless there is real choice based on real alternatives. Such a choice cannot exist where the only alternative to assistance by a partner or relative at home is residential care.

Feminist research which incorporated the experiences of disabled and older people might also raise the question of the meaning of the word 'home', separating this out, in a conceptual and political sense, from the feminist critique of the family. Disabled feminists should be able to assert their right to live in their own home without being accused of supporting the oppression of women within the family.

Feminist research on caring emphasises that most carers are women. There are in fact 2.5 million male carers and 3.5 million female carers, although women are more likely to be full-time carers (Green, 1988). It is of fundamental concern to (particularly heterosexual) disabled women to challenge the assumption that men will not 'care for' in a 'caring about' relationship.

This assumption is often experienced as oppressive by disabled women, confronted by health and social services professionals who undermine the ability of such women to sustain heterosexual relationships. For example, it seems to be common for married women entering spinal injury units, particularly if they are tetraplegic, to encounter a negative attitude towards the chances of their marriages surviving their disability (Morris, 1989, p. 83).

If men are carers they are most likely to be caring for their wives. In

1986, 46 per cent of British women in the 45–64 age group reported long-standing illness and for 28 per cent their illness limited their activities (General Household Survey, 1989, p. 147). We need to know more about the experiences of the significant number of women in both this age group and in older age groups who rely on their husbands for care.

Roughly the same levels of long-standing illness are found amongst men in these age groups, which must mean that there are many households where both partners require some level of care. Amongst the elderly population there is evidence that significant numbers of carers are also in need of care. We need to know what factors enable or prevent women from getting the care they need.

Feminist research tends to draw very distinct lines between carers and those who are cared for so the extent to which older and disabled women are also carers is obscured. Research on women who have experienced spinal cord injury found that 'women are primarily the carers within a family and most of us continue in this role. Yet too often it is assumed that we will be the passive recipients of care' (Morris, 1989, p. 188).

The failure of feminist researchers and academics to identify with the subjective experience of those who receive care has meant that they have studied caring situations where there are seemingly very clear distinctions between the person who cares for and the person who receives care. The most common source of identifying potential interviewees has been organisations to whom people have identified themselves as carers. However, a situation in which one party to a relationship has a clear identity as a carer while the other is clearly cared for can only represent one type of caring relationship. It may be that in other situations the roles are blurred, or shifting. We may also want to expand our definition of caring for to encompass not just physical tasks but also the emotional part of caring-for relationships. Research carried out by disabled feminists would, therefore, focus not so much on carers as on caring.

Disabled people would join with non-disabled feminists in rejecting the way that 'community care' too often means 'family care'. But we would assert our own political demand – a demand for the right to live within the community in a non-disabling environment with the kind of personal assistance that we would choose. In doing this, we are not only pursuing the human rights of disabled and older people but also launching an attack on the form that caring currently taxes. Such a strategy should therefore also be clearly supported by feminists who wish to undermine women's dependency within the family.

References

Begum, N. (1990) *The Burden of Gratitude*, University of Warwick and SCA, Warwick.

Brisenden, S. (1989) 'A charter for personal care', *Progress*, 16, Disablement Income Group.

Dalley, G. (1988) *Ideologies of Caring: Rethinking Community and Collectivism*, Macmillan, London.

Finch, J. (1984) 'Community care: developing non-sexist alternatives' *Critical Social Policy*, Vol. 9.

Finch, J. and Groves, D. (eds) (1983) *A Labour of Love: Women, Work and Caring*, Routledge and Kegan Paul, London.

Graham, H. (1983) 'Caring: a labour of love', in Finch, J. and Groves, D. (eds) *A Labour of Love: Women, Work and Caring*, Routledge and Kegan Paul, London.

Green, H. (1988) 'Informal Carers', *General Household Survey 1985*, Supplement A, HMSO, London.

Keith, L. (1990) 'Caring partnership', *Community Care*, 22 February 1990.

Morris, J. (1989) *Able Lives: Women's Experience of Paralysis*, Women's Press, London.

Morris, J. (1991) *Pride Against Prejudice: Transforming Attitudes to Disability*, Women's Press, London.

Shearer, A. (1982) *Living Independently*, CEH and King's Fund, London.

Ungerson, C. (1987) *Policy is Personal*, Tavistock, London.

Part III

POLICY

19

Introduction

This section provides material on the policy aspects of community care. It begins with an anthology of extracts from a variety of documentary sources since the early nineteenth century. Following the anthology are a series of articles that draw attention to recent policy debates. Peter Townsend's 'The structured dependency of the elderly' was a key paper of the early 1980s which anticipated many discussions a decade later. A more recent exploration of a case management approach to working with older people is then provided by David Challis and his colleagues. Alan Walker, within his general discussion of the emergence of community care policy, draws heavily on work about older people. This chapter provides the reader with a good overview of recent policy debates and points to key questions about cost containment and citizenship. Another review of the development of community care policy is offered by Joan Busfield, but this time the emphasis is on people with mental health problems. Professional and organisational questions are raised in this article in relation to policy formation. Martin Bulmer's article then summarises the importance of support networks outside professionally delivered services. Turning to people with learning difficulties, Joanna Ryan and Frank Thomas discuss an important policy influence – the campaign for principles of ordinary living – which values people who were previously institutionalised. Finally, looking to the future, David Pilgrim, rehearses some arguments, based on recent research, about user-led rather than professionally dominated mental health services.

20

*Anthology: Policy**

Compiled by DAVID PILGRIM

This anthology of extracts from official documents starts with the 1834 Poor Law, which enunciated the principle of 'less eligibility'. This ensured that those not in work were inevitably going to be poor, as they had to receive less than the lowest-paid worker. The Law also ushered in the end of outdoor relief and the central regulation of Poor Law institutions. The latter were workhouses for sane, able-bodied adults, or specialist institutions for others. The Poor Law administrators conceived of five groups in need of special provision: children, the sick, the insane, the 'defective' and the 'infirm and aged'. Gradually other legislation (like the 1845 Lunacy Act) formalised the separation of these groups after the general principle of segregation was announced by the Poor Law.

The sections from the Radnor and Wood reports demonstrate the interplay between a segregative policy in the first part of this century and prevailing eugenic ideas. These included the notion that a variety of groups – pauper lunatics, criminals and mental defectives – were a product of a 'tainted' genetic stock, which threatened the quality of the British race.

The extracts from the mid-twentieth century give some sense of the transition from the old segregative policy to one moving out to the community. The moral and political arguments for desegregation intensified following the Second World War in the wake of the Nazi concentration camps and in the context of an egalitarian ethos associated with the new National Health Service.

The material from the 1980s reveals a strong consensus in documents from and for government, as well as those from trade unions and voluntary bodies, about a positive approach to care in the community. Even the Wagner Report, which points to a new version of residential care as part of community care, strongly marks itself off from the old segregative philosophy. However, the role of enforced segregation is still apparent within this consensus. Examples of this are shown in sections of the 1983 Mental

---

*Comparisons of public policy documents applying to England, Wales, Scotland and Northern Ireland are made in the following texts: D.J. Hunter and G. Wistow, *Community Care in Britain: Variations on a Theme*, King's Fund, London 1987; M. Titterton, 'The missing Scottish dimension in social care policy', in *Scottish Government Yearbook*, Edinburgh University Press, 1989.

Health Act and the 1989 Children Act. The powers of the 1948 National Assistance Act quoted are also still in force. (Its revision, in 1951, actually increased the speed at which local authorities can effect segregation.) Thus, by the end of the twentieth century, legislation prescribes both continuing local state *powers* to segregate people but also *obligations* to provide services for those defined to be in need, whether they are at home or not.

Extract from the **English Poor Law** *1834. Here less eligibility is recommended and the notion that the benefit to the individual has to be weighed against that of the 'country at large'.*

. . . in the administration of relief, the public is warranted in imposing such conditions on the individual relief, as are conducive to the benefit either of the individual himself, or of the country at large, at whose expense he is to be relieved. The first and most essential of all conditions, a principle which we find universally admitted . . . is that his situation on the whole shall not be made really or apparently so eligible as the situation of the independent labourer of the lowest class. . . . Every penny bestowed, that tends to render the condition of the pauper more eligible than that of the independent labourer, is a bounty on indolence and vice. . . . All relief whatever to able-bodied persons or to their families, otherwise than in well-regulated workhouses . . . shall be declared unlawful.

From the **Report of the Royal Commission on the Care and Control of the Feebleminded** *(***The Radnor Commission***), HMSO, London, 1908. This made recommendations which informed the 1913 Mental Deficiency Act.*

The Royal Commission devoted much attention to the causation of mental defect, and arrived at the conclusion that feeblemindedness is largely inherited; that prevention of mentally defective persons from becoming parents would tend to diminish such persons in the population; and that consequently there are strong grounds for placing mental defectives from each sex in institutions where they will be retained and kept under effectual supervision as long as may be necessary.

From the **Report of the Wood Committee**, *HMSO, London, 1929. This shows the continuing eugenic influences even after the First World War to reinforce the control of the fertility of segregated groups.*

If we are to prevent the racial disaster of mental deficiency we must not deal merely with the mentally defective person but with the whole subnormal group. . . . Primary amentia may be, and often is, an end result – the last stage of the inheritance of degeneracy of this subnormal group. The relative fertility of this group is greater than that of normal persons.

From the **National Assistance Act** *1948. Under this legislation, which is still in force, those threatening their own or others' health can be removed from the community. Section 47 of the Act allows for the removal to hospital or elsewhere of:*

persons who are (a) suffering from grave chronic disease or being aged, infirm or physically incapacitated are living in insanitary conditions and (b) are unable to devote to themselves and are not receiving from other persons proper care and attention.

50,000 Outside the Law, *National Council for Civil Liberties, London, 1951. This document, which describes the scandalous way in which 'mental defectives' were treated, exemplifies growing demands at the time to abandon a segregative social policy.*

This pamphlet tells a grave story! And this story belongs not to the England of the novels of Dickens, but to the England of 1951. Let us briefly summarise what it discloses:

1. Wrongful certification and detention takes place on a far from small scale. . . .
2. Breakdown of legal safeguards through failure of [the 1913 Mental Deficiency] Act to provide adequate machinery of appeal . . .
3. Exploitation of defective labour. . . .
4. Growth in interests which may cause unconscious bias to be developed in favour of retaining high grade patients under certification. . . .
5. Archaic conceptions of treatment in institutions and on license. . . .

Social welfare has been side-tracked from these people, who while certified remain a race apart. The community must accept responsibility for them – changing the concept of permanent segregation for that of integration within the community.

The Royal Commission on the Law Relating to Mental Illness and Mental Deficiency (The Percy Report), *HMSO, London, 1957. This informed the 1959 Mental Health Act and stressed the need to move towards community rather than hospital-centre care, which required more financial resources.*

There is increasing medical emphasis on forms of treatment and training and social services which can be given without bringing patients into hospital as in-patients, or which make it possible to discharge them from hospital sooner than was usual in the past. It is not now generally considered in the best interests of the patients who are fit to live in the community that they should be in large or remote institutions such as the present mental and mental deficiency hospitals. Nor is it a proper function of the hospital authority to provide residential accommodation for patients who do not require hospital or specialist services. . . . The local authorities should be responsible for preventative services and for all types of community care for patients who do not require in-patient hospital services or who have had a period of treatment of training in hospital and are ready to return to the community.

Social Workers: Their Role and Tasks **(The Barclay Report)** *on the role of the social worker, produced for the Government by the National Institute for Social Work, Bedford Square Press, London, 1982, recognised the need to rely on informal carers.*

The bulk of social care in England and Wales is provided not by the statutory or voluntary social services agencies, but by ordinary people who may be linked into informal caring networks in their communities. . . . Sharing social caring [with these networks] is a way both of promoting the better care and more care in the community, and of distributing the burden of caring for the disadvantaged more fairly. At present it often falls most heavily upon close relatives.

The 1983 Mental Health Act. *These sections highlight the continuing dual role of the state in prescribing duties of care as well as powers to remove threatening people from the community.*

After care. Section 117 (2). It shall be the duty of the District Health Authority and of the local social services authority to provide in cooperation with relevant voluntary agencies, after-care services for any person to whom this section applies until the District Health Authority and the local social services authority are satisfied that the person concerned is no longer in need of such service. . . .

Mentally disordered persons found in public places. Section 136. If a constable finds in a place to which the public have access a person who appears to him to be suffering from mental disorder and to be in immediate need of care and control, the constable may, if he thinks it necessary to do so in the interests of that person or for the protection of other persons, remove that person to a place of safety.

Residential Care: a Positive Approach (The Wagner Report), *produced for the government by an independent committee based at the National Institute for Social Work, 1988.*

People who move into a residential establishment should do so by positive choice. A distinction should be made between need for accommodation and need for services. No one should be required to change their permanent accommodation in order to receive services which could be made available to them in their own homes. Living in a residential establishment should be a positive experience ensuring a better quality of life than the resident could enjoy in any other setting. . . . [They] should continue to have access to the full range of community support services [and] leisure, educational and other facilities offered by the local community. . . . Residential staff are the major resource and should be valued as such. The importance of their contribution needs to be recognised and enhanced.

————————

Community Care – Which Way Forward? Confederation of Health Service Employees, London, 1990. COHSE and other trade unions resisted many changes in hospital-based services during the 1970s. However, during the 1980s they rapidly began to endorse a positive approach to community care, as shown here.

COHSE wishes to see a community care system which is fair, universal and under democratic control, which empowers the service users, values service workers and actively involves in promoting high standards, and which genuinely meets the neets of people. In particular we recommend:

1. Regular, uniform and nationwide assessment of need which involves consultation with service users.
2. Adequate funds, administered through the revenue support grant, specially reserved for community care. Redistribution of funds between rich and poor areas of the country. In addition, local authorities should not be prohibited from raising further funds through local taxes.
3. A framework of rights and entitlement aimed at enabling citizens to control the way their needs are defined and met.
4. Service users to have access to independent living advocates to help them put their views across.
5. Protection for staff moving between employers. The involvement of staff in consultation and decision making. Minimum staffing levels, determined nationally, for workers in residential homes and domiciliary and other community-based care.

6. Purchasing authorities to use contracts to specify adequate pay and conditions for service workers.
7. An independent inspectorate, whose job it is, firstly, to ensure high standards of care and, secondly, to ensure cost-effectiveness – in all forms of community care.
8. A concerted national strategy to ensure that people who are mentally ill are not kept in hospital unnecessarily, nor discharged into the community without proper care facilities and support being available for them.
9. To prevent the wholesale commercialisation of the independent sector and its 'swamping' by the values and tactics of profit-making business, a range of strategies should be considered e.g.:
   – the state to retain ownership of capital assets;
   – quality control mechanisms, imposed by contract, to insist that suppliers put quality of care before cost-control;
   – encouragement of not-for-profit suppliers;
   – encouragement of the advocacy and innovative work of the voluntary sector.
10. Positive policies to ensure that minority communities are properly consulted, and their special needs recognised and met, and that sufficient members of ethnic minorities are employed in community care.
11. The concept of asylum to be incorporated into locally based community mental health services.
12. Integration of housing policies with community care policies.
13. Special training for carers and other volunteers in community care, as well as for paid carers in the independent sector.
14. Improved arrangements for joint planning between health authorities and local authorities.

Waiting for Community Care, MIND, London, 1990. Major charities like MENCAP, MIND, Barnardos and the Spastics Society joined in the call during the 1980s for ordinary living for disabled children and adults. MIND's position is given here as an example.

In MIND's view a policy framework is required which directs community care developments towards specified goals including:
– To transform the mental health service from one centred on unpopular institutions to one based on the actual wishes and needs of people who use the service.
– To move towards a comprehensive local mental health service in each area, offering nationally consistent standards. The service should

address the diversity of people's needs, for instance, work, housing, emotional support and sanctuary.
- To create a climate which encourages people with mental distress to pursue ordinary, non-specialist options where possible: for instance, secure housing and work in the open market.
- To pursue change through a major resource transfer from institutional to community services, coupled with a gradually increased allocation to mental health.

The 1989 Children Act. *Whilst the key objectives about government intentions on community care were set out by the Griffiths Report and the White Papers preceding the 1990 National Health Service and Community Care Act (see later), these paragraphs from the Children Act also provide policy for a particular client group in the community.*

Part III, Section 17   Provision of services for children in need, their families and others.

1. It shall be the duty of every local authority . . .
   (a) to safeguard and promote the welfare of children within their area who are in need; and
   (b) so far as is consistent with that duty, to promote the upbringing of such children by their families. . . .

(10) For the purposes of this Part a child shall be taken to be in need if –
   (a) he is unlikely to achieve or maintain, or have the opportunity of achieving or maintaining, a reasonable standard of health or development without this provision for him of services by a local authority under this Part:
   (b) his health or development is likely to be significantly impaired, or further impaired, without the provision for him of such services; or
   (c) he is disabled. . . .

Section 18   Day care for pre-school and other children

1. Every local authority shall provide such day care for children in need within their area who are –
(a) aged five or under; and
(b) not yet attending schools

as is appropriate. . . .

5. Every local authority shall provide for children in need within their area who are attending any school such care or supervised activities as is appropriate –
   (a) outside school hours; or
   (b) during school holidays. . . .

Section 31   Care and supervision orders

1. On the application of any local authority or authorised person, the court may make an order –
   (a) placing the child with respect to whom the application is made in the care of a designated local authority; or
   (b) putting him under the supervision of a designated local [389] authority or of a probation officer.

2. A court may only make a care order or supervision order if it is satisfied –
   (a) that the child concerned is suffering, or is likely to suffer, significant harm; and
   (b) that the harm or likelihood of harm, is attributable to –
      (i)   the care given to the child, or likely to be given to him if the order were not made, not being what it would be reasonable to expect a parent to give him; or
      (ii) the child being beyond parental control.

Community Care: Agenda for Action (*The Griffiths Report*), 1988. *Here are key points of philosophy that were to be incorporated, in the m ain (barring the call for a minister for community care), by the government when constructing Caring for People (see below) and its consequent community care legislation.*

Central government should ensure that there is a Minister of State in DHSS, seen by the public as being clearly responsible for community care. . . . Local authorities should, within the resources available: assess the community care needs of their locality, set local priorities and service objectives and develop local plans in consultation with health authorities in particular (but also others including housing authorities, voluntary bodies and private providers of care) for delivering those objectives; identify and assess individual needs, taking full account of personal preferences (and those of informal carers), and design packages of care best suited to enabling the consumer to live as normal a life as possible; arrange the delivery of packages of care, building first on the available contribution of informal carers and neighbourhood support, then on the provision of domiciliary and day services or, if appropriate, residential care; act for these purposes as the designers, organisers and purchasers of non-health care services and not primarily as direct providers, making the best possible use of voluntary and private bodies to widen consumer choice, stimulate innovation and encourage efficiency.

Caring for People: Community Care in the Next Decade and Beyond, CM 849, *Department of Health, HMSO, London, 1989. This was the White Paper, along with* Working for Patients, *which built on the Griffiths Report and prefigured the National Health Service and Community Care Act 1990.*

The Government believes that for most people community care offers the best form of care available – certainly with better quality and choice than they might have expected in the past. These changes . . . are intended to:

- enable people to live as normal a life as possible in their own homes or in a homely environment in the local community;
- provide the right amount of care and support to help people achieve maximum possible independence and, by acquiring or reacquiring basic living skills, help them achieve their full potential;
- give people a greater individual say in how they live their lives and the service they need to help them do so.

Promoting choice and independence underlies all the Government's proposals. . . . [T]he key components of community care should be: services that respond flexibly and sensitively to the needs of individuals and their carers; services that allow a range of options for consumers; services that intervene no more than is necessary to foster independence; services that concentrate on those with the greatest needs.

The Government's proposals have six key objectives for service delivery:

- to promote the development of domiciliary, day and respite services to enable people to live in their own homes wherever feasible and sensible. . . .
- to ensure that services providers make practical support for carers a high priority. . .
- to make proper assessment of need and good case management the cornerstone of high quality care . . .
- to promote the development of a flourishing independent sector alongside good quality public services . . .

- to clarify the responsibilities of agencies and so make it easier to hold them to account for their performance . . .
- to secure better value for taxpayers' money by introducing a new funding structure for social care.

21

The Structured Dependency of the Elderly: A Creation of Social Policy in the Twentieth Century*

PETER TOWNSEND

Retirement has become a social phenomenon of vast importance in the short span of the last fifty years. According to statistics published by the International Labour Office, between 40 per cent and 70 per cent of men 65 and over in all industrial countries were still economically active in the 1930s. But by the mid-1960s, with the exception of Japan, where the percentage had declined only slightly, the proportion had shrunk dramatically to between 10 per cent and 40 per cent with the mean about 20 per cent. The reduction has continued during the 1970s, though not so rapidly. This change cannot be attributed to changes in the risk of ill-health or disability, or the masking of disability in periods before substitute pensions were available. It is attributable to changes in the organisation of work and in the kind of people wanted for work. Bigger work organisations, with more pronounced hierarchies, have become established and career promotion through the successive tiers of these hierarchies is regarded as normal and to be expected. The objectives of economic growth, productivity and increasingly rapid replacement of skills have been adopted within these organisational settings and, as a direct consequence, more workers at older ages have found themselves

---

*The original complete version of this article referred to substantial empirical evidence to support the arguments summarized here. It was first published in *Ageing and Society*, Vol. 1, No. 1, March 1991, pp. 5–28.

misplaced. In the late 1970s another factor has become all-important. The development of multi-national corporations and improvements internationally in transport and communication have led to a deliberate shifting of manufacturing production to poor countries where the work-forces can be paid very low wages. In 1975 the workforce of the overseas subsidiaries of German manufacturing industry represented 20 per cent of the manufacturing workforce in Germany itself.

Problems arise for companies and unions which can only be resolved by a kind of mass redundancy, which retirement has become. Retire-ment is in a real sense a euphemism for unemployment. The phenome-non has ben enforced and is being enforced in a number of industrial countries at earlier ages and yet is, paradoxically, being represented as a social achievement in capitalist and state socialist societies alike. The spread of retirement is interpreted as reflecting the success of campaigns on behalf of the rights of workers when they have 'earned a rest', and is associated with the rights of old people to peace and dignity. But many older, especially active, people deplore the termination of economic activity. People reaching retirement age do not welcome it as warmly as they had thought they would. Many who *have* retired deeply regret their inactivity or loss of status. The satisfaction which is expressed by some retired people is more what they think is expected of them, and more an assertion of hope, than a true representation of what they feel. Closer historical examination of retirement as a social institution shows that its adoption has also been associated with pressures to shed moral if not contractual obligations to loyal workers and to exclude certain groups of workers from the bargaining process. The public are encouraged to accept the lessened value to the economy of workers past certain ages. Changing technology and the successive adoption of forms of training and educational qualifications have encouraged over-valuation of the productive capacity of older workers. This has affected other priorities. Less consideration tends to be given in sickness and disability at older than at younger ages and, indeed, retirement is cavalierly associated with failing health and capacity. Thus the combined effects of industrial, economic and educational reorganisation are leading to a more rigid stratification of the population by age.

While the institutionalisation of retirement as a major social phenome-non in the very recent history of society has played a big part in fostering the material and psychological dependence of older people, the institu-tionalisation of pensions and services has also played a major part. The propensity to poverty in old age could be said to be a function of low levels of resources, and restricted access to resources, relative to youn-ger people. Secondly it is due to restricted access to the new styles and modes of living being promoted in the community. In Britain there is official evidence for the last 15 years of about 10 per cent being in poverty, as defined by the state, and another 30 per cent or 40 per cent being on the margins in the sense that they are living at the state's standard or within 40 per cent of that standard. [. . .] Independent measures suggest the first of these figures (10 per cent in poverty) is understimated because of methodological shortcomings. [. . .] Restriction of resources is determined by different causal factors. State pensions and other cash benefits administered centrally comprise the most important source of income for the elderly in most advanced industrial societies and the initial rate of state pensions after retirement, and the amount of substitute or supplementary benefits which are paid, after the pensionable age or upon retirement, tend to be low relative to the earnings of younger adults. In Britain, various studies put the net incomes of single or widowed retired people, allowing for dependents, at about a third, and of married couples less than half, of younger non-retired people. [. . .] State help is offered on condition that people retire from paid employment and this status is imposed upon elderly people at a fixed chronological age, or they are persuaded to accept it as a social norm. Pension levels are defined in relation to subsistence needs, and are usually pitched considerably below net earnings during the period of paid employment. The initial rates of private or occupational pensions, with some exceptions, are also low relative to the earnings of young adults. Provisions for widows under the terms of these schemes have generally been poor and this fact, together with the failure of many such pensions to keep pace with inflation, explains why so many people formerly associated with non-manual occupations, certainly in Britain, descend, along with their working-class counterparts, into poverty or near-poverty after retirement. Lacking access to many of the positions where sectional interests can be properly represented, the elderly find their position in a rapidly evolving economy getting worse. Their resources fail to keep pace in value with the resources of other groups in society; either certain forms of assets held, such as household goods and equipment and certain types of income from savings, and occupational pensions, depreciate in value absolutely or relatively to the rise in living standards, with increasing length of retirement, or many do not have, and have not in the past had, an opportunity of obtaining types of resources which are newly becoming available to younger people. What is more, greater exposure to certain forms of social desolation and isolation, brought about by the death of a spouse, the loss of close relatives or friends, and the decay of industries or city centres, as well as by retirement, tends to deprive the elderly of access to alternative or subsidiary resources and sometimes leads to additional costs. Liability to disablement restricts access to resources and, in the absence of compensating cash benefits and services, leads to additional costs for many which outweigh the savings consequent upon retirement.

There is a sharp contrast between the low status in which old people are held publicly and the regard in which they are held privately in their families. In the family age is of secondary importance. People are grandparents, parents, brothers or sisters and friends or neighbours first and foremost. Retirement from familial roles is a much more flexible contingency, dependent primarily upon health or disablement. In some respects the family also provides escape from the psychological and social bruises which can be inflicted externally, and up to a point provides meaningful activity and genuine respect. The positive contribution to the welfare of grandchildren and children of many elderly women is greatly underestimated just as their labour specifically on behalf of their husbands and in general on behalf of the economy throughout adult working life goes largely unrecognised. Capital and state separately or in combination, may have fostered the dependency of women within the family but, paradoxically, has created an independent system of interdependence, occupation, mutual respect and loyalty. The defensive and restorative mechanisms of the family temper the dependency created by the state. [. . .]

21.1 The effects of residential care in creating dependency

Rich societies have still to come to terms with the engineering of retirement and mass poverty among the elderly in the twentieth century. These two are of course linked and they have been pre-eminent in creating the social dependency of the elderly. But their connection with the development of residential and community care is too frequently overlooked. When we turn to examine the part played by these two trends in fostering dependency it is important to understand how the assumptions of all the participants are already greatly affected by the facts of retirement and poverty. Not only do they materially restrict life chances. They govern the attitudes and not only the actions of professional staff, on the one hand, and elderly clients or residents, on the other.

A review of the history of residential developments and of the characteristics of the inmate populations shows that the institutions have been, and are, serving major functions other than those for which formally they were and are supposed to exist. In particular they have inhibited appeals in times of major stress for public help from the individual and the family, have operated as a cheap (because selective) substitute for public housing and community services, and have regulated public ideas of the lengths to which the family is expected to carry the burden of care. [. . .]

Socially, institutions are structured to serve purposes of controlling inmates. The type and level of staffing, amenities and resources have been developed not only in relation to the characteristics, including the perceived capacities, of inmates but also the roles staff expect inmates to play. Staff tend to resist any increase in the number or proportion of inmates requiring a great deal of attention. They become conscious of the value of inmates who perform large and small tasks in the organisation and tend to give excuses rather than rational grounds for the presence in the institution of these inmates. On the other hand, the roles are distinguished from those played by staff by their subordinate and even menial status and the derisory forms of payment which accompany them. Occupational roles are clearly distinguished partly to maintain the lower status and presumed dependency of inmates. The majority of residents in homes are placed in a category of enforced dependence. The routine of residential homes, made necessary by small staffs and economical administration, and committed to an ideology of 'care and attention' rather than the encouragement of self-help and self-management, seems to deprive many residents of the opportunity if not the incentive to occupy themselves and even of the means of communication. [. . .]

The maintenance and even increase of the share of resources going to hospitals and to residential institutions has been something of a paradox. Despite the powerful movements in favour of community care the emergence of that sector cannot be said to have properly materialised. This is not easy to explain. The failure to achieve a shift in priorities has to be explained partly in relation to the powerful vested interests of certain branches of the professions, unions of hospital staffs and certain sections of the administration. The brute fact is that the majority of medical staff and the vast majority of nursing staff work in residential homes. The failure to shift the balance of health and welfare policy towards community care also has to be explained in relation to the function of institutions to regulate and confirm inequality in society, and indeed to regulate deviation from the central social values of self-help, domestic independence, personal thrift, willingness to work, productive effort and family care. Institutions serve subtle functions in reflecting the positive structural and cultural changes taking place in society.

The numbers of bedfast, severely incapacitated and infirm old people living in the community dwarfs the number in institutions and there are real dangers in the present situation of committing available resources for the care of a few at the expense of the much larger number living in the community who require only modest forms of support to live independently with their families. [. . .] Our object must be a renewed attempt to replace institutional care by increased and new forms of support in the home. While the costs of care in residential institutions are not always easy to compare with the costs of providing alternative services when old people are living at home (depending on levels of disablement as well as the types of benefit or service included in the measurement) most of the studies that have been carried out have concluded that the costs of care at home are smaller. [. . .]

In this chapter I have argued that the concepts of retirement, pensionable status, institutional resident and other passive forms of community care have been developed in both capitalist and state socialist countries in ways which have created and reinforced the social dependency of the elderly. Such 'structured' dependency is a consequence of twentieth-century thought and action, and especially of the management of modern economies and the distribution of power and status in such economies. The severity and extent of that dependency cannot be justified by appeal to certain major types of evidence. Empirical studies of capacity and desire for productive occupation, reciprocation of services, and familial and social relationships, as well as self-care, challenge the assumptions which prevail. There is clearly room for an alternative interpretation of the roles to be payed by the elderly whereby many more of them continue in paid employment, find alternative forms of substantial and productive occupation, have rights to much larger incomes, and have a much greater control over the place and type of accommodation where they live, and the kind of community services to which they contribute as well as have access.

22

Case Management in the Care of the Aged: The Provision of Care in Different Settings

DAVID CHALLIS, JOHN CHESTERMAN, ROBIN DARTON and KAREN TRASKE

Within the diverse patterns of provision of care for elderly people in different countries, a major area of concern has been the extensiveness and appropriacy of admissions to institutional care. This reflects the problems of rising costs, apparent misplacement and consumer preferences (Evers, 1991). Linked to this has been a concern to strengthen the range of home care services, to enable frail elderly people to remain at home, despite the difficulty of achieving coordination caused by fragmentation arising from different providers of care and different sources of funding (Audit Commission, 1986). These factors underlie problems of lack of effectiveness and efficiency in the provision of long-term care. Case management has been identified as a potential coordinating mechanism for providing enhanced home care as an alternative to institutional care, and recent UK policy statements describing the objectives of community care policy have stressed the need 'to make proper assessment of need and good case management the cornerstone of high quality care' (Department of Health, 1989). This policy has been influenced by a series of studies of case management in the care of elderly people undertaken at the University of Kent. The first of these was undertaken in a retirement area in Kent (Challis and Davies, 1980, 1985, 1986; Davies and Challis, 1986), run by the local authority social services department. Subsequent studies have developed the original Kent model, and involve case management for frail people based both in social care and in primary health care (Gateshead) and in geriatric care

(Darlington). The evaluation of this series of studies has been under-taken using quasi-experimental designs, in which cases receiving the experimental services have been compared with similar individuals receiving the existing range of services (Davies and Challis, 1981; Challis and Darton, 1990).

22.1 Case management in social care (Kent and Gateshead)

22.11 The Kent scheme: the initial model

The model of case management that was developed was designed to ensure that improved performance of the core tasks of case management – case-finding and screening, assessment, case planning, and monitor-ing and review (Steinberg and Carter, 1983) – could contribute towards more effective and efficient long-term care. (For more details on the relationship between the core tasks of case management and efficiency see Challis and Davies, 1986, chapter 1; Davies and Challis, 1986, chapter 2; Davies *et al.*, 1990, chapters 6, 13.) Through the devolution of control of resources to individual social workers, acting as case mana-gers, it was designed to permit more flexible responses to needs and the integration of fragmented services into a more coherent package of care to provide a realistic alternative to institutional care (Table 22.1).

The scheme was targeted on the most frail elderly people, whose needs placed them on the margin of entry to long-term institutional care. The case managers had small caseloads (about 25–30 cases) and were recruited as being more trained/experienced than is usual in work with elderly people, reflecting the needs and problems of these clients, the responsibility of the work and the cost consequences of inappropri-ate decisions. Qualifications and experience in social work were seen as providing a suitable background (Central Council for Education and

TABLE 22.1   The community care approach: operational features

1   Clear and continuing case responsibility
2   Targeted caseload; elderly people on margin of institutional care
3   Smaller caseloads
4   Trained and experienced fieldworkers
5   Decentralised budget, with clear expenditure limits
6   Knowledge of unit costs of services
7   Service packages costed
8   Systematic records for assessment and monitoring
9   Closer health care linkages, both formal and informal

Training of Social Work, 1991). The case managers controlled a budget that could be used to purchase or develop additional services beyond those currently available to permit a wider range of responses to clients' needs. In making care decisions they were aware of the unit costs of other services, since the overall weekly cost of an individual package of care was limited to two-thirds of the cost of a place in a residential home, reflecting the approximate 'care costs' of that setting. Higher expenditure on individual cases was allowed but required management approval. This was designed to permit flexibility within an overall framework of accountability. The record system had three main elements aimed at enhancing accountability and supplementing ongoing case notes: assessment information covering the need circumstances of clients; the use of a structured case review at least four times a year covering case manager activities, client problems and the range of resources deployed; and weekly costings of the care packages for each client. The records permitted summary feedbacks to be given about caseloads, the mix of client problems, case manager activities and costs (Challis and Chesterman, 1985).

The findings of the initial Kent study indicated that case managers with devolved budgets could significantly improve the effectiveness of social care for very frail elderly people (Challis and Davies, 1980, 1985, 1986; Davies and Challis, 1986). For such individuals, lower rates of institutionalisation were observed for those receiving case management (Table 22.2), and the quality of life of elderly people and their carers improved compared with people receiving existing services (Table 22.3). These effects appeared to involve no greater cost than the existing services (Table 22.4). These changes were designed to enable effective case management within an accountable organisation and thereby contribute to greater efficiency in social care.

22.12 The Gateshead scheme

The approach was further developed in Gateshead (Chalis *et al.*, 1988, 1990), providing a basis for testing the portability of the model in an urban setting. A matched group of elderly people receiving the usual range of services from adjacent areas within Gateshead provided a comparison group for the evaluation. Ninety matched pairs of cases were identified for comparison. Both groups of elderly people and their carers were interviewed upon identification and followed up a year later. The costs of service were monitored over a one year period for both groups.

Case management in the Gateshead social care scheme

Referrals and targeting. During the period of monitoring the scheme, 101 cases were referred and accepted as appropriate, 40 per cent of which were from National Health Service sources, particularly general practitioners, hospitals and community nurses, and 31 per cent were from informal sources: family, friends or neighbours. These cases constituted a frail group with an average age of 81, who were predominantly female (87 per cent), rather more dependent than those in Kent and three-quarters lived alone. Incontinence and confusion afflicted one-third of the cases, while immobility and risk of falling affected a higher proportion. Most required help with key activities of daily living and all needed help with household chores. Over two-thirds had an identifiable informal carer, of whom two-thirds were seen as under stress. The average age of the carers was 55, and 42 per cent were over 60. Three-quarters were female, the largest single group being daughters or daughters-in-law, but only 14 per cent of all carers actually lived with the elderly person.

Assessment. A comprehensive assessment was central to the scheme's aim of creating individual, flexible packages of care which were responsive to changes in need. It was evident that the possible greater flexibility of response available through a devolved budget encouraged more detailed assessments, less constrained by existing services (Challis and Davies, 1985, 1986). The process of assessment was aided by the use of a detailed assessment form, which was completed during the first two visits, and a monitoring chart, which helped to give a breakdown of an elderly person's daily activities and the support they received during a usual week (Challis and Chesterman, 1985).

Care planning and organising services. An individual care plan was based on the detailed assessment, and took into account the choices expressed by the elderly person and their carers. This approach overcame the more common response of a hastily constructed and uncoordinated package developed in response to different demands over time. New forms of help were developed using the budget under the case managers' control. In common with the Kent scheme, a group of local 'helpers' who could work flexibly were employed, and paid on a sessional basis, to undertake a wide variety of tasks that often do not fall within the remit of traditional services. The range of tasks undertaken by helpers was very wide, involving such activities as ensuring an adequate diet, providing personal care, helping to manage incontinence, giving social support, and assisting people with dementia through reassurance and reality orientation (Holden and Woods, 1982). On occasions, helpers worked to improve mobility following a stroke, under the supervision of a physiotherapist.

Monitoring care.   As well as monitoring care through their contact with the care network, case managers completed formal case reviews at four-monthly intervals, identifying problems encountered, the present situation, changes to be aimed for over the next period, case manager activities and contacts with agencies (Challis and Chesterman, 1985; Challis *et al.*, 1988).

The outcome and cost of care

Destinational outcomes.   Table 22.2 shows the destinational outcomes at one year for the 90 matched pairs of elderly clients. Whereas 63 per cent of those who received the scheme remained in their own homes, only 36 per cent of the control group clients did so. Not dissimilar numbers of each group were in long-stay hospitals, although there was a very marked difference in the rate of admission to residential homes, 1 per cent compared with 39 per cent. There was no significant difference in the death rates or length of survival between the two groups. Over one year those receiving the scheme remained in their own homes on average for 43 weeks, compared with only 33 weeks for those receiving the usual range of services ($p<0.001$).

Quality of life and quality of care for clients.   Table 22.3 shows the outcomes, which were observed over one year, on a range of quality of life and quality of care indicators for the elderly people. For all of the social and

TABLE 22.2 Destinational outcomes for matched cases at one year (Kent and Gateshead)

	Kent social care		Gateshead social care		Gateshead health and social care	
	Project (%)	Control (%)	Project (%)	Control (%)	Project (%)	Control (%)
Own home	69	34	63	36	64	21
Local authority home	4	22	1	37	4	50
Private or voluntary home	8	5	0	2	4	0
Hospital	4	5	7	4	0	4
Died	14	33	28	20	28	25
Moved away	1	1	1	1	0	0
No. of cases	74	74	90	90	28	28

Source: Challis and Davies (1986); Challis *et al.* (1990).

TABLE 22.3   Outcomes for elderly people and their carers: mean change scores over one year (Kent and Gateshead)

	Kent social care			Gateshead social care		
	Project	*Control*	*p-value*	*Project*	*Control*	*p-value*
ELDERLY PEOPLE						
Social and emotional needs						
Loneliness	−1.46	0.36	<0.001	−1.1	−0.4	0.001
Depressed mood	−0.68	−0.17	<0.01	−4.1	−1.9	<0.05
Morale	2.99	−1.00	<0.001	2.1	1.66	ns
Dissatisfaction with life development	−0.38	0.23	<0.05	−0.5	−0.3	<0.05
Felt capacity to cope	5.03	0.66	<0.001	5.3	2.9	<0.001
Going out/social visits	5.66	−0.77	<0.001	1.0	−0.9	<0.001
Quality of care						
Need help with						
rising and retiring	−0.58	0.13	<0.05	−2.3	−0.5	<0.001
personal care	−9.47	−1.29	<0.001	−41.3	−8.6	<0.001
daily housework	−6.68	−1.71	<0.001	−16.5	−5.4	<0.001
weekly housework	−4.77	−1.94	<0.001	−7.3	−3.8	<0.001
Need for extra services	−2.44	0.69	<0.001	−6.4	−2.3	<0.001
CARERS						
Stress and burden indicators						
Lifestyle effects	−2.5	−1.74	ns	−2.1	−1.39	0.05
Subjective burden	−1.12	−0.33	<0.03	−0.60	−0.33	<0.05
Mental health difficulties	−0.82	−0.25	0.09	−0.60	−0.16	<0.001
Level of strain	−1.24	−0.5	0.09	−1.18	−0.41	<0.001

Source: Adapted from Challis and Davies (1986); Challis *et al.* (1990).
Note: ns = not significant

emotional need indicators, except the overall morale indicator, there was a significant positive advantage for those who received the scheme. They were more likely to have improved in terms of depressed mood, loneliness, satisfaction with life (a component of morale) (Lawton, 1975), their level of social activity and perception of their capacity to cope. For the measures of quality of care, a minus sign indicates improvement, a reduction in the level of need. Reductions of need were consistently significantly greater for those receiving the scheme than for the comparison group. Thus, for this highly dependent population the standard range of domiciliary services appears to be insufficient to meet some of their practical and emotional needs.

TABLE 22.4 Costs for different parties over one year (Kent and Gateshead)

	Case management scheme	Control group	p-value[1]
Kent social care (1977 prices)			
Social services department	639	702	ns
National Health Service	778	708	ns
Social opportunity cost	2670	2498	ns
Gateshead social care (1981 prices)			
Social services department (revenue net cost)			
Non-inner city	1609	1793	ns
Inner city	2008	1535	
National Health Service (Assuming 5% capital allowance)			
Non-inner city	1798	1588	ns
Inner city	1505	483	
Social opportunity cost (capital elements discounted at 5%)			
Non-inner city	5220	5203	ns
Inner city	5333	3847	
Gateshead health and social care (1981 prices)			
Case management team	1570	–	–
Other social services department (revenue net cost)	606	1899	–
Other National Health Services (Assuming 5% capital allowance)	1162	1584	–
Case management team, SSD and NHS	3338	3483	ns
Social opportunity cost (capital elements discounted at 5%)	5159	5070	ns

Note:
[1] F-test. ns = not significant.
Source: Challis and Davies (1986); Challis *et al.* (1990).

Outcomes for carers.   There were no differences between the two groups of carers on key factors such as age, relationship and whether or not they lived with the elderly person. For problems of lifestyle, which consist of such factors as effects on domestic routine and social activities, the scheme significantly reduced the stresses on carers. Similar conclusions may be drawn about the level of strain experienced by carers and the extent of expressed burden. In terms of mental health problems, the scheme significantly reduced the stresses for carers in such areas as guilt and anxiety, compared with existing services (Table 22.3).

The costs of care.   Costs have been analysed at a 1981 price base, the year in which the scheme commenced. Table 22.4 shows the average annual costs per case incurred by the social services department, the National Health Service and society as a whole. The National Health Service costs include an allowance for capital at a discount rate of 5 per cent (Dwight *et al.*, 1981; Challis and Davies, 1986; Davies and Challis, 1986). Costs to society as a whole consist of the costs borne by the social services department and the National Health Service, together with the identifiable financial costs borne by informal carers, resources consumed by the elderly person and an allowance for the cost of their housing. Costs analyses also examined whether or not the person was an inner-city resident, since the delivery of community care in inner cities may be more costly, and possibly require different patterns of resources to other districts. There was no significant difference between the costs to the social services department, National Health Service or society as a whole between the community care scheme and standard provision. However, irrespective of whether the client received the scheme or standard provision, the health service costs were lower in the inner city, due to the lower utilisation of acute hospital beds.

22.2 Case management in primary health care (Gateshead)

Despite the clear evidence of marked improvements in the care and support provided to elderly people as a result of the social care scheme in Gateshead, further progress was constrained by the complexity of the health care needs of some severely disabled elder persons, in particular incontinence, immobility and episodes of acute illness. It was considered that these difficulties could be most effectively tackled by working more closely with staff who had medical, nursing and paramedical expertise (Challis *et al.*, 1990).

Additional funding provided for a full-time senior nurse, a part-time junior doctor and 25 per cent of the time of a physiotherapist to complement the team, as well as additional resources to be spent on the care of elderly people in a flexible way, as in the original social care scheme. The costs of care purchased by the team were shared equally between the social services department and the National Health Service. This service was designed to focus upon the even more frail elderly, and drew its clients from the patients of a large general practice.

Organisationally, building on the established social care scheme, the existing team leader took responsibility for team management. In order that staff of different backgrounds could develop a team ethos, they were located within the existing team's office within the social services department. The nurse adopted a case management role, comparable with that undertaken by the social workers, while the doctor and physiotherapist were principally concerned with the functions of assessment and monitoring. As the nurse took on the full-time role of case manager, the practical nursing functions were undertaken by existing nurses working in the community.

Resources did not permit a detailed experimental evaluation of this scheme, but it was monitored closely using assessment, case review and costing information completed by the case managers themselves. This made it possible to compare the destinational outcomes and costs of elderly people receiving this scheme with a subset of the control group cases used in the social care evaluation. This provided a comparison between 28 matched pairs.

Case management in primary health care

Referrals and targeting.   The referral sources to the scheme were unrestricted, although most came from general practitioners, district nurses and the social services department. The main criteria for referral included the presence of multiple health and social care needs, carers suffering stress, and that home care was a possible means of enhancing quality of life for the elderly person. On the whole, the cases were more dependent than their counterparts in the social care scheme. In particular, all the informal carers appeared to be stressed, and a higher proportion, about one half, of elderly people suffered from incontinence and confusional states.

Assessment.   Either the nurse or a social worker, acting as the case manager, would make the first visit, often depending on the major presenting problem, and over a period of up to six weeks the elderly person would be seen by each member of the team. The case manager would be responsible for completing the assessment and setting up an initial care plan, which would be reviewed at an informal case conference. The assessment schedule was based on that used in the social care scheme, with additional medical and mobility assessments, which on occasions identified problems unknown to general practitioners, including the effects of poor eyesight, diabetes, thyroid deficiency and inadequate fluid intake.

Care planning and organising services. The inclusion of staff from different disciplines and agencies within the team made it possible to provide a wider range of services, using both health and social services resources. A social activity group organised around meal-times was set up in a sheltered housing unit to provide stimulation, companionship and activity to about ten or twelve elderly people once a week. The team physiotherapist took part in this group and organised a series of simple exercises to music for the elderly people, in order to improve mobility and also to monitor their progress. It is unlikely that such a simple but flexible use of resources would have occurred in the absence of an integrated team. As previously, the input of local helpers formed a major part of the care provided. However, with training and supervision from team members, helpers undertook more personal care tasks, such as managing incontinence and assisting with dressing, as well as more work in the care of confused elderly people.

Monitoring care. Again, close and regular monitoring of the elderly person's well-being, the carer's ability to cope and the adequacy and effectiveness of services were crucially important. The usual pattern was one where the case manager, through close contact with the helpers, was able to monitor the situation, and this was supplemented by regular visits to the elderly person, and intervention if there were any difficulties.

The outcome and cost of care

Destinational outcomes. Whereas 64 per cent of those receiving the scheme were at home after twelve months, for the comparison group this was only 21 per cent (Table 22.2). The effect on the prevention of unnecessary admission to residential care was very marked and length of stay in acute hospitals was reduced. The average period of time spent living at home for those receiving the scheme was 39 weeks over one year, compared with 24 weeks in the comparison group.

The costs of care. Table 22.4 indicates the costs of care at 1981 prices, estimated as in the social care scheme, for the social services department, National Health Service and society as a whole. The costs of the case management team and its budget have been separated from other costs incurred by the social services department and the National Health

Service, as well as aggregated. Financial costs borne by informal carers were not included due to the lack of specific research interview data. The annual costs borne by the social services department, other than those of the case management team, were significantly less for those elderly people receiving the scheme. This was due to a much lower rate of admission to residential care. Costs to the National Health Service and society as a whole were not significantly different between the two groups.

22.3 Case management in geriatric care (Darlington)

The project in Darlington was planned to provide home care to physically frail elderly people who would otherwise require long-stay hospital care. The project sought to extend the case management approach described earlier into a geriatric multi-disciplinary team, using multi-purpose care workers (home care assistants) to reduce overlap between personnel (Challis *et al.*, 1989, 1991a,b). The project team, employed by the social services department, consisted of a project manager, three service managers whose role was to act as case managers, and a team of home care assistants. The service managers had to cost the service they provided to clients, working to an average budget of two-thirds of the cost of a long-stay hospital bed. The case managers were members of the geriatric multi-disciplinary team, through which all referrals were directed.

The study compared individuals receiving services from the project with a similar group of patients identified in long-stay wards of an adjacent health district, which was seen as providing a reasonably similar style of geriatric service. Their informal carers were also interviewed, focusing on the experience of care and degree of burden, and compared with a third group of carers of elderly people receiving the usual range of health and social services while living in the community.

Case management in the geriatric care scheme

Referrals and targeting.   Thirty-six males and 65 females were discharged from hospital to the project and their average age was 80 years (Challis et al., 1991b). Most patients had been in hospital for two years or less, 96 per cent of the projected clients and 90 per cent of the control group. However, the mean length of stay for the project clients was 123 days, compared with 305 days for the control group, because a small number of control group patients had been in hospital for a substantially longer time, three years or more. Thirty-eight project clients were discharged to live alone; 42 returned to live with a spouse; 16 were discharged to live with other relatives or friends; three were placed with families; and two were placed in a group-living home. The most common cause of impairment was stroke, which afflicted over one-third of the clients. Most clients had severe mobility and self-care problems, and about two-thirds experienced problems in maintaining continence. Minor psychiatric disorder, in the form of depression or anxiety, appeared to be evident in the majority (88 per cent) of the group and nearly one-third suffered from confusional states. On the basis of the Behaviour Rating Scale (BRS) from the Clifton Assessment Procedures for the Elderly (CAPE) (Pattie and Gilleard, 1979), the project clients were similar to patients in an acute medical ward. The project clients and the control patients were similar on each of the CAPE BRS subscales, with the exception of social disturbance, on which the control group had a higher average level of impairment.

Assessment.   Clients who were to receive the service were assessed by the geriatric multi-disciplinary team, comprising medical staff, hospital and community nursing staff, social workers, paramedical staff and the service managers from the project. The service managers coordinated the assessments of the elderly persons from the different professionals in the multi-disciplinary team and took responsibility for assessing the family and the potential support network. In about half the cases a home visit was undertaken with the elderly person, so that the suitability of the person's home environment could be assessed.

Care planning and organising services.   Each service manager was allocated a budget for their caseload of about 20 clients. A large percentage of this budget was allocated to home care assistant time, but resources were also spent on paying for additional services from members of the community, and the input of other health and social services resources was also costed. Home care assistants were instructed and used by a variety of different professionals, in an attempt to integrate much of the work of several different 'hands-on' providers into the activities of one single care worker. Thus the functions of a home help, auxiliary nurse or an aide to an occupational group were combined in one person. It was the responsibility of the instructing service providers to satisfy themselves that a particular home care assistant was competent to perform any identified task.

Monitoring care.   The service managers' prime function was, in consultation with the multi-disciplinary team, to develop, coordinate and regularly review a package of care, linking together all the necessary resources from a range of different providers, formal and informal. As well as the tasks of monitoring, liaison and coordination, this role also required the service manager to give considerable amounts of emotional support and advice to elderly people and their families, complementing the activities of informal carers, and to provide support for the home care assistants and resolve conflicts in the care network.

The outcome and cost of care

Destinational outcomes. About two-thirds of the experimental group were still in their own homes after six months, and only three people were in institutional care, the remainder having died during the period (Table 22.5). After 12 months, over 50 per cent were still at home. Although there was a significantly higher death rate in the project group after six months, this is not evident at twelve months, after allowing for a higher proportion of project clients who were terminally ill. Over the first six months (182 possible days), project clients were at home for an average of 137 days, and the number of days in any form of institutional care was very small.

Qualify of life and care for clients. The effects of the project were measured by examining the differences between interview data collected before hospital discharge and six months after discharge, and equivalent measures were derived for the control population. Comparisons between the change scores were made using analysis of variance, and the initial difference in social disturbance in the two groups was statistically controlled using covariance analysis. For indicators of subjective well-being (Table 22.6), there was a statistically significant improvement in overall morale (Lawton, 1975; Challis and Davies, 1986) and a nearly statistically significant improvement in a measure of satisfaction with

TABLE 22.5 Destinational outcomes at six and twelve months (Darlington)

Location	Project group		Control group	
	6 months (%)	12 months (%)	6 months (%)	12 months (%)
At home	66	56	12	9
Institutional care	3	4	78	60
Dead	31	40	11	31
No. of cases	101	101	113	113

Note:
Overall χ^2-tests: at 6 months χ^2 = 123.7 ($p<0.001$); at 12 months χ^2 = 89.9 ($p<0.001$).

TABLE 22.6   Client well-being: mean change scores over six months (Darlington)

	Project Group	Control Group	p-value[1]
Subjective well-being			
General satisfaction	0.79	0.08	0.056
Satisfaction with life development	0.18	0.10	ns
Morale	1.74	0.21	0.037
Depression	−2.88	−1.05	<0.01
No. of cases (minimum)[2]	41	72	
Behavioural indicators (CAPE BRS)			
Physical disability	0.19	0.17	ns
Apathy	−0.62	0.12	0.014
Communication difficulties	0.07	0.11	ns
Social disturbance	0.60	0.09	ns
BRS total score	0.33	0.56	ns
No. of cases	66	99	
Quality of care indicators			
Need for improvement in level of care	−4.94	−0.22	<0.001
Social activity level	6.48	2.08	0.011
No. of cases (minimum)[2]	42	76	

Note:
[1]F-test. ns = not significant
[2]Minimum number of cases for which a comparison could be made, due to variable non-response to individual questions, losses due to deaths and missing initial data for project clients who entered the project at the beginning.

their current life situation, and a reduction in depression (Goldbert, 1972), for the elderly people receiving the Darlington project, compared with the control group. On most of the behavioural indicators (Pattie and Gilleard, 1979), no marked changes were observable, except for a significant reduction in apathy for project clients, compared with the hospital patients. This is not surprising, since it is unlikely that such changes would occur as a result of discharge from hospital. In terms of more practical indicators of quality of care, the Darlington clients experienced greater benefits than controls, with a significantly reduced need for additional care, and they also experienced a significant gain in the number of social activities in which they participated, compared to the long-stay patients.

Effects on carers.   Research interviews were carried out with three groups of carers. 'Project carers', whose relative received the Darlington project, were seen on two occasions, about two weeks after discharge

TABLE 22.7 Stress and burden indicators for project carers, day-hospital carers and control group hospitalised carers: mean scores (Darlington)

	Project	Day hospital	Hospital	p-value[1]	Significant group differences[2]
Behavioural and burden indicators					
Care tasks undertaken	6.7	7.9	n/a	<0.05	n/a
Elderly person's behaviour	13.5	18.4	14.8	ns	–
Burdens experienced	4.6	6.3	5.3	ns	–
No. of cases	68	29	27		
Subjective indicators					
Distress – care tasks	4.6	9.9	n/a	<0.001	n/a
Distress – behaviour	12.8	24.1	17.6	<0.001	a, b
Distress – burdens	4.6	7.3	5.6	<0.05	a
Malaise score	6.0	7.4	8.9	<0.05	c
No. of cases	68	29	27		

Notes:
[1] F-test. ns = not significant.
[2] Using Newman–Keuls procedure (Snedecor and Cochran, 1980):
a = project vs day hospital significant at 0.05 level;
b = day hospital vs hospital significant at 0.05 level;
c = project vs hospital significant at 0.05 level;
n/a = not applicable.

and again after six months. There were two comparison groups: 'day-hospital carers', whose elderly relative attended the day hospital in Darlington but otherwise received traditional service support at home; and 'hopspital carers', who were carers of elderly people forming part of the client 'control group'. These latter two groups were interviewed on one occasion. Hence the effects of caring for an elderly person have been examined in a cross-sectional comparison of the three groups of carers studied. The effect of the higher level of social disturbance in the control groups has been controlled statistically using covariance analysis. The objective tasks, the elderly person's behaviour and other burdens of caring were measured where applicable, as were the carers' subjective reactions to these (Platt, 1985). Project carers carried out significantly fewer care tasks than day-hospital carers, and were significantly less subject to distress associated with the performance of these tasks (Table 22.7). Although their elderly relative's behaviour was not seen as significantly different by the three groups of carers, the day-hospital carers were significantly more distressed by the elderly person's behaviour than either of the other two groups. Differences in the practical burdens of daily living experienced by carers in the three groups do not reach an acceptable level of statistical significance, but the project carers were significantly less distressed than the day-hospital carer group. Psychological stress, or malaise (Rutter *et al.*, 1970), was signficantly lower for project carers than for those carers whose elderly relative remained in continuing hospital care. This supports the observations of other studies which suggest that admission to institutional care may reduce the practical burdens experienced by carers, but not necessarily the feelings of anxiety and guilt associated with such an admission (Brane, 1986). Follow-up interviews with carers of Darlington project clients after the elderly person had been discharged for six months indicated no change in the levels of burden or subjective distress.

The costs of care. Table 22.8 indicates the costs of care over a six-month period, at 1986–7 prices, for the main cost accounts, estimated as previously: the Darlington project itself, including case managers, home care assistant time, budget and overheads; the National Health Service; the social services department; and social opportunity costs. Two different figures are given for National Health Service costs since long-stay beds for elderly people in Darlington were mainly provided in an acute hospital, whereas elsewhere beds would be in a lower cost setting, reflected in the second cost estimate, based on the costs of the control group hospital.The total service costs to the two main agencies and to the project were approximately £195 per week, compared with £402 per week in the control group (Table 22.8). Social services costs, except for project services, were very low. Even using the lower unit cost for

TABLE 22.8   Costs for different parties, 1986–7 prices (Darlington)

	Project cases		Control cases	
	Over 6 months (£)	Per week alive (£)	Over 6 months (£)	Per week alive (£)
Community care project	2,850	143	–	–
Other SSD (revenue net cost)	30	1	115	4
Other NHS (5% capital allowance)				
1 DMH base	870	51	9,838	398
2 Geriatric base	659	39	6,205	251
Total agency cost				
1 DMH base	3,750	195	9,953	402
2 Geriatric base	3,539	183	6,320	255
Total social opportunity cost				
1 DMH case	4,977	254	10,493	424
2 Geriatric base	4,766	242	6,859	277

Notes:
[1]Long-stay hospital costs at Darlington Memorial Hospital level.
[2]Long-stay hospital costs at geriatric hospital level.

hospital care, the apparent cost advantage for the project was £72 per week, £183 compared with £255 per week. Social opportunity cost figures, using the lower unit cost for hospital care, were estimated as £242 per week for project cases and £277 for the control group.

22.4 Concluding observations

The findings from this series of case management in the homecare of frail elderly people would seem to be remarkably consistent. In all of the studies there was a reduction in the use of institutional care facilities, and all the available data indicate that the quality of life of elderly people and their carers receiving these case management services improved significantly more than those receiving the usual services. In all the studies these gains were achieved at no greater cost than existing services, indicating improved efficiency in care provision. On average, the cost of care management varied from between 14 and 19 per cent of the social services department costs and remained around 10 per cent of the joint health and social services costs, a relatively low percentage cost for better co-ordianted and planned care. However, it would seem unwise to generalise these findings to the care of less frail elderly people where the opportunity for substitution of institutional by community provision is less. Individuals whose needs fall just below that of institutional care currently receive relatively low levels of provision, and case management with more detailed assessments could well lead to increased expenditure beyond that currently made. Indeed, it would seem that careful targeting is one of the factors associated with the positive results of these studies from the experience of large-scale case management schemes elsewhere (Kemper, 1988).

As well as the importance of targeting, these studies indicate two other important facets relevant to the development of case management services in the care of vulnerable elderly people. These are the role of financial devolution and the style of case management. The findings from these studies indicate that control over resources proved to be an important factor in enabling case managers to respond more effectively to the varied individual needs of elderly people. At worst, in the absence of resource control, the case manager can only request resources from the providers of the services, but has relatively little power to ensure that services are sufficiently responsive to adequately meet clients' needs. It would seem to be the capacity to use resources to influence both the type and content of services that permits genuine individualisation of care (Hodgson and Quinn, 1980; McDowell, 1990). In relation to the style of case management, there is a debate between what may be characterised as 'administrative' and 'clinical' case management approaches (Kenter, 1989; Harrris and Bachrach, 1990). It would seem that some agencies have perceived the core tasks of case management more as administrative activities than requiring staff with human relations skills. However, the present studies indicate that case management has been successful in performing the core tasks through the use of human relations skill, including counselling and support, not only to carers and users but also to hands-on workers. Such a style would not be deemed integral to an administrative model of case management which might see these skills as extra rsources to be purchased where necessary and might therefore not confer the benefits described here (Davies *et al.*, 1990).

In view of the kinds of changes in community care provision that are desired, and policy-makers' expectations of case management as one of the processes to achieve these changes, clarity about target populations, models of case management and degrees of flexibility within these models is required. Without such clarity, investment in case management systems could run the risk of being a more expensive response that fails to produce major changes in patterns of provision.

References

Audit Commission (1986) *Making a Reality of Community Care*, HMSO, London.
Brane, B. (1986) 'Normal ageing and dementia disorders – coping and crisis in

the family', *Progress in Neuropsychopharmacology and Biological Psychiatry*, 10, pp. 287–95.

Challis, D., Chessum, R., Chesterman, J., Luckett, R. and Traske, K. (1990) *Case Management in Social and Health Care: the Gateshead Community Care Scheme*, Personal Social Services Research Unit, University of Kent, Canterbury.

Challis, D., Chessum, R., Chesterman, J., Luckett, R. and Woods, R. (1988) 'Community care for the frail elderly: an urban experiment', *British Journal of Social Work*, Vol. 18 (supplement), pp. 13–42.

Challis, D. and Chesterman, J. (19085) 'A system for monitoring social work activity with the frail elderly', *British Journal of Social Work*, Vol. 15, pp. 115–32.

Challis,D. and Darton, R. (1990). 'Evaluation research and experiment in social gerontology', in Peace, S. (ed.) *Researching Social Gerontology*, Sage, London.

Challis, D., Darton, R., Johnson, L.,Stone, M., Traske, K. and Wall, B. (1989) *Supporting Frail Elderly People at Home: the Darlington Community Care Project*, Personal Social Services Research Unit, University of Kent, Canterbury.

Challis, D., Darton, R., Johnson, L., Stone, M. and Traske, K. (1991a). 'An evaluation of an alternative to long-stay hospital care for frail eldelry patients: part II: Costs and effectiveness', *Age and Ageing*, Vol. 20, pp. 245–54.

Challis, D. and Davies, B. (1980). 'A new approach to community care for the elderly', *British Journal of Social Work*, Vol. 10, pp. 1–18.

Challis, D. and Davies, B. (1985) 'Long-term care for the elderly: the community care scheme', *British Journal of Social Work*, Vol. 15, pp. 563–79.

Challis, D. and Davies, B. (1986) *Case Management in Community Care*, Gower, Aldershot.

Central Council for Education and Training of Social Work (1991) *Assessment, Care Management and Inspection in Community Care: Towards a Practice Curriculum*, CCETSW, London.

Davies, B., Bebbington, A., Charnley, C., Baines, B., Ferlie, E., Hughes, M. and Twigg, J. (1990) *Resources, Needs and Outcomes in Community Based Care*, Gower, Aldershot.

Davies, B. and Challis, D. (1981) 'A production-relations evaluation of the meeting of needs in the community care projects', in Goldberg, E.M. and Connelly, N. (eds) *Evaluative Research in Social Care*, Heinemann, London.

Davies, B. and Challis, D. (1986). *Matching Resources to Needs in Community Care*, Gower, Aldershot.

Department of Health (1989) *Caring for People: Community Care in the Next Decade and Beyond*, CM 849, HMSO, London.

Evers, A. (1991) 'Concluding remarks on the significance of existing policy frameworks and planned reforms: similarities and differences in problems, perceptions and concepts', in Kraan, R.J., Baldock, J., Davies, B., Evers, A., Johansson, L., Knapen, M., Thorslund, M. and Tunissen, C. (eds) *Care for the Elderly*: Significant Innovations in Three European Countries, Campus/ Westview, Boulder, CO.

Goldberg, D.P. (1972) *The Detection of Psychiatric Illness by Questionnaire*, Oxford University Press, Oxford.

Harris, M. and Bachrach, L. (1990) *Clinical Case Management*, New Directions for Mental Health Services No. 40, San Francisco, Jossey-Bass.

Hodgson, J.M. and Quinn, J.L. 'The impact of the TRIAGE health care delivery system on client morale: independent living and the cost of care', *Gerontologist*, Vol. 20, pp. 364–71.

Holden, U.P. and Woods, R.T. (1982). *Reality Orientation: Psychological Approaches to the 'Confused' Elderly*, Churchill Livingstone, Edinburgh.

Kanter, J. (1989) 'Clinical case management: definition, principles, components', *Hospital and Community Psychiatry*, Vol. 40, pp. 461–8.

Kemper, P. (1988) 'The evaluation of the national long term care demonstration–10: Overview of findings', *Health Services Research*, Vol. 23, No. 1, pp. 161–74.

Lawton, M.P. (1975) 'The Philadelphia Geriatric Center morale scale: a revision', *Journal of Gerontology*, Vol. 30, pp. 85–9.

McDowell, D. (1990) 'Comments on the Australian situation: a US view', in Howe, A., Ozanne, E. and Selby Smith, C. (eds) *Community Care Policy and Practice: New Directions in Australia*, Public Management Institute, Monash University, Victoria, Australia.

Pattie, A.H. and Gilleard, C.J. (1979) *Manual of the Clifton Assessment Procedures for the Elderly*, Hodder and Stoughton, Sevenoaks.

Platt, S. (1985) 'Measuring the burden of psychiatric illness on the family: an evaluation of some rating scales', *Psychological Medicine*, Vol. 15, pp. 383–93.

Rutter, M., Tizard, J. and Whitmore, K. (1970) *Education, Health and Behaviour*, Longmans, London.

Snedecor, G.W. and Cochran, W.G. (1980) *Statistical Methods* (seventh edition), Iowa State University Press.

Steinberg, R.M. and Carter, G.W. (1983) *Case Management and the Elderly*, D.C. Heath, Lexington, MA.

Wright, K., Cairns, J. and Snell, M. (1981) *Costing Care*, Social Services Monographs: Research in Practice, University of Sheffield.

23

Community Care Policy: From Consensus to Conflict

ALAN WALKER

23.1 Introduction

The purpose of this chapter is to review some important contemporary developments in government community care policy. It focuses on policy changes since 1979 and looks forward to the implications of these changes for the provision of community care services in the 1990s. Towards the end of the chapter the government's approach to community care is contrasted with an alternative one based on user empowerment.

The main argument advanced in the chapter may be stated simply: community care policy underwent a significant transition during the 1980s, from a position in which there was a consensus, albeit precarious, about the central role of local authority socials services departments (SSDs) in the provision of formal services to one in which policy is directed towards residualising (or minimising) their role. Thus the main object of community care policy during this period was the reduction in the role of local authorities as direct service providers while, at the same time, the growth of informal, voluntary and private welfare was encouraged, often under the guise of promoting a 'mixed economy of welfare'.

Before proceeding with the main analysis it is necessary to make two qualifications. First, the culmination of policy developments during the 1980s was the National Health Service and Community Care Act 1990. This legislation is currently being phased in over the period 1991/2 to 1993/4 (though at the time of writing some doubts were being expressed in official circles about whether it would ever be fully operational). This means that whether or not the *outcome* of stated policy objectives actually does represent a decisive break with the past must await a later assessment.

Second, while it is being argued that government policies during the 1980s represented a departure from the post-war consensus, the meaning of community care as it is experienced by the majority of older people, people with learning difficulties and others in need changed very little, if at all. Thus there is a continuity in their *experience* of the formal sector of community care, as a casualty or last-resort service in which users have very little say in the organisation and delivery of services and which leaves the vast bulk of care needs to be met within the informal sector, largely by female kin (Walker, 1982; 1991; Finch and Groves, 1983; Qureshi and Walker, 1989). So, this chapter is concerned with the shift from consensus to conflict in the policy arena. This is not to imply that there ever was consensus between policy-makers, service providers and users; indeed I have argued elsewhere that community care policy has always been underpinned by conflict between people in need of care and their carers, on the one hand, and the state on the other (Walker, 1983). Therefore this assessment of community care developments during the 1980s and early 1990s concentrates on their impact or likely impact on service users and potential users.

23.2 The end of the consensus on community care

The post-war party political consensus on community care policy was sustained, in part, by the symbolic nature of the term 'community care' and its wide appeal in the policy system. To paraphrase Edelman (1977), the words succeeded magnificently but the policy failed miserably. Not surprisingly the consensus was a precarious one, relying on ambiguity and uncertainty of purpose in policy and the absence of strategic planning; the maintenance of the family as the main provider of care with SSDs occupying a very restricted and junior role; and the subordination of community care services to institutional interests in both the health and social services.

None the less there was a consensus among policy-makers on both the secondary role of the formal sector to the informal sector and on the premise that when services were provided *in* the community the most appropriate location for the planning, organisation and delivery of these services was SSDs. It must be said, however, that beyond this general support on the part of policy-makers for the value-laden and idealistic concept of community care, the primacy of the family and the leading role of SSDs in service provision, there was no deeper consensus even among policy-makers (Titmuss, 1968; Walker, 1986a). For example, over the whole of the post-war period there was (and remains) a wide divergence between local authorities in the levels of their service provision (see, for example, Webb and Wistow, 1987, pp. 160–85). Moreover the failure to extend social services provision in response to rising need (created largely by demographic change) has resulted in a growing 'care gap' between the need for care and the provision of domiciliary services (Walker, 1985).

So, after 30 years of community care policy, by the late 1970s the burden of care in the informal sector was increasing and institutional budgets continued to dominate both health and social services (Gray *et al.*, 1988). Then on to the stage came urgent economic pressures, stemming initially from the fiscal crisis of the mid-1970s but given the added impetus of strong ideological commitment following the election of the Thatcher government in 1979. These produced severe budgetary and resource constraints and the cost-effectiveness imperative, which, combined with a major expansion of need for care particularly among very elderly people, created the political will to overcome both the policy inertia and power struggle between sectional interests that lay behind the precarious consensus on community care. But the policy itself departs significantly from the previous consensus. Thus the emphasis in policy has been shifted away from care *in* the community by local authority personnel towards a confusing mix of care *by* the community itself and private care, regardless of whether in domiciliary or institutional settings.

Signs that the post-war consensus on community care policy was about to be destroyed became apparent soon after the election of the first Thatcher government. In contrast to its predecessors it was characterised by an overt neo-liberal (or new right) ideology and this remained the driving force behind policy throughout the 1980s. The government's first public expenditure White Paper (Treasury, 1979) combined with a speech by the Secretary of State for Social Services (Jenkin, 1979) marked a radical break with the past – the ending of protected status for personal social services (PSS) spending, the abandonment of the coordination and monitoring of local service provision and the increasing reliance on non-statutory forms of welfare (Webb and Wistow, cited in Walker, 1986b) – a trend that was confirmed subsequently by a series of official reports and statements culminating in the National Health Service and Community Care Act 1990. The rest of this section is devoted to outlining the three main dimensions of the new policy that unfolded during the 1980s.

23.2.1 Promoting the private sector

While the primary intention of community care policy during the 1980s and early 1990s appears to have been the negative one of reducing the role of health and social services authorities in the provision of care, the 1980s also witnessed for the first time the active official encouragement of the private sector. This new policy direction was signalled early on in the life of the first Thatcher government when, soon after coming to power, the Department of Health and Social Security (DHSS)[1] moved to encourage a switch in the provision of residential care from the public sector to the private sector.

It did so, first of all, by reducing the resources available to local authorities, by 4.7 per cent in 1979/80 and 6.7 per cent in 1980/1 (Walker, 1986b, p. 17). Although cuts in PSS expenditure were carried out in the mid-1970s these fell particularly on capital, with some limited protection (2 per cent real growth per annum) being offered to current spending. In fact what happened in practice in response to government policy in the early 1980s is that many local authorities took steps to protect their PSS spending, that is until the introduction of the block grant system in 1981/2 and the subsequent imposition of rate-capping and poll-tax-capping considerably reduced their room for manoeuvre (Walker, 1986b, p. 27).

Second, while the public sector received the stick the private sector was given the carrot. The DHSS agreed not only to meet the full cost of care in private residential and nursing homes for those on income support (then supplementary benefit) but it also allowed local offices to set limits on such board-and-lodging payments as were deemed appropriate for their area. As a result the number of places in private residential homes for older people and people with physical and mental disabilities nearly doubled (97 per cent) between 1979 and 1984, and by 1990 had risen by 130 per cent since 1979. The parallel story of expenditure on both residential and nursing homes was that of a rapid increase, from £6 million in 1978 to £460 million in 1988 and to £1.3 billion in 1991. The proportion of people in private residential homes receiving help with their fees through income support payments increased from 14 per cent in 1979, to 35 per cent in 1984 and, by 1988 had reached 56 per cent (Bradshaw and Gibbs, 1988, p. 4; National Association of Citizens Advice Bureaux, 1991, p. 6).

Since this growth in spending conflicted with the government's policy of reducing public expenditure the DHSS acted to stem the flow of resources, first by freezing local limits in September 1984 and then, in April 1985, by imposing national limits for board-and-lodging payments. These limits, at the time of writing, are £150 for residential and £200 for nursing homes for older people and £175 and 215 respectively for homes for people with mental disabilities, and, therefore, still represent a major source of income to the private sector. In addition many local authorities use private homes on an agency basis to house some of their residents. The picture sometimes painted of government ministers being taken by surprise by the unplanned expansion of the private residential sector sits rather uneasily with the purposeful encouragement given to it and the government's antagonism towards local authority spending.

Some policy analysts (see, for example, Day and Klein, 1987) have mistakenly viewed the growth of the private sector of residential care as beneficial in terms of increasing choice in an expanding 'mixed economy or welfare'. Indeed the appeal to increased choice has proved an important source of popular legitimation for the fast expansion of the private sector. However, while it is true that there has been a rapid multiplication of private homes – estimated by the Audit Commission to be doubling in size each year – genuine choice requires a range of alternatives: public sector homes, day care, the chance to remain in an ordinary home with community support. But, ironically, this choice has been restricted by the 'perverse incentive' (Audit Commission, 1986) provided by social security. Furthermore, when it comes to entering a residential home the concept of 'choice' is rarely appropriate. The need for residential care usually arises because of a crisis of care in the informal sector, leaving little time to 'shop around' for alternatives. Thus, as Bradshaw (1988) has confirmed, the promise of choice held out by the supporters of the private sector is illusory.

A study of the private sector by the Centre for Policy on Ageing found that only one-quarter of residents exercised any choice about the home they were admitted to, while nearly one-quarter said that their admission resulted from unsolicited arrangements by a third party (Bradshaw, 1988, p. 18). Choice between private homes is severely restricted by factors such as geographical location, waiting lists and ability to pay. There is, for example, a clear north–south divide in the public/private mix of welfare. Private nursing-home beds in the south-west outnumber those in the northern region by seven times. In two regions, South-East and South-West Thames, the private sector was providing more than half the total unit health care for older people by the mid 1980s (Larder *et al.*, 1986). According to the Audit Commission (1986) a more equitable distribution of resources for health and social services, sought through the National Health Service (NHS) Resource Allocation Working Party and Department of the Environment Grant Related Expenditure Assessment (GREA) calculations, was being offset by board-and-lodging payments for private care.

Within local areas choice can be restricted by the admission criteria applied by private homes, often excluding confused or demented people or those who are difficult to control. Thus an Association of Directors of Social Services (1985) survey found a tendency for private homes to select the less severely disabled older people, leaving the more severely disabled for the public sector. Also, private homes often levy charges above the income support limits, requiring top-up payments, or make supplementary charges for single rooms or items such as laundry. This problem worsened after the government imposed national limits on board-and-lodging payments in 1985 and then failed to raise the benefit ceilings in line with increases with residential and nursing-home charges. As a consequence, and despite the high cost of these payments to the Exchequer, more and more older residents found their benefits inadequate to cover the fees charged. According to August 1988 DSS figures (the latest at the time of writing), 42 per cent of private residents on income support were paying fees above the national limits (Social Services Committee, 1990a).

The research evidence also suggests that residents are not able to exercise much choice once they are inside private homes. A study of homes in North Yorkshire found that 21 per cent had undergone a change of ownership in the previous 18 months (Bradshaw, 1988, p. 19). Residents have no say in such changes and are not always informed before they happen, nor do they have any choice about other changes in the character of their home:

> Residents entering small homely homes may find them enlarged. Residents have no control over the mix of residents or who shares their bedroom. As charges move ahead of [income support] limits residents may find themselves shifted into double or treble rooms, required to commit their pocket money to supplement the [income support] allowance or being subsidised by relatives – often without their knowledge.
>
> (Bradshaw, 1988, pp. 19–20)

Questions have not only been raised about the distributional consequences of the government's policy of promoting their private sector; considerable doubts have also been voiced about the quality of the care provided. As the private residential sector mushroomed, evidence mounted of abuse, misuse of drugs, fraud, lack of hygiene and fire hazards in some homes (Harman and Lowe, 1986; Holmes and Johnson, 1988). Some of the worst cases of abuse were documented by the media, such as Yorkshire Television's 1987 programme 'The Granny Business'. Evidence of abuse in the private sector inevitably invites comparison with the public sector and there are similar instances of ill-treatment to be found there (see, for example, Gibbs *et al.*, 1987). However, concentrating on this sort of comparison of rogues diverts attention from the key issues: the operation of power in a residential setting, regardless of whether it is publicly or privately run, and which of the two sectors can be sufficiently regulated to ensure that no abuse of power occurs. I shall return to these issues later.

So far this discussion has concentrated on private care from the perspective of service users, partly in order to dispel the myth of choice that is usually associated with the private sector. But, while the quality of care is substandard in some private homes, there is also plenty of evidence to show that the pay and conditions of staff working in some of them is well below their public counterparts. There are documented examples too of untrained and low-paid staff having to bear high levels of responsibility for the care of vulnerable people and being threatened with dismissal if they join a trade union (Holmes and Johnson, 1988, pp. 82–105).

23.2.2 Care in the community

At the same time as imposing severe resource constraints on local authorities and encouraging the rapid growth of private residential and nursing homes, the government embarked on a radical programme of mental health hospital closure. The policy of hospital run-down, particularly of mental illness facilities, dates back to the Hospital Plan of 1962. However, prior to 1987 no major hospital had been closed (Social Services Committee, 1985, p. xix).

There has been a steady decline in the number of patients in both mental illness and mental handicap hospitals. For example, in the 10 years to 1986 the average number of daily occupied beds in mental illness hospitals fell from 109,000 to 82,500 and in mental handicap hospitals from 59,000 to 42,500. But the decline accelerated during the 1980s as the governmmment's discharge programme took effect.

The 1981 Care in the Community initiative (Department of Health and Social Security, 1981a, 1983) was specifically intended to promote the discharge of long-stay hospital patients by enabling district health authorities to transfer their funds (above and beyond joint finance) to local authorities and voluntary organisations in order to support ex-patients in the community. In addition, during the early 1980s the DHSS exerted considerable pressure on health authorities to close hospitals within specified time limits (Social Services Committee, 1985, p. xii). This contrasts with the earlier consensus period of community care policy as exemplified by the 1976 DHSS document on priorities in the health and social services: 'The closure of mental illness hospitals is *not* in itself an objective of Government policy, and the White Paper stresses that hospitals should not encourage patients to leave unless there are satisfactory arrangements for their support.' (Department of Health and Social Security, 1976, p. 55).

Although the radical Conservative welfare policy has succeeded, where previous consensus policies had failed, in overcoming institutional inertia and professional interests in the promotion of community care, the main motivation for doing so has been cost-efficiency, with the effectiveness of care received in the community taking second place. This was the main thrust of the trenchant critique by the government's community care policy towards people with mental disabilities by the all-party House of Commons Social Services Committee (1985), one of the most authoritative of several similarly critical reports to be issued over the last decade.

The Social Services Committee focused attention on the disaster course that had been set by forcing a closure programme without sufficient planning, preparation and consultation and, furthermore, without any agreed understanding of what the intended community care would actually entail. It was especially mindful of the danger that community care is perceived as a cheap option. In the Committee's own words:

> A decent community-based service for mentally ill or mentally handicapped people cannot be provided at the same overall cost as present services. The proposition that community care should be cost neutral is untenable. . . . We are at the moment providing a mental disability service which is under-financed and understaffed in its health and social aspects.
>
> (Social Services Committee, 1985, p. xiv)

The official rhetoric surrounding government policy may be community care, but the reality is actually more like decanting and de-hospitalisation coupled with an increase in both public and private residential placements. For example, between 1976 and 1985 there was an increase of 70 per cent in mentally handicapped people in local authority staffed homes and 154 per cent in private homes. The bulk of the increase (133 per cent) in the numbers in private homes occurred between 1981 and 1985, while most of the increase (47 per cent) among those in public sector homes took place between 1976 and 1981. So the result of hurried de-hospitalisation in the face of the underfunding of community-based services is that many people with mental disabilities are merely being shifted from one institution to another, smaller, one. People are ending up in residential homes when they do not need to because there is no realistic alternative and private sector places are subsidised by DSS board-and-lodging payments.

The Social Services Committee summed up the irresponsible nature of the government's care in the community policy in its now famous sentence: 'Any fool can close a long stay hospital: it takes more time and trouble to do it properly and compassionately' (Social Services Committee, 1985, p. xxii). In trying to bring some sense to bear the Committee attempted to establish the basic principles of a community care policy and insisted that the statutory health and social services are central to the provision of community care, both of which fell on deaf ears because they harked back to the pre-1980s consensus, though the government did act in response to the Committee's cricitisms and ordered the slow down of the discharge programme (Department of Health and Social Security, 1985). Moreover in the 1989 White Paper it was stated that 'Ministers will not approve the closure of any mental hospital unless it can be demonstrated that adequate alternatives have been developed' (Department of Health, 1989, p. 56). However, the Social Services Committee (1990b, p. 31) subsequently questioned whether the government was monitoring adherence by health authorities to this modified policy and whether the government had an operational definition of 'adequate alternatives'.

23.2.3 Residualising the Social Services

A series of what seemed, as they occurred, to be separate policy developments over the past 12 years may, with the benefit of hindsight, be seen as part of an evolving government strategy aimed at turning local authority social services from the main providers of formal care into something far more limited: the provider of those residual services that no-one else could or would take on.

In 1980, in a speech to directors of SSDs, the then Secretary of State, Patrick Jenkin, outlined a supportive and decidedly residual role for the social services: 'a long-stop for the very special needs going beyond the range of voluntary services (Jenkin, 1980). In 1981 the White Paper on services for older people asserted, in a widely quoted phrase, 'care in the community must be increasingly mean care *by* the community' (Department of Health and Social Security, 1981a, p. 3). The previous year, when giving evidence before the House of Commons Social Services Committee, Jenkin had justified the cuts in PSS expenditure and the closure of long-stay hospitals (outlined above) on the, unsubstantiated, assumption that the informal and voluntary sectors would expand:

> When one is comparing where one can make savings one protects the Health Service because there is no alternative, whereas in personal social services there is a substantial possibility and, indeed, probability of continuing growth in the possibility of voluntary care, of neighbourhood care, of self help.
>
> (Social Services Committee, 1980, pp. 99–100)

This aim of placing greater reliance on quasi-formal voluntary help and informal support was reflected in the Care in the Community (1981) and the Helping the Community to Care (1984) initiatives.

But it was Jenkin's successor as Secretary of State, Norman Fowler, in a speech to the 1984 Joint Social Services Conference in Buxton, who provided the clearest and most detailed outline of the new residual role proposed for social services. He argued that there are 'three paramount responsibilities' of SSDs: to take a comprehensive strategic view of all the sources of care available in the area; to recognise that the direct provision of services is only part of the local pattern and that in many cases other forms of provision are available; to see a major part of their function as promoting and supporting the fullest possible participation of the other different sources of care. The fundamental role of the state, according to Fowler, was 'to back up and develop the assistance which is given by private and voluntary support' (Fowler, 1984, p. 13).

The Audit Commission's inquiry into community care came to the same conclusion as countless previous independent studies:

> Joint planning and community care policies are in some disarray. The result is poor value for money. Too many people are cared for in settings costing over £200 a week when they would receive a more appropriate care in the community at a total cost to public funds of £100–£130 a week. Conversely, people in the community may not be getting the support they need.
>
> (Audit Commission, 1986, p. 3)

Later the Griffiths Report was to echo exactly the same criticisms of government policy. The Audit Commission proposed various organisational changes aimed primarily at clarifying the overlapping responsibilities of health and social service authorities. For example, in the case of the physically and mentally disabled, local authorities were to be given 'lead' responsibility for their long-term care in the community, except for the most severely disabled who would remain the responsibility of the NHS. The long-term care of older people in the community would be financed from a single budget established by contributions from the NHS and local authorities. The budget would be under the control of a single manager who would purchase services from the appropriate public or private agency. Health authorities were to be given lead responsibility for the care of the mentally ill in that community (Audit Commission, 1986, p. 4).

The Audit Commission's critical report was much more influential with the government than any previous one had been, including the authoritative analysis by the House of Commons Social Services Committee. The Secretary of State had been promising, for two years, the publication of a Green Paper on the personal social services. This did not materialise, and instead, in response to the debate following the Audit Commission report, Sir Roy Griffiths was appointed, in March 1986, to examine problems in the arrangements for community care between the NHS and local authorities and to explore the option of putting the whole service for older people 'under the control of a manager who will purchase from whichever public or private agency is appropriate'. (Sir Roy Griffiths had conducted a similar inquiry into the management of the NHS in 1983, which led to the appointment of general managers at district level.) The report of the Griffiths enquiry was published in March 1988, the White Paper, *Caring for People*, followed in November 1989 and, within days, the National Health Service and Community Care Bill was published.

Together these policy developments, taken with those reviewed earlier, suggest a strategy aimed at residualising the social services. The issue of how far the Griffiths Report and the White Paper chime with this strategy will be discussed in the next section. For the moment the three main dimensions to the policy of residualisation may be summarised.

In the first place, the provision of community care is being deliberately *fragmented*. Though sometimes presented as promoting a more mixed economy of welfare, the main motivations here have been to curtail the monopoly role of local authorities in the delivery of formal care – an aim that, as we have seen, has already been achieved in several parts of the country with regard to the residential care of older people – and to encourage the growth of cheaper sources of informal and quasi-formal care. Sir Kenneth Stowe, the former permanent secretary of the DHSS, described this new approach as 'letting a hundred flowers bloom'.

The first of the Thatcher Secretaries of State for Social Services, Patrick Jenkin, had hoped for the expansion of voluntary help, self-help and informal care (see above) and, to encourage the development of these alternative forms of provision, a series of special initiatives, including the Care in the Community and the Helping the Community to Care programmes, were introduced. Indeed, with the Department of the Environment so effectively controlling local authority expenditure by means of the block grant, the main influence exerted by the DHSS over community care has been the promotion of these initiatives and the targeting of research resources on projects designed to extend informal and voluntary help, such as the Kent community care scheme. One result of this policy of fragmentation was the advent, in the 1980s, of a wide range of precarious, often short-life, projects relying on grant aid and government training schemes. Thus, for example, in September 1986 there were some 66,459 community programme workers engaged in providing direct services to social welfare clients.

Second, there is *marketisation*. As we have seen, while finances for local authority services have been tightly controlled, the private sector has been encouraged to expand by the open-ended provision of social security board-and-lodging subsidies. Contracting out, or purchases of service contracting, has a long history in the personal social services but it has been used primarily in relation to the voluntary sector (Webb and Wistow, 1987, p. 89). So far, direct privatisation has not affected the social services to the same extent as the NHS. But the Local Government

Act 1988 gave the secretary of State for the Environment powers to add to the list of services that must be contracted out.

Some policy analysts have taken the view that the expansion of the private sector at the expense of the public sector is simply an extension of welfare pluralism, leading to increased choice and efficiency, and in any case, a reduced role in the provision of services could be balanced by an increased regulatory role (Day and Klein, 1987). The extent to which the private sector promotes choice has already been discussed. In addition marketisation may be seen as one among many examples of the new right's antagonism towards the decommodifying aspects of the welfare state. It is intended to challenge the extent, albeit limited, to which the social services intrude on market values and threaten their reproduction by promoting citizenship rights and needs-based priorities. It is this idealogical driving force behind the expansion of the market, and the simplistic assumptions it is derived from concerning the effectiveness of the market, that proponents of regulation tend to overlook. Regulation hinders the efficient operation of the market and this might endanger the government's primary goal of expanding private provision.

Third, the government has pursued a twin-track policy of *decentralising* administration and operations, while *centralising* control over resources. This is one manifestation of the general new right strategy of rolling back the frontiers of the state while centralising state control (Gamble, 1986). The process of centralising control over social services resources began early in the life of the first Thatcher administration with the introduction of the block grant and, within it, detailed GREAs for the different elements of the personal social services (Walker,1985, p. 27). This approach was translated into poll tax Standard Spending Assessments in 1990 (1989 in Scotland) and is likely to survive the abolition of the poll tax. But responsibility for the operation of social services within centrally determined budgets remains with local authorities. A similar policy has been implemented with regard to housing benefit and the health service. In theory the decentralisation of operations offers the prospect of greater user involvement. But this is unlikely to be realised unless resources and responsibility are also devolved.

The cumulative impact of these three sets of policy developments is a strategy aimed at further residualising the role of local authorities providing community care. This was the process envisaged by the chief architects of the present community care policy, Patrick Jenkin and Norman Fowler, and echoed by senior DHSS officials in public statements. For example, in 1980, the head of the social work service observed: 'I do not [therefore] have difficulty in accepting the role of the State as residual – the voluntary sector must to some extent return to providing and paying for services which we have come to expect from the state.' (Utting, 1980). Although some aspects of these policies were to be found under former governments – for example, the 1977 Good Neighbour Scheme was the forerunner of the 1980s' DHSS initiatives – a concerted strategy of this sort has not been identifiable previously. Of course, in relation to the totality of care, both formal and informal, the social services have never been anything other than residual. The essence of the Thatcher and Major governments' approach towards community care, however, is that it is attempting, with some success, to reduce the role of local authorities as providers within the formal sector. Furthermore, it is intended to fill this artificially created care gap with a mixtue of private, voluntary and informal care. The likely impact of this policy is considered in the next section.

23.3 Community care in the 1990s

The provisions in the National Health Service and Community Care Act represent the culmination of the previous decade of policy, as outlined above, and establish a new framework for services. The Act was based on the White Paper *Caring for People* (Department of Health, 1989), which, in turn, was derived in large measure (80 per cent according to the ministerial statement on 12 July 1989) from the recommendations of the Griffiths Report (Griffiths, 1988).The Act received the royal assent on 29 June 1990 and was due to be implemented in full on 1 April 1991. However, on 18 July 1990 the Secretary of State announced a delay in the implementation of the main financial provisions of the Act until April 1993. The government explained this delay in terms of its lack of confidence in local authorities to introduce the new system of community care within reasonable cost boundaries. But it would appear that, while the local authorities were prepared to implement the Act, the government itself had no idea what the cost would be and was, therefore, rather nervous about the implications of the charges for poll-tax levels (Henwood *et al.*, 1991).

What are the main changes in policy that will flow from the implementation of the Act? The White Paper defined four key components of community care which together reflected the emphasis on promoting choice by policy developments over the previous decade as well as being cast in the language of consumerism. They are: services that respond flexibly and sensitively to the needs of individuals and their carers; services that intervene no more than is necessary to foster independence; services that allow a range of options for consumers; and services that concentrate on those with the greatest needs (Department of Health, 1989, p. 5). In the White Paper 'choice' is defined as 'giving people a greater individual say in how they live their lives and the services they need to help them' (Department of Health, 1989, p. 4). This is to be achieved in two mains ways: a comprehensive process of assessment and care management, which 'where possible should induce [the] active participation of the individual and his or her carer', and a more diverse range of non-statutory providers among whose benefits is held to be 'a wider range of choice of services for the consumer' (Department of Health, 1989, pp. 19, 22).

The main policy changes are as follows: local authorities became responsible, as lead agencies, for assessing individual need, designing care arrangements and ensuring services are delivered. Thus the provision of services is separated from their purchase (as under the NHS reforms) and it is expected that SSDs make maximum use of private and voluntary services. Local authorities are to produce and publish plans for the development of community care services. A new funding structure was established for this with public support in non-statutory residential and nursing homes (though the changes do not apply to those in residence up to April 1993). Resources are to come from a single unified budget, in the hands of local authorities, comprising existing social services resources *plus* the care element of social security board-and-lodging allowances deemed likely to be necessary by the government for new users. There is a new specific grant to promote the development of social care for people with a mental illness and, in this case only, health authorities are to act as the lead agencies.

The revised timetable for the implementation of the Act meant that the new specific grant with regard to mental illness came into effect on 1 April 1991 with the complaints procedures and 'arm's length' local inspection units for residential care. After 1 April 1992 local authorities must publish their first community care plans, and after 1 April 1993 the new funding arrangements commence, with local authorities taking full responsibility for funding community care. At the time of writing questions have been raised as to whether these proposals will ever be fully implemented because of their cost implications. Moreover, in March 1991 the government announced a review of the organisation of local government, as part of its strategy to replace the poll tax, and this could entail major changes in responsibility for social services funding and delivery. However, for the purposes of this discussion, it is assumed that the package outlined above will be introduced. Certainly the cost of funding private residential and nursing homes is rising rapidly and the government will be forced to do something to curb the perverse incentive it has created.

Some controversy surrounded the award of lead agency status to SSDs following the publication of the Griffiths Report. It was conjectured that the report's release on the day after the 1988 Budget and the long-delayed response to it signalled the government's displeasure with this central recommendation. On the face of it too this proposal (now enacted) is completely at odds with the residualisation strategy set out in the first part of this chapter. However, Griffiths made a clear distinction between responsibility for ensuring that care is provided and actual provision: 'the role of the public sector is essential to ensure that care is provided. How it is provided is an important but secondary consideration' (Griffiths, 1988, p. vii). This places the Griffiths Report, White Paper and 1990 Act firmly in the mainstream of government community care policy stretching back to 1979. The role established for local authorities is the management of care not its provision. As managing agents they will oversee the further residualisation of public sector provision while encouraging the expansion of the private and voluntary sectors.

The only significant difference between the government's proposals and the Griffiths Report concerned the mechanism by which resources will be allocated to local authorities. Griffiths had recommended an earmarked (or ring-fenced) grant but the government rejected this in favour of maintaining the present system whereby resources are channelled through the general Revenue Support Grant to local authorities. Indeed so determined was the government that it overturned a House of Lords amendment to the National Health Service and Community Care Bill in order to prevent ring-fencing.

23.3.1 Implications for users of the community care proposals

What are the likely implications for users of these radical developments in the organisation and delivery of services? In making such an assessment it must be remembered that the Griffiths Review, from which the White Paper was derived, was designed from its inception as a top-down managerial appraisal intended to tackle the problems identified by the Audit Commission. Not surprisingly, therefore, the outcome was management-oriented. In turn the main justification for change provided in the White Paper was financial rather than, for example, the needs of people with disabilities or the quality of care. Thus it is impossible to imagine a document like the White Paper (or the Griffiths Report) being prepared by a group of service users and their carers. The official documents are management-oriented rather than user-oriented; their primary concern is cost not the quality of care. It is for this reason that the promises of wider choice and the opportunity for service users to exercise some influence over the care packages they receive are unlikely to be realised.

In the first place, despite the political rhetoric concerning choice and user involvement accompanying the White Paper, neither the Act nor the policy guidelines accompanying it contain any concrete proposals for user involvement or empowerment. In the absence of clear guidelines for such involvement it is likely that professional opinions will continue to dominate. This is evident to some extent in the language employed: 'managers of care packages', 'case managers' and 'caring *for* people'. Thus, rather than determing their own packages of care, service users are apparently still seen as passive receivers of care. Similarly with the prominence given to care (or case) management. This can be either administration-centred or user-centred. In the context of the goals of value for money and efficiency case management is likely to prove to be primarily an administrative tool for cost management.

Second, also as a result of the ideological context of these changes, a premium is placed on non-state forms of provision. So local authorities will be expected to employ competitive tendering or other means of marketing the production of welfare. This gives a rather biased meaning to 'packages of care' or the 'mixed economy of care'. For example, the White Paper suggested that one of the ways in which SSDs could promote a mixed economy of care is by 'determining clear specifications of service requirements, and arrangements for tenders and contracts' (Department of Health, 1989, p. 23). But evidence from the US indicates that competitive tendering may actually *reduce* the choice available by driving small producers out of contention (Demone and Gibelman, 1989). This is likely to affect specialist provision for some minority group needs, such as those of black people and particularly disability groups.

There are two further important implications of the continued residualisation of SSDs as direct service providers. As the private sector 'creams-off' the less severely disabled, less costly users, leaving a rump of the most severely disabled in the public sector this will pose very difficult staff morale problems in the latter. Griffiths had recommended that the government create a 'level playing-field' between public, voluntary and private home funding, but this was rejected and, instead, residents in non-public-sector homes are to receive an additional subsidy in the form of income support and housing benefit entitlements. This gives a financial incentive to local authorities to privatise their residential homes and blows apart the idea that these changes were designed to increase choice. People with proven need will, in effect, be prevented from choosing to enter a publicly owned home. The continued reduction in the service provision role of local authorities is likely to curtail the progress that some have been making towards equal opportunities policies and anti-oppressive practice. It will be difficult to sustain such policies under the new funding regime and in a world in which local authorities have very little influence over the terms and conditions of day-to-day service delivery in contracted agencies.

Third, the government's professed aim of increasing choice and sensitivity to user requirements is likely to be inevitably compromised by the process of assessment that is required to ration resources. Thus no-one is to receive public funding for residential care after April 1993 unless they have been assessed and recommended by case managers. This process is bound to limit individual choice and user influence while, conversely, enhancing the power of bureau-professionals. Moreover users do not have a right to elect to be assessed and there are no safeguards – such as an appeals procedure – for those who disagree with professional assessments.

Fourth, despite the rhetoric concerning the needs of carers there are no proposals designed to ensure that their needs are taken into account. In the absence of such guarantees, of course, there is a danger that, under financial pressure, they will be ignored. Furthermore, the fact that there might be a conflict of interest between carers and cared-for is not recognised by the government. But this is a very real problem facing people with disabilities, their carers and service providers. The failure to address this dilemma stems from the assumption underlying both the White paper and the Griffiths Report that the family should in all circumstances be the primary source of care. However, research has shown that this confidence in familism is sometimes misplaced: family care can be both the best *and* the worst form of support (Qureshi and Walker, 1989). If policy-makers continue to assume that it is always the soundest basis for care they will overlook inherent conflicts in the caring relationship and be guilty of imposing some destructive relationships on both carers and cared-for.

Finally, as well as opportunities the new system of organising community care heralds dangers for the voluntary sector. In a world of competitive tendering it will be difficult for voluntary agencies to maintain their autonomy and act as independent representatives of the groups they serve. Financial pressures may limit the extent of user participation that voluntary agencies can sustain. Moreover, since contracts will be between the local authority purchaser and the service provider, rather than with the individual service *receiver*, users are bound to be excluded.

Of course, the precise impact of the proposed changes rests on resources, but so far the financial details of the community care package have not been revealed. The Ministerial Statement on 12 July 1989 made it clear that there would not be any extra money and, even worse, that what there was would be cash limited. This means that, in line with the government's twin-track centralisation/decentralisation policy, local authorities will be given responsibility but without a guarantee that they will be provided with adequate funds to support the necessary growth in home care services. It is also clear that service users themselves will have to contribute increasingly towards the financing of services and the expectation is that a means-test will follow the assessment process (Department of Health, 1990, p. 29).

23.3.2 From consumerism to empowerment?

Underlying these deficiencies in the new community care arrangements
– especially when viewed from the perspective of service users – are the
legacy of antagonism towards public welfare provision discussed earlier
and a very restricted conception of user involvement (Walker, 1991).

The Griffiths Report, White Paper and National Health Service and
Community Care Act all derive from the limited form of supermarket-
style consumerism which assumes that, if there is a choice between
'products', service users will automatically have the power of exit from a
particular product or market. Of course, even if this is true in markets
for consumer goods, in the field of social care many people are mentally
disabled, frail and vulnerable; they are not in a position to 'shop around'
and have no realistic prospect of exit.

Underlying the consumerist model of social care are two questionable
assumptions. It is assumed that monopolies only operate in the public
sector. Also it is assumed that the private sector can adequately substitute for the public sector. But, as far as, for example, an older person
currently resident in either a public *or* a private home is concerned, her
provider *is* the monopoly power because she has no alternative. Having
a range of theoretical alternatives will not make the consumer sovereign
if she cannot exercise effective choice. Moreover, a financial transition
does not necessarily mean the bestowal on the purchaser of either
influence or control over the provider. Furthermore, unlike markets for
consumer durables, in the field of social care if the private producer goes
out of business this will not only have immense human consequences
but the public sector will be expected to pick up the pieces. In other
words, the private sector exercises equivalent power over users to public
providers but it does not necessarily carry the same responsibility.

The only way that frail and vulnerable service users can be assured of
influence and power over service provision is if they or their advocates
are guaranteed a 'voice' in the organisation and management of services. This would, in turn, ensure that services actually reflected their
needs. In practice the weak form of consumer consultation pursued
under the 1990 Act could consist of no more than an occasional survey
among users together with minimal individual consultation at the point
of assessment. (This is certainly the model being offered to local authorities by private management consultants and the signs are that many are
adopting it.) Thus despite the rhetoric concerning 'packages of care' and
making services more responsive to users, in practice the government's
proposals are silent on how user involvement can be ensured and are
characterised by old-style paternalism.

In contrast to the consumer-oriented model, the user-centred or
empowerment approach would aim to involve users in the develop-

ment, management and operation of services as well as in the assessment of need. The intention would be to provide users and potential users with a range of realisable opportunities to define their own needs and the sorts of services they require to meet them. Both carers and cared-for would be regarded as potential service users. Where necessary the interests of older people with mental disabilities would be represented by independent advocates. Services would be organised to respect users' rights to self-determination, normalisation and dignity. They would be distributed as a matter of right rather than discretion, with independent inspection and appeals procedures, and would be subject to democratic oversight and accountability.

What changes in policy are necessary if community care services are to move beyond consultation to empowerment? In the first place it is necessary to recognise that while the private and voluntary sector may extend choice in social care they cannot substitute for the public sector. Only the public sector can guarantee rights to services. Moreover the motivations of a for-profit private producer are quite different from those of a public sector provider. Although both may provide opportunities to exploit vulnerable people it is only in the public sector that a direct line of enforceable public accountability exists (Walker, 1988). It must be said too that, as far as Britain is concerned, the public sector of care is notably more successful at involving users than its private counterpart.

Second, change is necessary in the organisation and operation of formal services. The concept of social support networks is particularly helpful in emphasising the need for formal and informal helpers to cooperate, share tasks and decision-making and 'interweave' (Whittaker and Garbarino, 1983). In addition SSDs must develop explicit strategies for the involvement of service users, carers and potential users. The essential ingredients of such a strategy are positive action – to provide users and potential users (or their advocates) with support, skills training, advocacy and resources – so that they can make informed choices, and access – the structures of the agency must afford opportunities for genuine involvement. According to Croft and Beresford (1990, p. 14): 'Unless both are present people may either lack the confidence, expectations or abilities to get involved, or be discouraged by the difficulties entailed. Without them, participatory initiatives are likely to *reinforce* rather than overcome existing race class, gender and other inequalities.' Thus user involvement must be built in to the structure and operations of SSDs and not bolted on.

Third, change must be initiated in professional values and attitudes within the formal sector so that co-operation and partnership with service users is regarded as a normal activity. This does *not* mean that service provision must be deprofessionalised if user involvement is to flourish; rather that the role of professionals must change in order to share power with users. This means challenging, to some extent, the traditional basis of professional status and providing for the input of informed user knowledge and preferences, which means finding ways for community members themselves to take part in the development of community care policy – in short, power sharing.

Fourthly, the previous two points suggest a major transformation in training and retraining for social services personnel. Thus the emphasis would shift away from autonomous expertise and individual diagnosis towards skills for working in partnership with service users and their carers, and encouraging community participation.

Finally, user involvement is not a cheap option; it is usually time-consuming and costly. Therefore there is a need for increased resources in the social services not only to improve the choice and quality of services but also to ensure that they provide sufficient space for the direct involvement of users.

Thus if significantly greater reforms were made available it would be possible for some of the reforms contained in the National Health Service and Community Care Act 1990 to be implemented in a progressive way. For example, assessment could be operationalised as an open process designed to explore and create options rather than ration resources. It could be carried out by users themselves or in partnership with social services professionals. Contracts could be used to ensure high standards are maintained, rather than high prices, and that agencies have equal opportunities employment policies and anti-oppressive forms of practice. Quality could be guaranteed by granting users *rights* in terms of both standards and levels of services. But, arguably these sorts of development would alter the main thrust of current community care policy and, therefore, would first require a change of political direction.

23.4 Conclusion

Looking back over the post-war period it is clear that the precarious political consensus on community care held together because of the remarkable gulf between rhetoric and action and the interests of the most powerful groups involved in sustaining it. The consensus began to break down in the mid-1970s under economic and external International Monetary Fund pressures, but there was still a commitment to publicly provided domiciliary services. The serious challenge to the consensus came after 1979, when the government set about a radical shift in policy, towards an increasing use of private and informal care and the residualisation of the social services. The debate following the publication of the

Griffiths Report, culminating in the 1990 Act, could have marked a watershed in raising public consciousness about community care and provided a basis for the development of policies aimed at user involvement and empowerment. Unfortunately that opportunity was wasted and the measures currently being implemented are directed at cost-containment and the run-down of public social services.

Note

1. The DHSS was split into two departments, Health (DH) and Social Security (DSS), on 25 July 1988.

References

Association of Directors of Social Services (1985) *Who Goes Where?* ADSS, London.
Audit Commission (1986) *Making a Reality of Community Care*, PSI, London.
Bradshaw, J. (1988) 'Financing private care for the elderly', Department of Social Policy and Social Work, University of York.
Bradshaw, J. and Gibbs, I. (1988) *Public Support for Private Residual Care, Avebury, Aldershot.*
Croft, S. and Beresford, P. (1990) *From Paternalism to Participation*, Open Services Project, London.
Day, P. and Klein, R. (1987) 'The business of welfare', *New Society*, 19 June, pp. 11–13.
Demone, H. and Gibelman, M. (1989). *Services for Sale: Purchasing Health and Human Services*, Rutgers University Press, London.
Department of Health (1989) *Caring for People: Community Care in the Next Decade and Beyond*, Cm 849, HMSO, London.
Department of Health (1990) *Community Care in the Next Decade and Beyond*, Department of Health, London.
Department of Health and Social Security (1976) *Priorities for Health and Personal Social Services in England*, HMSO, London.
Department of Health and Social Security (1981a) *Care in the Community*, HMSO, London.
Department of Health and Social Security (1981b) *Growing Older*, Cmnd. 8173, HMSO, London.
Department of Health and Social Security (1983) *Explanatory Notes on Care in the Community*, DHSS, London.
Department of Health and Social Security (1985) *Response to Second Report from the Social Services Committee*, Cmnd. 9674, HMSO, London.
Edelman, M. (1977) *Political Language*, Academic Press, New York.
Finch, J. and Groves, D. (eds) (1983) *A Labour of Love*, Routledge and Kegan Paul, London.

Fowler, N. (1984) 'Speech to Joint Social Services Annual Conference', 27 September, DHSS, London.

Gamble, A. (1987) *The Free Economy and the Strong State*, Pluto Press, London.

Gibbs, J., Evans, M. and Rodway, S. (1987) *Report of the Inquiry into Nye Bevan Lodge*, Southwark Council, London.

Gray, A.M., Whelan, A. and Normand, C. (1988) *Care in the Community: a Study of Services and Costs in Six Districts*, Centre for Health Economics, University of York.

Griffiths,Sir R. (1988) *Community Care: Agenda for Action*, HMSO, London.

Harman, H. and Lowe, M. (1986) *No Place Like Home*, House of Commons, London.

Henwood, M., Jowell,T. and Wistow, G. (1991) *All Things Come (to Those Who Wait?)*, King's Fund Institute, London.

Holmes, B. and Johnson, A. (1988) *Cold Comfort*, Souvenir Press, London.

Jenkin, P. (1979) 'Speech to Social Services Conference', Bournemouth, 21 November.

Jenkin, P. (1980) 'Speech to the Conference of the Association of Directors of Social Services', 19 September.

Larder, D., Day, P. and Klein, R. (1986) *Institutional Care of the Elderly: the Geographical Distribution of the Public/Private mix in England*, University of Bath.

National Association of Citizens Advice Bureaux (1991) *Beyond the Limit*, NACAB, London.

Qureshi, H. and Walker, A. (1989) *The Caring Relationship*, Macmillan, London.

Social Services Committee (1980) *The Government's White Papers on Public Expenditure: the Social Services*, Vol. II, HC 702, HMSO, London.

Social Services Committee (1985) *Community Care*, HC 13–1, HMSO, London.

Social Services Committee (1990a) *Community Care: Future Funding of Private and Voluntary Residential Care*, HC 257, HMSO, London.

Social Services Committee (1990b) *Community Care: Services for People with a Mental Handicap and People with a Mental Illness*, HC 664, HMSO, London.

Titmuss, R.M. (1968) *Commitment to Welfare*, Allen and Unwin, London.

Treasury (1979) *The Government's Expenditure Plans 1980/81*, Cmnd 7746, HMSO, London.

Utting, B. (1980) 'Changing ways of caring', *Health and Social Services Journal*, 4 July, p. 882.

Walker, A. (ed.) (1982) *Community Care: the Family, the State and Social Policy*, Blackwell/Martin Robertson, Oxford.

Walker, A. (1983) 'Care for elderly people: a conflict between women and the state', in Finch, J. and Groves, D. (eds) *A Labour of Love*, Routledge and Kegan Paul, London, pp. 106–28.

Walker, A. (1985) *The Care Gap*, Local Government Information Service, London.

Walker, A. (1986a) 'Community care: fact and fiction', in Willmott, P. (ed.) *The Debate About Community*, PSI, London, pp. 4–15.

Walker, A. (1986b) 'More ebbs than flows', *Social Services Insight*, 29 March, pp. 16–17.

Walker, A. (1988) 'State of confusion', *Community Care*, 3 March, pp. 26–7.

Walker, A. (1991) 'Increasing user involvement in the social services', in Arie, T. (ed.) *Recent Advances in Psychogeriatrics*, Vol. 2, Churchill Livingston, London.

Webb, A. and Wistow,G. (1987) *Social Work, Social Care and Social Planning: the Personal Social Services Since Seebohm*, Longman, London.

Whittaker, J.K. and Garbarino, J. (eds) (1983) *Social Support Networks: Informal Helping in the Human Services*, Aldine, New York.

Managing Madness: Changing Ideas and Practice*

JOAN BUSFIELD

The post-war policy shift towards community care has been explained in a number of different ways. A standard account, often favoured by psychiatrists, relates it to the therapeutic developments of the post-war 1950s, and, to a lesser extent, to the impact of the sustained and vocal critiques of institutional care that come from both within and outside psychiatry during the same decade.[1] The chemically synthesised drugs of the 1950s permitted, it is contended, a greater number of patients to be treated outside the hospital and facilitated the earlier discharge of those who did have to be admitted. This, together with an increasing recognition of the anti-therapeutic nature of institutional care led, it is argued, to general support for policies of shifting care away from the mental hospital towards the community.[2] Put simply we can characterise the policy change and the explanation that is offered of it in terms of the simple model set out in Figure 24.1.

There are, however, a number of problems with this explanation of the shift to community care, grounded as it is in the liberal-scientific view of medical work, as Scull in his book *Decarceration*, and others, have indicated.[3] First, it is defective on grounds of timing. The decline in the size of the resident population of psychiatric beds was apparent in national statistics for this country and in the US in the mid-1950s and in the statistics for particular hospitals from at least the beginning of the 1950s, yet the chemically synthesized drugs were only just beginning to be introduced in the mid 1950s.

_____

*This is an abridged extract from Chapter 10, 'Community Care', of *Managing Madness: changing ideas and practice*, Unwin Hyman, 1986, pp. 326–343.

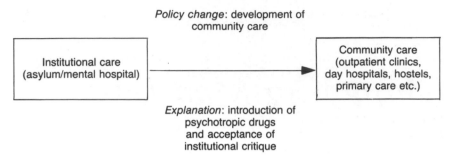

Figure 24.1

Scull presents a second objection to the thesis: that there is little evidence that the psychotropic drugs have been very effective in curing mental disorders. In his words there is 'a growing volume of evidence which suggests that claims about the therapeutic effectiveness of so-called 'anti-psychotic' medication have been greatly exaggerated.'[4]

Scull has presented us with an alternative description of the policy transition and an alternative explanation that questions the benevolent assumptions of the liberal explanation. For Scull, the key policy change is a negative one: the rejection of the asylum; he uses the term decarceration as a 'shorthand for a state-sponsored policy of closing down asylums, prisons and reformatories', a policy more commonly described as deinstitutionalisation.[5] According to Scull this represents a movement away from what he calls 'an institutionally based system of segregative control'.[6] He measures the adoption of this policy by the decline in the number of resident patients in state mental hospitals in the US and the UK since the mid-1950s, a decline more substantial in the US than in the UK and one that he recognizes is far from complete in either country. The results, he contends, are, however, clear enough. There has been a run down of facilities provided for the mentally ill and an indifference to their problems that has often been far from benign:

Clearly a certain proportion of the released inmates are able to blend unobtrusively back into the communities from whence they came. After all, many of those subjected to processing by the official agencies of social control have all along been scarcely distinguishable from their neighbours who were left alone, and presumably they can be expelled from institutions without appreciable additional risk. But for many other ex-inmates and potential inmates, the alternative to the institution has been to be herded into newly emerging 'deviant ghettoes', sewers of human misery and what is conventionally defined as social pathology within which (largely hidden from outside inspection or even notice) society's refuse may be impressively tolerated. Many become lost in the interstices of social life, and turn into drifting inhabitants of those traditional resorts of the down and out, Salvation Army hostels, settlement houses, and so on. Others are grist for new, privately-run, profit-oriented mills for the disposal of the unwanted – old age homes, halfway houses, and the like. And yet more exist by preying on the less agile and wary, whether these be 'ordinary' people trapped by poverty and circumstance in the inner city, or their fellow decarcerated deviants.[7]

Scull's description of the transition is not, therefore, of a move from mental hospital care to community care but from segregation in the asylum to neglect and misery within the community. This description of the nature of the transition generates its own explanation: that the main reasons for the adoption of the new policy were economic. Decarceration was introduced because 'segregative modes of social control became, in relative terms, far more costly and difficult to justify'.[8] For him the anti-institutional ideology of the 1950s may have facilitated decarceration but was not in itself sufficient to account for its adoption. As evidence he points to the critique of institutional care in the nineteenth century, which he asserts had little real impact. Portrayed graphically, Scull's interpretation of decarceration and its explanation is shown in Figure 24.2.

Like the liberal–scientific explanation he rejects, his own account is defective on grounds of timing. The fiscal crisis of the state to which he refers is a phenomenon of the early 1970s and later, and not of the 1950s, when, although public expenditure was increasing, rapid economic growth and greater prosperity helped to ensure that there was comparatively little anxiety about the increase.[10] In addition his explanation ignores the changes that have occurred in the pattern of mental health service expenditure during this century. In particular it ignores the development and expansion of psychiatric services outside the mental hospital, especially in the field of primary care. While, therefore, Scull is right to draw attention to the dangers attendant on a policy of community care that can hide a failure to make provision for the mentally ill under a gloss of the apparent humanity of putting people back in the

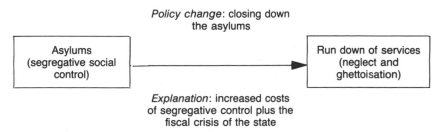

Figure 24.2

communities to which they belong; and while he is right to point out that during the last two decades or more there has been a mystification and distortion of a reality of neglect and lack of resources to those discharged from mental hospitals; nevertheless he cannot account for the introduction of the policy of running down mental hospitals in the 1950s and 1960s in simple economic terms.[11] Scull's argument fits events of the mid-1970s onwards much better than it does those of the 1950s and 1960s.

The move towards community care has been associated with a significant reorientation of services away from the chronic long-stay patients, towards those with less serious, shorter-term problems, who were formerly little catered for by public mental health services. It is not, therefore, that all mental health services have been run down under the guise of community care, rather that resources have largely gone into selected community services, those for acute, less serious mental disorders, and not into those dealing with chronic, more serious complaints. As a result aggregate expenditure on mental health services has increased, but this has largely been at the expense of those in need of some form of residential support, whether in a mental hospital or 'in the community'. Community services for the acute and milder forms of mental illness have by and large expanded over the post-war period. Community services for chronic, long-term mental illness, which have always been meagre, have not.[12] Hospital provision for them has been reduced, and little has been put in its place. The issue is not therefore of a reduced overall expenditure on the mentally ill to be accounted for by governmental reluctance to increase or maintain particular levels of public expenditure, though there is plenty of recent evidence of this in the last decade, but of the direction and form that expenditure has taken in the post-war period. Scull, in his concern to account for decarceration in economic terms fails to attend to the ideas, beliefs and objectives of those who formulate and implement policy, which have structured and mediated the economic concerns of the state.

24.1 The policy of community care

The first official use of the term community care apparently came in the 1930 Annual Report of the Board of Control when it was used to refer to a policy then being put forward, of making provision for the mentally handicapped to live outside hospitals wherever possible.[13] This policy paralleled that advocated by a number of nineteenth-century critics of asylums of making provision through the Poor Law system for chronic and incurable cases by boarding them out with friends or relatives under supervision. The National Association for the Promotion of Social Science had pointed to the advantages of such policies when discussing the treatment of pauper lunatics in 1869:

> Now . . . the question may properly be asked, whether . . . we cannot recur, in some degree, to the system of home care and home treatment; whether, in fact, the same care, interest, and money which are now employed upon the inmates of our lunatic asylums, might not produce even more successful and beneficial results if made to support the efforts of parents and relations in their humble dwelling. . . . If only one-twentieth of inmates of our asylums could by any machinery whatever, be restored to their relations, we should have strengthened the bonds of family affection and enlarged the sphere of individual liberty. Moreover, such a mode of treatment would form a fitting extension of the non-restraint system.[14]

Underlying these suggestions was the concern for the swelling numbers of asylum patients and the way in which chronic and incurable cases blocked up the asylums and stopped them from being real hospitals. However, in the second half of the nineteenth century the asylum was still the preferred locus of therapeutic intervention; care outside the hospital was to be a supplement to the asylum, freeing it for its proper role, not providing an alternative to it.

The policy of community care that developed in the twentieth century not only sought to free the hospital for its proper therapeutic purposes but no longer viewed the hospital as the ideal locus of treatment: the community was to be the place where treatment should take place wherever possible.The Report of the 1954–7 Royal Commission on the Law Relating to Mental Illness and Mental Deficiency (the Percy Report) marks the turning point in official policy concerning mental health services from a hospital to a community-based system of care and therapy.[15] The Commission's report, published in 1957, extended and developed the arguments of the earlier commission that a mentally disordered person should be treated where possible like a person with a physical illness. Its starting point was not, however, an assertion of the close interconnection of mental and physical illness, but the related claim that mental disorder was an illness and should be treated as such: 'Disorders of the mind are illnesses which need medical treatment.'[15]

The recommendations concerning the use of legal procedures followed from this assertion of the proper identity of mental disorder as an illness. The 1930 Mental Treatment Act had moved in the direction of treating the mentally ill on comparable terms to the physically ill by introducing the possibility of voluntary admission. But the act still required that those with mental disorder should 'be well enough to sign an application form expressing a positive wish to receive treatment'.[16] Such a formality was not required of the physically ill. The Percy Report urged, therefore, that 'the law should be altered so that whenever possible suitable care may be provided for mentally disordered patients with no more restriction of liberty or legal formality than is applied to people who need care because of other types of illness, disability or social difficulty.'[17] The Commission did not believe that compulsory powers could be entirely abandoned, but felt they should be used 'only when they are positively necessary to override the patient's own unwillingness or the unwilingness of his relatives, for the patient's own welfare or for the protection of others'.[18] They recommended, however, that the term 'certification' should no longer be used in connection with any legal procedures; instead the report spoke of 'formal' and 'informal' admission.[19]

The Commission's assertions about community care followed from the commitment to treating mental illness as an illness. Mental illness was seen as a broad category covering 'a much wider range of forms and degrees of mental disorder than the term of "unsound mind" (which it was to replace), and the appropriate form of treatment must be correspondingly diverse'.[20] As with sickness generally, in-patient treatment might not be necessary. 'The majority of mentally ill patients . . . do not need to be admitted to hospital as in-patients. Patients may receive medical treatment from general practitoners or as hospital out-patients and other care from community health and welfare services.[21] Such treatment outside the hospital was embraced under the loose term community care, a term which was not given any precise definition in the report but was used to refer to services and benefits provided by the state for the mentally ill, whether specific to them or not, which did not involve in-patient admission.

The hospital was no longer the ideal locus of care, and if admission were necessary, the patient should be discharged as soon as possible. In part this was a reiteration of the old argument of ensuring that hospitals should be used for their proper therapeutic purposes and not end up merely providing a home for those with no suitable place to live: 'Patients should not be retained as hospital in-patients when they have reached the stage sat which they could return home if they had reasonably good homes to go to.'[22] Local authorities should, therefore, take on the responsibility of providing residential accommodation for elderly mentally ill or infirm patients 'who need to be provided with a home and some help and advice but do not need psychiatric training or nursing care in hospital', as well as for others recovering from mental illness.[23] More importantly, however, the emphasis on community care involved a new model of therapeutic provision for the mentally ill in which the institution no longer had pre-eminence as the best place for the treatment. The new model of care aimed to provide services for every stage of the illness, and for prevention as well as cure: primary care facilities, acute hospital beds, hospital beds for chronic patients who still needed medical or psychiatric care, residential hostels, half-way houses, day hospitals, social work support as well as the health and welfare services more generally. This model of care contrasts very markedly with the model that underlay the establishment of the nineteenth-century asylums. It is not simply that the old asylum was now to be supplemented by a diverse range of public services that did not involve in-patient admission, but that the asylum was no longer considered the ideal therapeutic environment. Integration into the community rather than separation from it had become the new ideal.

In sum we can offer an alternative description of the policy change termed deinstitutionalisation, and an alternative explanation of it. It views the key policy change as the adoption of a new model of care for the mentally disordered, with services designed to cover all stages of the patient career and the full range of disorders, acute and chronic, severe and mild. This policy is in direct line of descent from the desire of medical reformers in the second half of the nineteenth century to encourage the early treatment of mental illness, and to transform the asylum into a mental hospital. A number of factors contributed to the adoption of this new model of care. First, the emergence of new medical ideas about the causes and treatment of mental illness undermined the support for and commitment to institutions as the desirable locus of care explicit in earlier environmentalist thinking about insanity. Second, the development of a broader range of state-funded services and benefits not only eliminated the institutional bias of the welfare system, but also increasingly made institutional care seem neither necessary nor appropriate. Third, the new model of care offered opportunities to psychiatrists for a fuller integration of their specialism with the rest of

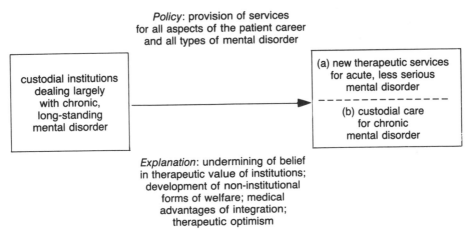

Figure 24.3

medicine and a close approximation of their practice to that of the parent discipline. Fourth, the therapeutic optimism generated by the therapeutic innovations of the 1930s, 1940s and 1950s made shorter stays in hospital and adequate outpatient care seem a practical proposition. The alternative description and explanation is set out in Figure 24.3.

Notes

1. See, for instance, Jones, K. (1960) *Mental Health and Social Policy*, Routledge and Kegan Paul, London, p. 166. Also Scull, A. (1977) *Decarceration*, Prentice-Hall, Englewood Cliffs, NJ.
2. Barton, R. (1959) *Institutional Neurosis*, John Wright, Bristol; Wing, J. (1962) 'Institutionalism in mental hospitals', *British Journal of Social and Clinical Psychology*, Vol. 1, pp. 38–51.
3. Scull, *Decarceration*, chapters 5 and 6.
4. *Scull, Decarceration*, p. 82.
5. Ibid., p. 1.
6. Ibid., p. 64.
7. Ibid., pp. 152–3.
8. Ibid., p. 135.
9. O'Connor defines a fiscal crisis as the 'tendency, for government expenditure to outrace revenues'; O'Connor, J. (1973) *The Fiscal Crisis of the State*, St James Press, London.
10. Ibid., p. 41.
11. A similar point is made by Sedgwick, P. (1982) *Psychopolitics*, Pluto Press, London, pp. 200–5.
12. Ibid., p. 213.
13. This claim is made by Hunter, R. and MacAlpine, I. (1974) *Three Hundred Years of Psychiatry*, Oxford University Press, p. 67.
14. Quoted in ibid., p. 66.
15. Royal Commission on the Law Relating to Mental Illness and Mental Deficiency (1957), p. 205.
16. Jones, *Mental Health.*, p. 128.
17. Royal Commission, pp. 3–4.
18. Ibid., p. 4.
19. Ibid., p. 133.
20. Ibid., p. 20.
21. Ibid., p. 5.
22. Ibid., p. 207.
23. Ibid., p. 211.

25

The Social Basis of Community Care*

MARTIN BULMER

'Community care' is concerned with the resources available outside formal institutional structures, particularly in the informal relationships of the family, friends and neighbours, as a means of providing care. Yet [. . .] 'community' is hardly a satisfactory term to convey the social basis of such care. No longer is its provision geographically confined to particular localities, however much this was so in the past. Some means is needed, all the same, to refer to the personal ties between those involved in informal relationships of one kind or another. The term 'social network' has come to be used extensively, as a means of relating abstract concepts such as institution or group to the activities and relations of actual people.

The concept of social network is particularly useful for the analysis and understanding of local level informal social ties, of what Clyde Mitchell in an early influential paper distinguished as personal relationships (1966, pp. 54–6). He contrasted these personal ties to institutionalised relationships at work, in a political party, a church, and so on, and to categorical relationships, as when members of different races (his examples were drawn from Southern Africa) met in the market-place and treated each other on the basis of perceived skin colour. Personal relationships are at the heart of informal care, but they are also a mainstay of local social relationships. The value of the term 'network' lies in avoiding the reification involved in talking about 'community', yet enabling one to talk about a wider set of informal relationships than just the family or the extended kin group. The set of relationships has broadened to include friends, neighbours and work associates. There has always been an analytical problem for the social scientist to find a means of portraying such relationships. 'Social network' seems to be a useful way of doing so.

*This is an abridged extract from The Social Basis of Community Care, Allen and Unwin, 1987, pp. 108–115.

'Community care', however, is a practical policy, not just a matter for detached academic debate. The pursuit of the policy has been hampered by confusing terminology, pre-eminently in the term 'community' itself. To what extent do 'social network' and associated terms such as 'social support' provide a way round these problems? This chapter examines some of these issues in the application of network analysis, and begins by looking at some instances of such use in the field of social welfare policy. This is a prelude to tracing the origins of the approach in social anthropology, and teasing out some of the analytic in sights which it can provide. Examples of applications in social welfare show that ideas of 'social network' and 'social support' have been taken up with enthusiasm, particularly but not exclusively in North America, so much so as to constitute what one recent observer has called 'a kind of romantic ideology for social work practice' (Specht, 1986, p. 219).

25.1 Social networks in community care

In discussions of provision of care and service delivery,the concept of 'social network' has come to be widely used. In Britain, the key source has been the Barclay Report on social work, published in 1982. Barclay defines 'community' as made up of 'local networks of formal and informal relationships, together with their capacity to mobilise individual and collective responses to adversity' (p. xiii). The majority of people in trouble turn first to their own families for support. If this is lacking or insufficient, people turn to wider kin, friends or neighbours, because seeking help from such informal networks is socially acceptable and seen as less of a blow than approaching officialdom. Thus help from kin, friends and neighbours is referred to as provided by informal caring networks, usually locally based.

Such usage is an application of the terminology by now common in anthropology and sociology, but it then takes on a life of its own. The Barclay Report recognised that informal networkss are complex and not always benign. If links are made between informal and formal care, formal carers need to develop detailed knowledge of informal networks and work in close understanding with them. Partnerships need to be developed between formal and informal carers. 'Caring networks in a community need to have ready access to statutory and voluntary services and to contribute their experience to decisions on how resources contributed by these services are used within their community' (Barclay Report, 1982, p. 202). The majority of social care in Britain is provided now by statutory or voluntary agencies but by individual citizens who are often linked into informal caring networks. These informal carers,

Barclay argued, need to be brought within the ambit of professional care.

Applied to social work, this meant that, although individuals or families with problems remained the centre of attention, the focus should be upon individuals within the networks of which they formed a part. 'The circle of vision is extended to include those who form, or might form, a social network into which the client is meshed. Social workers have to be able to take account of a variety of different kinds of network. These will vary in size and in the bonds which hold them together' (Barclay Report, 1982, p. 205). The social worker could make use of the networks in three ways. The first is the most obvious, moving out from an individual to the kin, friends and neighbours who constitute that person's network, to identify and map the most significant personalities in a client's life. Secondly, social workers could identify and build on the ties between those in a neighbourhood, residential home, day centre or hospital, to develop networks among people who live or spent time together. Thirdly, there was scope for developing networks among those sharing similar communities of interest or concern, for example, parents of mentally handicapped children.

The Barclay Report considered that a change was also needed in the orientation and role of social workers. What was pre-eminently required was an attitude of partnership.

> Clients, relations, neighbours and volunteers become partners with the social worker in developing and providing social care networks. We have already referred to the description of the relationship by one respondent as 'equal but different'; we might be prepared to go further and describe social workers as upholders of networks. This may make clear our view that the function of social workers is to enable, empower, support and encourage, but not usually to take over from, social networks.
>
> (Barclay Report, 1982, p. 209)

In its advocacy of community social work, Barclay was thus placing great reliance upon the notion of network and its potential for harnessing to community care. In doing so, it reflected earlier American enthusiasm for the potential of networks in promoting social care. An early paper was Collins and Pancoast's *Natural Helping Networks* (1976), which argued that natural helping networks had tremendous potential in social welfare.

> They exist as semi-permanent social structures in all cultures, in cities as well as villages, among people of every class. Their importance for social order and integration may increase rather than diminish as society becomes more complex. Networks are one of the most vital bridges between the individual and the environment. Helping networks are the informal counterpart to

organised social services, and in many areas carry the largest part of the service load.

(Collins and Pancost, 1976, pp. 28–9)

Collins and Pancost's focus was upon mutual aid, particularly among neighbours, and they saw what they called 'natural networks' as one of the key means of social support, absorbing the load which formal services could not cope with. Various techniques were suggested for harnessing these networks, one of the most important of which was the identification of what Collins and Pancost called 'central figures' or 'natural neighbours' in a locality. 'Central figures' possess sufficient psychic resources to be on top of their own life situations to be able to give to others and respond to the needs of others. Some may establish that role purely on the basis of informal personal ties – for example, the home-centred housewife who establishes links with other mothers and needy neighbours in the locality. Another way in which such nodal figures may emerge is through a particular occupational role – for example, local shopkeepers, meter readers for public utilities, local hairdressers and bar staff.

It is then suggested that social workers involved in neighbourhoods should seek to recruit such 'natural neighbours', through whom the social worker could work in the locality to draw on existing informal networks and extend them as a means of support. 'Central figures' would be encouraged to enlarge their social circle to increase the effectiveness of the social network used to provide informal care. This would bring in others previously unknown either to professionals working locally or to the 'central figure', both through personal efforts and referrals from other professionals, alongside whom the 'central figure' works. Social workers may refer other professionals to the 'central figure' to effect such introductions. Though the 'central figure' remains part of the informal system, the social worker recruiting such a person must be satisfied as to his or her competence and responsibility, for example in respecting the confidentiality of information acquired in the course of the work. In *Natural Helping Networks* both the notion of a network and the position of an individual at a key position in such a network assume central significance.

Such an approach to the analysis of informal care was taken further in work by Charles Froland and others at the Regional Research Institute for Human Services in Portland, Oregon. Their work uses the term 'helping network' more broadly

to describe a wide range of informal helping activities that staff in the agencies we studied have sought to identify, support and reinforce. . . . Emphasizing informal helping within the context of a *network* of relationships has distinct conceptual advantages to more traditional ways of viewing social relationships. The concept of network in its most general form draws our attention to the *structure* of relationships among a set of actors as well as the specific *exchanges* which take place among them and the *roles* they play with each other. Networks describe social relationships in fairly concrete terms. . . . Even the most socially isolated individuals and the most anomic communities seem to have a few relationships of this sort. We all use our networks when we need information or special assistance. In turn, our networks influence us by channeling and shaping the kinds of information we take in. They also require certain forms of reciprocation as well as the ongoing effort of maintaining the linkages. Networks are part of a sense of who we are.

(Froland *et al.*, 1981, pp. 19–20).

In an analysis of the work of social welfare agencies in providing social support through building upon networks, they identify five different strategies which may be followed. (1) A *personal networks* strategy is used by a professional worker to build upon the client's personal ties with kin, friends and neighbours, involving these signficant others in the client's problems and their resolution. In some circumstances, attempts may be made to expand the client's range of social ties and support. (2) A *volunteer linking* strategy, on the other hand, may be invoked in situations where there is limited personal support. Here, an attempt is made to match the client with volunteer supporters, not previously known to him or her, who have had personal experience of the problem the client faces or who are willing to provide help. For example, help for the physically disabled was provided in one scheme by recruiting people who could advise upon the problems of independent living in the community.

(3) *Mutual aid networks*, as a third type, aim to build peer support by bringing together people who have experienced similar problems or have comon interests. Similar in aim to self-help organisations, they are, however, informal without a charter or formal programme. Such networks may sustain existing efforts, develop new sources of support, or, in some circumstances, serve an advocacy role. Such networks can be used to promote a sense of normalisation and social integration among clients such as ex-mental patients, and in them members may give and derive support without feelings of stigma or dependency.

The last two types of network build upon geographical propinquity. (4) In *neighbourhood helping networks* agencies they seek to identify and form relationships based upon existing local networks among neighbours, key figures, and local influential people such as clergy. Their aim is to help isolated individuals, promote local mutual aid, identify local issues and promote informal social organisation, often with particular client groups in mind such as the housebound elderly, the disabled or discharged mental patients. Consultative relationships are stablished to work with neighbours to identify problems, and to encourage local residents to become involved in helping activities. It is in this type of network that the role of 'central figure' or 'natural neighbour' is most salient. It is claimed that 'staff may effectively reach an entire community through a manageable number of individuals who are central linking and referral agents within the informal social organisation of a community' (Froland *et al.*, 1981, p. 79).

Finally, (5) *community empowerment networks* aim to establish local action groups to meet local needs and provide community forums through which local opinion may be articulated and represented to policy-makers. Such an emphasis is more directly political, and involves working with neighbourhood leaders (who are not necessarily or even usually 'central figures' in informal networks), with local voluntary associations, and with opinion leaders in local business, trade unions and churches. An example is given of an agency who used such a strategy in an inner city Polish Catholic working-class neighbourhood to seek better mental health services. The aim is both to articulate the need for formal services and to show how they could, if provided, be integrated with the informal network existing in the locality.

In each of the five types of strategy, the concept of 'network' is central, as a means for understanding the informal ties that it is sought to tap or to create, and in characterising the way in which formal and informal provision can be combined. The term is central; without it the strategies could not be adequately described or contrasted with each other. The typology is useful because it broadens the reference covered by the term, and avoids equating social support with particular forms of helping such as 'natural helping networks'.

A different approach to the same set of issues, particularly salient in North American literature on mental health, is the use of networks in providing social *support*, with the emphasis upon support rather than network. A social support network may be defined as 'a set of interconnected relationships among a group of people that provides enduring patterns of nurturance in any or all forms, and provides contingent reinforcement for coping with life on a day-to-day basis' (Whittaker, 1983, p. 55).

The notion of social network has been pushed to its furthest extreme by American enthusiasts in the social work field who use the term 'networking' to refer to 'a purposeful process of linking three or more people together and of establishing connections and chain reactions among them' (Maguire, 1983, p. 13). It involves professionals working with informal helping networks in the manner described above, except that the process is conceived more actively and in more prescriptive terms.

People whose relationships or linkages with potentially helpful family and friends are tenuous can be tremendously helped by an informal networker.

The social network analyses that allow us to define clearly who should be involved in the helping network, as well as what that person can provide and when it should be provided, are all available. By learning how to analyse a network, help make connections, and support constructive chain reactions, one need not leave to chance what must be done.

(Maguire, 1983, p. 23)

Maguire suggests that the active networker starts off with the insights and tools provided by social science to map existing networks and grasp the factual situation, before adding his or her own human judgement or clinical experience to develop a practical strategy which will work in the context of a fluid system of social ties. The technique of personal networking, for example, involves phases of identification, analysis and linking, by which networkers identify potential networks, analyse them and then link the person and the network into a more dense, caring and knowledgeable support system. The networker is the intermediary between the individual and his or her network.

These are some of the more direct applications in the field of community care. Yet an immediate difficulty is apparent: what does the term 'network' actually refer to? Does it not itself become a blanket term, equivalent to saying that all people have some personal ties and close relationships, but tending to tautology? If we are all members of such networks, what is the particular significance of such networks for care? Some of the uses of 'network' just discussed raise serious problems. These difficulties become apparent if one compares these applications to the original uses of this mode of analysis in the social sciences.

References

Barclay Report (1982) *Social Workers: Their Role and Tasks*, National Institute for Social Work/Bedford Square Press, London.

Collins, A.H. and Pancoast, D.L. (1976) *Natural Helping Networks: a Strategy for Prevention*, NASW, Washington.

Froland, C., Pancoast, D.L., Chapman, N.J. and Kimboko, P.J. (1981) *Helping Networks and Human Services*, Sage, Beverly Hills.

Maguire, L. (1983) *Understanding Social Networks*, Sage, Beverly Hills.

Mitchell, C. (1966) 'Theoretical orientations in African urban studies', in Banton,M. (ed.) *The Social Anthropology of Complex Societies*, Tavistock, London.

Pilisuk, M. and Minkler, M. (1985) 'Social support: economic and political considerations', *Social Policy*, Vol. 16, No. 3, pp. 6–11.

Specht, H. (1986) 'Social support, social networks, social exchange and social work practice', *Social Service Review*, Vol. 60, No. 2, pp. 218–40.

Whittaker, J.K. (1988) 'Mutual helping in human service practice', in Whittaker, J.K., and Gabarino, J. (eds) *Social Support Networks: Informal Helping in the Human Services*, Aldine, New York.

26

Concepts of Normalisation*

JOANNA RYAN and FRANK THOMAS

From quite different sources an ideology of 'normalization' has become current, emphasising the importance of the total environment and how institutional environments particularly contribute greatly to the burden of being handicapped. The so-called 'normalisation principle' has become the guiding philosophy of those who argue that mentally handicapped people should not live in hospitals of any kind. This principle would, according to one of its leading Scandinavian proponents, make available to all mentally handicapped people 'patterns of life and conditions of everyday living which are as close as possible to the regular circumstances and ways of society'. Similarly, CMH [Campaign for People with Mental Handicaps, now called Values Into Action] argues that the aim of services for mentally handicapped people should be to enable them to lead 'as normal a life as possible'. This includes a normal rhythm of days, weeks and years, normal-sized living units, adequate privacy, normal access to social, emotional and sexual relationships with others, normal growing-up experiences, the possibility of decently paid work, choice and participation in decisions affecting their future.

The needs of mentally handicapped people are seen as basically similar to those of ordinary people, with the difference that they may not be able to meet these needs unaided or as independently as other people can, and that they may have additional special needs, such as specific medical or therapeutic requirements. It is argued that these additional needs do not mean that mentally handicapped people have to live separately from others, or that the special services they need must be provided in the place where they live (as in hospital) but could be met through the general medical and social services, as are other people's special requirements.

*This is an abridged extract from the *Politics of Mental Handicap*, Free Association Books, London, 1987, second revised edition, pp.128–136.

'Normalisation' can mean many different things to different people and it has other advocates who see it as quite compatible with a sufficiently reformed hospital life. Doctors and psychologists arguing for changes within the hospital system often adopt such a position. Thus, Gunzburg, an influential advocate of moderate change, propounds the idea of the hospital as a normalising environment: 'An intensive training environment which whilst not normal in itself will nevertheless help to normalise people.' He sees the mentally handicapped as having 'deficiencies in living skills'. In providing them with 'normal living experiences', both formally and informally, the hospital should enable them to practise 'normal skills of living' and thus become more acceptable outside.

Another advocate of hospital reform, Day, says: 'Normalisation of the physical environment is essential to a personalized approach to care and a normal living routine, and it is now accepted that residents of all ability levels should live in small groups in a substitute home environment.' Behind this approach to the physical environment lies the philosophy that 'treating the mentally handicapped person as an individual is a most important aspect of the normal approach to care' – an acknowledgement that to date the mentally handicapped have not been treated as individuals. Day sees this normalisation being achieved not just by a much greater flexibility of ward regimes, but also by the increased development of mentally handicapped people as the consumers of goods and leisure activities – clothing and television, for instance – an idea which crudely encapsulates contemporary notions of the value and functioning of the lifestyle in society.

A similar commitment to a normal lifestyle 'within the community' is one of the principles on which the recent Jay report is based, the other principles being their right to be treated as individuals, and their right to obtain additional help from the community in which they and from professional services. From these principles come the recommendations for a flexible system of small-group living, and an end to the domination of nursing care.

These views of 'normalisation' entail a much greater degree of integration of mentally handicapped people with the rest of society than exists now. From such a standpoint life in a hospital can never be normal.

In examining the arguments for extensive normalisation of the lives of mentally handicapped people, it can be seen that the common basis is a claim to humanity which they share with the non-handicapped. Nirje, for example, states as part of his argument for the 'normalisation principle' that 'A person is a person first, the handicap is secondary.' Another advocate of normalisation maintains '. . . these are ordinary people who must have rights and duties similar to those of every other citizen.' And a popular pamphlet published by CMH and MIND claims:

The important thing is that mentally handicapped people are *people*. Everyone enjoys being with friends and joining in what's going on as far as they can. Everyone gets sad and bored and angry if they feel alone. Mentally handicapped people don't feel any differently just because their brains learn more slowly.

Statements such as these are conspicuously missing from the proposals of various professional-interest groups, such as doctors and nurses, who tend to see mentally handicapped people much more in terms of their abnormalities and needs for special services. It is true that the normalisation arguments run a risk of idealising the common humanity which, it is claimed, exists between mentally handicapped people and the rest of society. Insufficient attention is paid to the difficulty of recognising, valuing and sharing this common humanity. However, it is not the case, as some critics argue, that these arguments deny the existence of any handicap at all; the CMH proposals, for example, demonstrate a full understanding of the special problems that mentally handicapped people may encounter and of particular kinds of help and treatment they may need (for example, assistance with money for those earning wages, help with choices, wheelchair access to buildings, support in confronting a difficult and hostile world, special technical aids, advice about relationships).

26.1 Rights to normality

A frequent claim is made by those arguing for various forms of 'normalisation' is that mentally handicapped people have a *right* to normality. Given the degree of exclusion from society that mentally handicapped people have suffered, the abnormality that has been forced upon them, gaining this right in a concrete way would be a momentous achievement, and one which we are very far from achieving. However, 'normalisation' and the 'right to normality' cannot be accepted uncritically. Such arguments often have a very unquestioning attitude to the normality that is proclaimed as a right. Conventional and conformist lifestyles can be imposed on mentally handicapped people in the name of normality, standards that are almost an exaggeration of normality. Thus 'normalisation' within the hospital is often seen as recreating the family: 'Residents are encouraged to undertake the roles they would have in a normal family, the women doing the domestic chores and assisting in the day-to-day care of the children and the men going out to work.'
Normalisation can mean much greater pressure on mentally handicapped people to adjust to prevailing customs and standards. Nirje describes it as involving a better adjustment to society'. It does not necessarily mean that 'normality' will adjust to fit them. Many of the

normalization arguments are very humane, in the sense that by the standards of the immediate past, they propose a great amelioration in the conditions of life for many handicapped people. What they seldom do, however, is raise the question of how we, the normal society into which mentally handicapped people are supposed to become more integrated, are likely to respond to this, or what changes are going to be demanded of us. The normalisation proposals simply suppose that as mentally handicapped people become more normal, or their lives resemble those of most other people more, they will be more acceptable and accepted. There is a very real basis for this supposition: sub-human living conditions make the people in them seem sub-human too, but the full implications of these proposals are seldom followed through. It is often left to those who are most hostile to the ideas of 'normalisation' to question whether the 'community' is willing to accept more mentally handicapped people amongst them or to do more than passively tolerate them.

The assertion that mentally handicapped people should have equal rights with all other citizens often has a hollow ring to it. The UN declaration of the rights of mentally handicapped people, which includes their right to special services and adequate care and treatment, simply poses the question: who is going to implement these rights and how? There is always a danger with equal rights arguments that existing material, psychological and cultural inequalities are overlooked. (For example, a right to equal pay for women is of little concrete benefit if there are no available jobs, or no adequate provision for child-care so that women could actually work at such jobs.) With mentally handicapped people, we have to ensure that they are actually able to use any improved opportunities that they are presented with. If, for example, their right to ordinary housing is accepted, if they are provided with ordinary houses and flats to live in, we also have to ensure that there is adequate human and social support for them to do so. If we try to make available a wider range of life-experiences for them, a greater degree of choice of occupation, of friends, of leisure activities, we have to ensure that these experiences are not overwhelmingly negative for them, that they are not teased, ignored or badly treated at work, on the street, in public places. Implementation of such rights would make great demands on the attitudes and responses of the increased number of people who would, either voluntarily or accidentally, come into contact with mentally handicapped people.

The implementation of these rights for mentally handicapped people would undoubtedly require more money being spent on them. This question of financial cost is one which many reforming groups have often dodged; some have tried to prove that their proposals would not cost any more than present arrangmeents. Others have argued that within the terms of welfare economics, increased investment in the

training of mentally handicapped people would bring long-term economic benefits from the wages they would eventually earn and their
contribution to the total economy thereby. It is not surprising that
people engage in such cost-effectiveness arguments, particularly in an
era of cuts in social welfare spending.

Whilst mental handicap services were made a relative priority within
the National Health Service in 1975, a recent statement by the minister
responsible, in an introduction to the NDG report on hospitals, is hardly
encouraging: he will support any changes that do not cost money. The
Jay report tackles this issue head on: their proposals would undoubtedly
cost more in the short term, since they require a doubling in the number
of staff needed.They argue that increased spending is essential if there is
to be any radical change at all, and that we should make a commitment
at the level of national priorities to this. Despite the figures provided by
this and other reports, they cannot be taken at face value as representing
the actual cost of implementing the various proposals. They do not take
into account any long-term economic benefits that might come from the
much greater participation of mentally handicapped people in the life of
the nation, and the savings in costs made by, for example, providing
adequate domiciliary support to the many families who now have to
hospitalise their children for lack of any other alternative. And models
that might take these consequences into account (like similar models of
the economics of education) are notorious for the large number of
untestable assumptions that have to be built into them.

These arguments also assume that mentally handicapped people will
accept the normalisation of their lives. There is little doubt, judging from
the expressed opinions of the people that have been asked, that they
would welcome a lessening of the enforced abnormalities and depriva-
tions in their lives, and a chance to experience at least some of the
choices that most ordinary people take for granted. However, we also
have to allow for the possibility that mentally handicapped people may
wish to question and reject some of the more exploitative and oppressive standards of our society, just as many non-handicapped people do.
Many people choose to live in various unconventional ways, for example, in communes in the country, or shared households in the city, to
reject certain standards of conventional dress and typical sex-role
behaviour, and mentally handicapped people may wish to do so too. If
the 'right to normality' is not to become a whole series of pressures on
mentally handicapped people to change and conform to other people's
standards, then this right must include both the right and the means to
question that normality, and to live a different life, one that is an
enrichment rather than an deprivation of 'normality'.

Mental Health Services in the Twenty-first Century: The User– Professional Divide?

DAVID PILGRIM

27.1 Introduction

By the turn of the twenty-first century, Western psychiatry will have endured forty years of sustained criticism. From internal professional dissenters and academics it will have been attacked for its crude and illogical illness model (Szasz, 1964; Boyle, 1990); its dehumanising prac- tices (Laing, 1967); its social control role (Basaglia, 1980); and its brain- damaging treatments (Hill, 1985). Its preferred hospital base will have been condemned as inhuman, degrading and disabling in its large institutional form (Goffman, 1961; Martin, 1985) and in its transformed guise of the district general hospital (DGH) acute psychiatric unit (Baruch and Treacher, 1978). All of these criticisms influenced, and were incorporated into, the emergent new social movements of critical patients in alliance with sympathetic professionals, in various countries, during the 1970s and 1980s: the Netherlands (Haafkens *et al.*, 1986); the USA (Chamberlin, 1990); Canada (Burstow and Weitz, 1988); Italy (Ramon and Giannechedda, 1988); and, eventually, Britain (Rogers and Pilgrim, 1991).

In the light of the above summary, psychiatry's crisis may be its users opportunity. What the split or tension between professional tradition and patient resistance highlights is that mental health services can be organised broadly to serve one but not the other group's interests. In this short article, I want to rehearse two possible futures: one that is user-friendly and one that instead serves the interests of professional power, social order and drug company profits. So that this is not merely yet another critique of, or polemic against, psychiatry, I first want to base my arguments on some empirical data. For reasons of space the latter can only be given in summary and selected form – literally as a list of key relevant findings. The list is taken from the People First survey I and others conducted in collaboration with national MIND in 1990. (A fuller version of the methodology and findings can be found in Rogers *et al.*, 1992. This provides numerous quotes from users which space does not permit here.)

The People First survey entailed sending a detailed (250-item) questionnaire out to 1,000 users of psychiatric services. About one-third of the items were open-ended questions generating qualitative data to augment and clarify the type of frequencies listed below. All of the 516 respondents who completed and returned the questionnaire had had one or more inpatient stays, with 120 of them having seven or more admissions. In other words, they were genuine users of the full range of services provided by psychiatry and its allied professions. For the purpose of this article the following findings are pertinent:

Hospital-centred practices. Hospital-based staff, supposedly helping the patient's return to the community, halved their contact following discharge. Even those staff specifically designated to work in the community (social workers and community psychiatric nurses) saw significantly less of patients out of hospital than in. Of patients' last day centre attendances 57 per cent had been on hospital site. And yet, the further away from hospital the interventions were the better they were rated by patients.

Professionals damned by faint praise. Only 11.8 per cent thought that the most helpful aspect of day-patient attendances was contact with staff (compared with 25.4 per cent most valuing contact with other patients). This trend was the same for attendance at occupational and industrial therapy. Inpatients found nurses the most helpful staff 30 per cent of the time and least helpful 10 per cent of the time. Psychiatrists were the least favoured, with respective figures of 11 and 21 per cent.

Poor informed consent. Nearly half the sample had been detained compulsorily at some time, with 83.3 per cent never having been offered an alternative to hospital. At admission, 56.6 per cent were not informed of their diagnosis and 63 per cent lacked a satisfactory explanation for why they were admitted. Forty-three per cent were given major tranquillisers against their wishes. Of those taking anti-depressants 71.5 per cent had never been asked their consent.

The dominance of physical treatments. Ninety-eight per cent had been prescribed drugs; 80 per cent had been prescribed major tranquillisers and 75 per cent anti-depressants. Nearly half had had electroconvulsive therapy (ECT), of whom 98.5 per cent complained of side-effects. Eighty-five had never been offered any alternative to the treatment they were given.

Lack of information. Only 38 per cent of those given major tranquillisers were told their purpose, and only 32 per cent were told of their potential side-effects. Of those taking anti-depressants 70 per cent had been told nothing about their potential side-effects (which were experienced by half of this group).

Poverty. Of the sample 83.6 per cent were on one or more welfare benefits. Only 16.3 per cent were in full-time employment. Nearly half of the sample had been on statutory benefits for more than five years.

27.2 Transporting the medical model into the community

Now that some of the main findings of the People First survey have been presented, let us consider what their implications are for the two competing futures I outlined at the outset.

The data suggest that whether or not they are liked by their recipients, late twentieth-century psychiatric interventions are centred on the hospital and are dominated by drugs and ECT. These are the very targets that professional and user critics of psychiatry have been shooting at since the Second World War. A related trend, which has also been the focus of criticism yet is clearly still strongly present in psychiatric practice, is the enforcement of treatment. Let us now consider these three features (the hospital, physical treatments and lack of informed consent) in more detail.

27.2.1 The role of the hospital

The data highlight the fact that despite the gradual removal of the large Victorian psychiatric institutions, comunity care has not actually diverted psychiatry much from its traditional patterns. The shift of resources from the large old Victorian hospital to making the district general hospital the focus of medical activity is symptomatic of psychiatry's inability to work without a territorial base. By moving to the DGH unit, psychiatrists have retained their power over clients by emphasising inpatient work. In many ways these units are more restrictive and repressive than the older hospitals. They typically have low ceilings and patients may be deterred from roaming on to general medical wards by having to wear pyjamas. (This actually compares unfavourably with the spacious grounds of the older institutions.) Also note from the data how even other services, such as day-patient appointments, have been dominated by hospital sites. The extent of hospital-centred funding of mental health services is highlighted by the fact that in 1979 12 pence in the pound of state finance on mental health was spent on non-hospital services. This had only risen to 15 pence in the pound by 1989 (Sayce, 1990). As far as mental health was concerned, by 1990 comunity care still meant hospital-orientated services.

27.2.2 Physical treatment

Despite modern textbooks suggesting to their readers that psychiatry has become more eclectic (for example Clare, 1977), the data above demonstrate that drugs and ECT are still the dominant responses to emotional distress. Perhaps the most worrying aspect of this is the lack of information and alternatives offered on average. Also the amount of polypharmacy (taking more than one drug concurrently) evident from the respondents provides evidence that patients are vulnerable to the side-effects of not only one set of drugs but many in interaction with one another. These interaction effects are understood by the medical profession to be dangerous, yet in practice psychiatrists commonly impose polypharmacy on patients (Edwards and Kumar, 1984; Johnson and Wright, 1990). Although ECT understandably causes anxiety and anger in many of its recipients, and prospective recipients, probably major tranquillisers represent the largest iatrogenic scandal in modern psychiatry. They are effective only in a minority of cases (Bentall *et al.*, 1988) and yet they expose all of their recipients to the dangers of irreversible movement disorders (tardive dyskinesia). The longer they are prescribed, the higher the chances of this iatrogenic effect occurring. For the many patients who are prescribed them on a long-term basis (as slow-release depot injections), the risk is very high.

27.2.3 Informed consent

The data describe two problems in relation to coercion. First, pressure from others is clearly widespread, even in those who are technically voluntary patients (in legal terms of 'informal status'). Second, the very fact that patients are so rarely given any alternatives to a hospital admission and physical treatments itself constitutes a form of coercion – one choice is no choice. The whole question of enforced treatment raised its head in 1988 when the Royal College of Psychiatrists sought, without success, to have the 1983 Mental Health Act modified to include the enforcement of 'community treatment orders'. The Act and its predecessors only permitted forced treatment in hospitals. The move to introduce the orders revealed the Royal College's attitude towards a respect for voluntary relationships with patients. The third dimension to this problem is shown in the data on satisfaction with information about treatment. Most patients were not happy about information given to them by psychiatrists. Generally medical practitioners rationalise this withholding of information on paternalistic grounds (that they want to avoid 'worrying the patient'). Were physical treatments effective and benign this paternalism would have its merits. However, as was discussed above, in psychiatry drugs are poorly effective yet they are highly dangerous. In such circumstances, full information to patients is particularly warranted.

The prospect of services dominated by the above three characteristics looks, at the time of writing, to be a distinct possibility for the twenty-first century. Resources and professional practices are still bound up with hospitals (as the figures quoted from Sayce earlier indicated). The dominant discourse of 'mental illness' still pervades the way not only professionals but also lay people think about emotional difficulties. The drug companies are still profiting greatly from the medical professions' virtual exclusive reliance on their products for treatment. However, this dominant picture remains problematic. Anti-psychiatry (the critique of coercive biological psychiatry by internal dissenters) in one sense is a thing of the past. In another sense its mantle and concerns have been taken over by disaffected users. The latter now seem to represent a permanent opposition to medical theory and practice and thereby constitute a 'new social movement' (Rogers and Pilgrim, 1991).

27.3 A user-friendly future?

In a recent critical review of mental health policy in Britain Goodwin (1990) makes the point that government after government has made the mistake of believing that psychiatric practice is sound and effective. The rise of the users' movement and the survey data signals clearly that Goodwin's conclusion is well founded. The point here is that, as with other aspects of health policy, if governments rely for their opinion on the medical profession then they will inevitably endorse medically preferred policies.

One of the paradoxes of the conflict about the long Conservative administration's attitude towards the National Health Service (between 1979 and 1991) is that a user-led ideology was introduced for the first time by government. For its part, the Labour opposition focused, as it had done since 1948, on the resourcing and ownership of the health care system. What Labour had not done was challenge medical experts. Quite the reverse – their position was to see medical professionals as harbingers of progress. By contrast, as part of a wider restructuring of welfare provision, a political project of the Thatcher administrations was to challenge or undermine traditional power elites, like the mature professions of medicine and law. The Conservatives of the 1980s wanted to bring these groups to heel, by strengthening their accountability to state managers on the one hand and deregulating their services on the other. Some doctors were given more powers in the government reforms. However, generally, as the British Medical Association reaction showed, the Conservative government was recognised by doctors for what it was: an enemy of traditional medical authority in health care decision-making (Strong and Robinson, 1990).

One consequence of the 'consumerist' emphasis from the right was that a new discourse emerged, which even political opponents had to join. By 1990 the cross-party talk was of 'user-friendliness' and 'quality assurance' in welfare provision. Whilst the Conservatives still pinned their hopes for this on the 'mixed economy' and the discipline of business and market principles to serve the consumer, Labour (in opposition) favoured democratic accountability and efficient manage- ment in a better financed state system. In particular regard to mental health, the Labour Party, after intense lobbying from users' groups, began to acknowledge the problems of psychotropic drugs and advo- cated the greater availability of psychological interventions.

This new political ambivalence about professionally defined policies creates an opportunity for a more user-friendly service. Our data sug- gest that such a service would have the following characteristics, which can be seen to be virtually the inverse of the first scenario above.

27.3.1   Ordinary living

The data make it clear that the further recipients are away from hospital, the more they like their lives. Hospital interventions are not user- friendly. They are associated generally with an oppressive or distressing experience. If patients and prospective patients are to live as normally as possible in the community, the implications are that service *options* should be available in that setting. These would include crisis houses, outreach work and 24-hour, seven-days-a-week crisis intervention teams, counselling, drop-in centres and day centres housing a variety of activities. The availability of a range of affordable housing options about which service users had genuine choice would be central to a non- hospital-based service. The data on welfare benefits show that mental health policy and employment and housing policy cannot be separated.

27.3.2 Benign treatment

Basically, users are tired of physical treatments being the typical offer made to them when they have problems. Drugs cause unwanted side-effects and do not solve or address personal or social difficulties in the patient's life. They may be convenient for doctors, but they are not welcomed by their recipients most of the time. What service users would prefer, in the main, is a sympathetic ear. Sometimes this is expressed as a need for formal counselling or psychotherapy as an alternative to drugs; at other times it is only a plea for the patient to be listened to and resepected. Respectfulness entails being taken seriously and having one's experience recognised as being meaningful. The traditional psychiatric interview often violates both of these principles. The patient's account is only taken in order to make a diagnosis or to check on whether or not prescribed drugs are working. By definition, the symptoms of mental illness are not recognised as meaningful because they represent pathology. For those distrustful even of psychological treatments, the service could provide the option of contact with other patients for fellowship as a worthy goal in itself. This could also involve facilities being used to house self-help groups.

27.3.3 Voluntary relationships

Psychiatric patients, being human, are no more welcoming of loss of liberty, or their bodies being interfered with without consent, than anybody else. A user-friendly service would minimise or eliminate coercion. It would also emphasise informed consent at every moment in a professional–patient relationship. Whenever professionals withhold information that is relevant to the patient's life, such as that concerning the dangers of prescribed drugs or psychological treatment, then the service is professionally led, not user-centred. Also, as was noted previously, voluntary relationships can only be encouraged in a context in which genuine choices are on offer to the patient. Where no choice exists, then the person is trapped by the sole offer being made by professionals.

Finally, there is the problem of predicting one or other of these two broad scenarios. Despite governments responsible for social policy formation now being sensitised to the 'view from below' of welfare clients, this is offset by other considerations. If medical–psychiatric dominance were to be subverted genuinely by government, then the advantages it has traditionally offered, particularly the role of policing the population and smoothing out infractions of rules in everyday life, would be jeopardised. Under the hammer of the Conservative administrations of the 1980s, medical elites were shaken and angered, but not broken. Their culturally accepted authority at all levels in society remains evident. Politicans of all hues still defer to doctors to identify the 'clinical needs' of 'their' patients. This reinforces the tradition of paternalism in welfare provision in which professionals 'know best' and patients are not expected to speak for themselves. As yet, there is only a weak sign that the national or local state is prepared to ask the people directly what their needs are. The users' movement has its work cut out at the turn of the century. In particular its success will hinge on allying itself successfully with that minority of professionals who themselves genuinely want to shift power to users.

References

Baruch, G. and Treacher, A. (1978) *Psychiatry Observed*, Routledge, London.

Basaglia, F. (1980) 'Breaking the circuit of control', in Ingleby, D. (ed.) *Critical Psychiatry*, Penguin, Harmondsworth.

Bentall, R.P., Jackson, H. and Pilgrim, D. (1988) 'Abandoning the concept of schizophrenia: some implications for validity arguments in studying psychotic phenomena', *British Journal of Clinical Psychology*, Vol. 27, pp. 303–24.

Boyle, M. (1990) *Schizophrenia: a Scientific Delusion*? Routledge, London.

Burstow, B. and Weitz, D. (eds) (1988) *Shrink Resistant: the Struggle Against Psychiatry in Canada*, New Star Books, Vancouver.

Chamberlin, J. (1990) *On Our Own*, MIND, London.

Clare, A. (1977) *Psychiatry in dissent*, Tavistock, London.

Edwards, S. and Kumar, V. (1984) 'A survey of prescribing of psychotropic drugs in a Birmingham psychiatric hospital', *British Journal of Psychiatry*, Vol. 145, pp. 502–7.

Goffman, E. (1961) *Asylums: Essays on the Social Situation of Mental Patients and Other Inmates*, Penguin, London.

Haafkens, J., Nijhof, G. and van der Poel, E. (1986) 'Mental health care and the opposition movement in the Netherlands', *Social Science and Medicine*, Vol. 22, No. 2, pp. 18592.

Goodwin, S. (1990) *Community Care and the future of Mental Health Srvice Provision*, Avebury, Aldershot.

Hill, D. (1985) *The Politics of Schizophrenia: Psychiatric Oppression in the United States of America*, University Press of America, Lanham.

Johnson, D. and Wright, N. F. (1990) 'Drug prescribing for schizophrenic outpatients on depot injections: repeat surveys over 18 years', *British Journal of Psychiatry*, Vol. 156, pp. 827–34.

Laing, R. D. (1967) *The Politics of Experience and the Bird of Paradise*, Penguin, Harmondsworth.

Martin, J. P. (1985) *Hospitals in Trouble*, Blackwell, Oxford.

Ramon, S. and Giannechedda, M. (eds) (1988) *Psychiatry in Transition: the British and Italian Experiences*, Pluto Press, London.

Rogers, A. and Pilgrim, D. (1991) ' "Pulling down churches": accounting for the British mental health users' movement', *Sociology of Health and Illness*, Vol. 13, No. 2, pp. 129–48.

Rogers, A., Pilgrim, D. and Lacey, R. (1992) *Experiencing Psychiatry: Users' View of Services*, Macmillan, London.

Sayce, L. (1990) *Waiting for Community Care*, MIND, London.

Strong, P. and Robinson, J. (1990) *The NHS Under New Management*, Open University Press, Milton Keynes.

Szasz, T.S. (1964) *The Myth of Mental Illness*, Harper and Row, New York.

PART IV

PRACTICE

28

Introduction

This section of the Reader brings together a collection of articles and documents that relate to community care practice. You will find charters of rights, programmes of action, accounts from paid workers in the statutory and voluntary sector, accounts from users and analyses of policies and projects. Some are personal accounts of problems solved and problems overcome. Some work through issues from a more detached stance, reviewing and discussing. What they all share is a focus on the dilemmas of resolving issues raised by the need for sensitive and acceptable provision of care and support for people living in the community.

'Good practice' sometimes raises the spectre of inadequacy and guilt feelings among workers and carers. None of the pieces included here has been selected for reasons of prescription. Our aim is to provide examples that can be drawn on as a basis for reflection as well as information. Susan Goff, a social worker, highlights the dilemma of deciding who is the client; in this case, is it an older woman, or is it her carer son? Christina Schwabenland, the director of a small voluntary organisation, takes us along the rocky path to becoming a contracted provider for a local authority. The process results in changes for her organisation, the users, the paid care staff and the local authority itself.

The anthology of charters includes demands for what sounds much like basic human rights: 'personal privacy' (Southwark Social Services residential and specialist day care); the right to 'lead their lives as and where they wish as full participants in their communities' (The Royal Association for Disability and Rehabilitation); 'Recognition of their contribution' ('A ten-point plan for carers'); and 'Full and free access to all personal medical records' (Survivors Speak Out). That they require formulation at all is at once recognition of the rights of users and, at the same time, recognition of the failure of many services to acknowledge issues of equity and choice in the delivery of care and support. Each raises issues for practice, for paid and unpaid carers as much as for other professionals and policy-makers.

Most of the samples of practice selected have a wider reference and significance. For example, Andrea Whittaker's approach to involving people with learning difficulties in meetings can be read from a number of points of view: from the user's perspective; from a chair-person's perspective; from an advocate's perspective; from the per-spective of an older person or a carer; from the perspective of some-one with hearing impairment; or from the perspective of a potential service purchaser. Paul Henderson and John Armstrong link com-munity care with community development in an article that has rele-vance for community workers, care professionals, care planners and care users.

Ann Macfarlane, in 'The right to make choices', takes over the role of broker herself. As a disabled person who feels that she has the right to manage her own affairs, she describes how she and her friend, Jane Campbell, hire their own personal assistance. Practical issues of repre-sentation, access to resources, personnel recruitment and budget man-agement are all confronted in her account. Her careful explanation will raise for other users the question of whether or not their solution is acheivable for everyone. For the wider community it raises the issue of choosing between cash or care.

Articles that provide a framework for comparison across a range of different contexts and practice situations include Lesley Hoyes and Robin Means', 'Markets, contracts and social care services: prospects and problems'. They discuss the outcomes of social care policies that focus on the market as the basis of provision. Their arguments raise questions about the implication of these policies for those who do not have equal access to market information or whose powers as consumers may be restricted by mobility or increasing frailty. In such cases the skills of brokers or care managers working in differing contexts may have to be well developed and sensitively used, or possibly exercised on behalf of someone, to provide the user with an advocate.

Tim Dant and Brian Gearing look at three different examples of case management projects. Their comparison raises issues for resourcing, advocacy and keyworking with vulnerable people living in the commun-ity.

The articles in this final section of the reader are led by Len Doyal's argument for 'Human need and the moral right to optimal community care'. This philosophical treatment introduces moral questions to debates around need and provision. At a time when community care decision-making tends to be framed by notions of targeting, budget management and cost-effectiveness, his humanistic perspective presents an encouraging refocus.

29

Anthology: Charters

Compiled by JOANNA BORNAT

This anthology includes criteria for good practice, statements of needs, a Declaration of Rights and a Declaration of Intent as well as charters. These different descriptions reflect the varied perspectives of users, activists, workers and professionals. Reading through these documents reveals common themes, formats and language. Rights, communication, support, consultation are just a few. At the same time, each statement demarcates a defined population, and its particular needs and demands. Inevitably it raises difficult issues, for example the tension between plurality and collective responsibility, the possible contradiction between different sets of demands. This sharing of common forms and language while at the same time fragmenting into a plurality of self-determining interest groups mirrors the image of community care practice and policy in the 1990s.

Survivors Speak Out is an organisation for people who use psychiatric services. The Charter of Needs was unanimously agreed at their 1987 national conference.

The national conference of psychiatric system survivors held on September 18–20 1987, unanimously agreed the following list of needs and demands:

1. That mental health service providers recognise and use people's first hand experience of emotional distress for the good of others.
2. Provision of refuge, planned and under the control of survivors of psychiatry.
3. Provision of free counselling for all.
4. Choice of services, including self-help alternatives.
5. A Government review of services, with recipients sharing their views.
6. Provision of resources to implement self-advocacy for all users.
7. Adequate funding for non-medical community services, especially crisis intervention.
8. Facility for representation of users and ex-users of services on

statutory bodies, including Community Health Councils, Mental Review Health Tribunals and the Mental Health Act Commission.
9. Full and free access to all personal medical records.
10. Legal protection and means of redress for all psychiatric patients.
11. Establishment of the democratic right of staff to refuse to administer any treatment, without risk of sanction or prejudice.
12. The phasing out of electro-convulsive therapy and psycho-surgery.
13. Independent monitoring of drug use and its consequences.
14. Provision for all patients for full written and verbal information on treatments, including adverse resarch findings.
15. An end to discrimination against people who receive, or have received, psychiatric services: with particular regard to housing, employment, insurance etc.

---

*Extract from the **Royal Association for Disability and Rehabilitation (RADAR) 1991 policy statements.** RADAR is a national organisation working with and for physically disabled people to remove architectural, economic and attitudinal barriers. RADAR is particularly involved in the areas of education, employment, mobility, health social services, housing and social security.*

Community care and independent living

Principles

1. Disabled people have the right to lead their lives as and where they wish as full participants in their communities.
2. Social Services Departments should be responsible for ensuring that co-ordinated programmes of support are available to disabled people.
3. Disabled people know best what their needs are and should therefore play an active role in drawing up their programme of support.
4. Disabled people have the right to use the services of an advocate or authorised representative.

In accordance with the above principles RADAR seeks to ensure that:

there is a structure of social service provision which enables disabled people to organise their lives as they wish and to receive the support they need in whatever environment they have chosen;
the Disabled Persons (Service, Consultation and Representation) Act 1986 is implemented in full;
comprehensive information is made available to disabled people concerning social and other community services and disabled people are enabled to make their own choices;

disabled people receive all the services to which they are entitled;
services are properly co-ordinated and that awareness of available services is
promoted by voluntary organisations.

---

*Southwark Social Services Residential and Specialist Day Care Charter of
Rights. The London Borough of Southwark Social Services Department has drawn
up its own Charter of Rights for residents and users of services.*

1. Residents have the right to control their own financial affairs.
2. Residents have the right to the same access to facilities and service in their surrounding community, as any other citizen.
3. Residents have the right to be given every opportunity of mixing with other people in the community.
4. Residents have the right to personal privacy.
5. Residents have the right to have their personal dignity respected.
6. Residents have the right to care for themselves.
7. Residents have the right to have their emotional, cultural, religious and sexual needs accepted and respected.
8. Residents have the right to look after their own medications.
9. Residents have the right to personal independence, choice and responsibility for their own actions.
10. Residents have the right to participate in a regular review of their needs at a period not exceeding 1 year.
11. Residents have the right to take a full part, in any decisions about daily living arrangements within the home.
12. Residents have the right of access to and where necessary assistance to contact:
    - the locally elected councillor
    - the local member of parliament
    - Age Concern
    - Help the Aged
    - Pensioners' Forum
13. Residents have the right to have any comments thoroughly investigated and resolved, to their satisfaction.
14. Residents have the right to request a move to another form of accommodation.

---

*A **Ten-point Plan for Carers** was drawn up by carers' organisations supporting the
King's Fund Carers' Project.*

Carers are people who are looking after elderly, ill or disabled relatives
or friends who cannot manage at home without help. They may be the

parents of a child with a mental handicap, a husband whose wife has a physical disability or a daughter looking after her frail elderly mother.

Carers come from all racial, ethnic and religious backgrounds. Their circumstances vary enormously, with the severity of the condition of the person cared for, their economic circumstances and the overall help and support available. The majority of carers are women and many carry out the tasks of caring completely on their own.

Carers are deeply concerned about the needs of the people they care for; services need to be planned for and with them.

Carers need

1. **Recognition of their contribution** and of their own needs as individuals in their own right.
2. **Services tailored to their individual circumstances,** needs and views, through discussions at the time help is being planned.
3. **Services which reflect an awareness of differing racial, cultural and religious backgrounds and values,** equally accessible to carers of every race and ethnic origin.
4. **Opportunities for a break**, both for short spells (an afternoon) and for longer periods (a week or more), to relax and have time to themselves.
5. **Practical help** to lighten the tasks of caring, including domestic help, home adaptations, incontinence services and help with transport.
6. **Someone to talk to** about their own emotional needs, at the outset of caring, while they are caring and when the caring task is over.
7. **Information** about available benefits and services as well as how to cope with the particular condition of the person cared for.
8. **An income which covers the costs of caring** and which does not preclude carers taking employment or sharing care with other people.
9. **Opportunities to explore alternatives to family care**, both for the immediate and long-term future.
10. **Services designed through consultation** with carers, at all levels of policy planning.

The National Pensioners' Convention Declaration of Intent. The National Pensioners Convention is an organisation of older people which includes amongst its affiliates the major pensioner organisations, charities, pressure groupos and trade-union-based pensioner organisations. The Declaration of Intent aims to improve the quality of life of retired people, and:

Declares that pensioners should have the right to:

1. an adequate State Retirement Pension of not less than one third of average gross earnings for a single person and one half for a married couple
2. live in accommodation which is appropriate to personal needs and circumstances with a reasonable degree of choice, including sheltered housing
3. be able to call on the full range of community and personal services to give full support as needs arises, e.g., Home Help, Meals on Wheels, chiropody, television and telephone
4. be able to use a national scheme of substantial concessionary facilities on all public transport in all parts of the country
5. have ready access to comprehensive free health care on demand.

The UK Declaration of the Rights of people with HIV and AIDS.

Preface

This declaration is made by people with HIV and AIDS and by organisations dedicated to their welfare. The Declaration lists rights which all citizens of the United Kingdom, including people with HIV and AIDS, enjoy under international law; the Declaration then prescribes measures and recommends practices which the writers of the Declaration believe are the minimum necessary to ensure that these rights are respected and protected within the United Kingdom.

The Declaration

All citizens of the United Kingdom, including people with HIV and AIDS, are accorded the following rights under international law:

- the right to liberty and security of person
- the right to privacy
- the right to freedom of movement
- the right to work

- the right to housing, food, social security, medical assistance and welfare
- the right to freedom from inhumane or degrading treatment
- the right to equal protection of the law and protection from discrimination
- the right to marry
- the right to found a family
- the right to education.

These rights exist in international treaties which the United Kingdom Government has agreed to uphold. But these rights, as they apply to United Kingdom citizens with HIV and AIDS, have not been adequately respected or protected. We therefore make a public Declaration of the Rights of people with HIV and AIDS and of our commitment to ensuring that they are upheld.

———————————

*The **National Council for Voluntary Organisation's Rural Unit** was set up to support voluntary action in rural areas. The **Ten-Point Plan** forms a basis for voluntary work that is effective and sensitive to the needs of people living in rural areas.*

1. **Promotion** of the valuable role of rural voluntary organisations in all walks of life.
2. **Representation** of rural voluntary organisations' concerns to public, private and voluntary agencies.
3. **Resources**, including a 'Rural Premium' to compensate for the extra cost of working in rural areas.
4. **Partnerships** between statutory, private and voluntary agencies.
5. **Support** in practical ways to enable voluntary action, such as meeting places, systems for shared work and collaboration.
6. **Information**, advice and training for those involved with rural voluntary action to ensure their effective work.
7. **Assistance** from the private sector with cash, help in kind, and training for rural voluntary action.
8. **Recognition** of the value of local, mobile and outreach services to reach small numbers of people in rural areas.
9. **Understanding** of the special qualities of rural voluntary action and their relevance to all parts of the country.
10. **Targeting** of the work of rural voluntary organisations to alleviate disadvantage.

———————————

Values Into Action (VIA) is the national campaign with people who have learning difficulties. Previously called the Campaign for People with Mental Handicaps, it has worked since 1971 for an end to the injustice and misunderstanding that have impoverished the lives of people with learning difficulties.

What does VIA believe?

VIA believes that people with learning difficulties –
- Have the same rights as other people, and should be allowed the same choices.
- Are just as important as other people, and should be treated with dignity and respect.
- Can live in the same way and in the same places as other people live, and should be given the help they need to make this possible.
- Should be allowed and, where necessary, helped to have the same opportunities in school, college, work, and leisure as other people.

These beliefs apply to all people with learning difficulties, however severe their disabilities.

Good Practices in Mental Health (GPMH) is a national charity set up to promote and assist the development of good mental health services through information services, consultation and developmental support to mental health agencies and users.

Defining good practice

GPMH have identified five principles of good practice which we believe should underpin all mental health services. We aim to promote services which reflect some if not all of our principles of good practice, which are:

Participation   Where service users participate collectively with service providers through discussion, decision-making and taking responsibility.
Respect   All people who have contact with mental health services are entitled to dignity and respect. This means being treated as a whole person and not as a collection of symptoms. An individual's right to privacy should be respected.
Information   Service providers have an obligation to inform and to listen to people who use their service, their relatives and friends. Information should be accessible, provided in non-medical language and in language appropriate to a local community. A consultation mechanism should exist to facilitate an exchange of information between professionals and users. Information should also be used to re-educate the public about mental health services and their users.

Choice   People should have the opportunity or power to consider alternative courses of action. Service users must be aware of all existing services from which they may choose and alternatives to existing services need to be made available, e.g. different types of housing, work and leisure opportunities.

Individuality   Services must recognise that each person is a unique individual with particular life experiences. Services should not treat users as a homogenous group with common needs nor assume that those needs can be elucidated or satisfied by standard approaches. It is especially important to recognise the individual needs of men and women from different racial and cultural backgrounds.

On 12–14 April 1989 representatives of disabled people from various European countries came together through support from the German Green Party via the **Strasbourg Independent Living Expert Seminar** *at the European Parliament. They drew up the statement below. The seminar led to the establishment of the European Network of Independent Living (ENIL) which has since become recognised as the Disabled Peoples' International (European Region) Independent Living Group.*

Preamble

We, disabled people from the Netherlands, UK, Denmark, Italy, Switzerland, Sweden, France, Austria, Finland, Belgium, USA, Hungary, Federal Republic of Germany and Norway have come together from April 12–14 1989 at the European Parliament, Strasbourg, France.

This conference has focussed on Personal Assistant Services as an essential factor of Independent Living, which itself encompasses the whole area of human activities, e.g. housing, transport, access, education, employment, economic security and political influence.

We, disabled people, recognising our unique expertise, derived from our experience, must take the initiative in the planning of policies that directly affect us.

To this end we condemn segregation and institutionalisation, which are a direct violation of our human rights, and consider that governments must pass legislation that protects the human rights of disabled people, including equalisation of opportunities.

We firmly uphold our basic human right to full and equal participation in society as enshrined in the UN Universal Declaration of Human Rights (extended to include disabled people in 1985) and consider that a key pre-requisite to this civil right is through Independent Living and the provision of support services such as personal assistant services for those who need them.

The recommendations of the UN World Programme of Action (S 115) specifically states that 'Member States should encourage the provision of support services to enable disabled people to live as independently as possible in the community and in so doing should ensure that persons with a disability have the opportunity to develop and manage these services for themselves'.

Resolution 1 of the 43rd UN General Assembly (1988) reaffirms the validity of the World Programme of Action, Resolution 2 stresses that 'special emphasis should be placed on equalisation of opportunities'.

Considering these and similar recommendations from both the European Community and the Council of Europe and to ensure that disabled people within Europe should have parity of equalisation of opportunities, we stress that these objectives must be achieved.

In support of the international movement of disabled people and of Disabled Peoples' International, which has a special commitment to setting up a network of initiatives for Independent Living as part of the implementation of equalisation of opportunities, we call on governments and policy makers to enforce the following principles:

Resolutions

1. Personal assistance services are a human and civil right which must be provided at no cost to the user. These services shall serve people with all types of disabilities, of all ages, on the basis of functional need, irrespective of personal wealth, income, marital and family status.
2. Personal assistance users shall be able to choose from a variety of personal assistance service models which together offer the choice of various degrees of user control. User control, in our view, can be exercised by all persons, regardless of their ability to give legally informed consent.
3. Services shall enable the user to participate in every aspect of life such as home, work, school, leisure, travel and political life etc. These services shall enable disabled people, if they so choose, to build up a personal and family life and fulfil all their responsibilities connected with this.
4. These services must be available long-term for anything up to 24 hours a day, seven days a week, and similarly on a short-term or emergency basis. These services shall include assistance with personal bodily functions, communicative, household, mobility, work and other related needs. In the assessment of need the consumer's view must be paramount.
5. The funding authority shall ensure that sufficient funds are available

to the user for adequate support, counselling, training of the user and of the assistant, if deemed necessary by the user.

6. Funding must include assistants' competitive wages and employment benefits, all legal and union-required benefits, plus the administrative costs.

7. Funding shall be a legislative right and payment must be guaranteed regardless of funding source or local government arrangements. Funding shall not be treated as disposable/taxable income and shall not make the user ineligible for other statutory benefits or services.

8. The user should be free to appoint as personal assistants whoever s/he choses, including family members.

9. No individual shall be placed in an institutionalised setting because of lack of resources, high costs, sub-standard or non-existent services.

10. There shall be a uniform judicial appeals procedure which is independent of funders, providers and assessors; is effected within a reasonable amount of time and enables the claimant to receive legal aid at the expense of the statutory authority.

11. In furtherance of all the above, disabled people and organisations controlled by them must be decisively involved at all levels of policy making including planning, implementation and development.

From **Community Life: a Code of Practice for Community Care**, *Centre for Policy on Ageing, 1990. This excerpt is edited from a document developed by the Centre for Policy on Ageing in response to policies outlined in the White Paper* **Caring for People: Community Care in the Next Decade and Beyond**. *It is aimed at the organisers, supervisors and users of community care schemes involving adults and attempts to 'codify the elements of community care', taking partnership as a key theme.*

It is recommended that, on behalf of these citizens, the social services department adopt a community care charter, embracing a number of interlocking component parts. It is . . . further recommended that representatives of consumers and carers be invited to participate in the drafting of such a charter. The charter should include the following elements:

Information

Published information should be in plain language, readily accessible and widely disseminated.

Written agreement

Individual consumers need to know what to expect and what is expected of them. The code, in supporting the notion of an agreement between provider and consumer, endorses the view that there are then rights and responsibilities on both sides.

These expectations should be expressed in the form of a written agreement. Written in clear language, it should give:

• details of the parties to the agreement
• essential information about providers and consumers
• details of the type of service or package of care agreed
• details, if appropriate, of the duration of the provision, any costs involved, and any date for due reassessment
• details of any complaints procedure, with encouragement to make use, if dissatisfied, of that process.

Consultation

The recommendations about assessment and reassessment and about a written agreement imply consultation. The code emphasises the value of consultation at all times. At all points in the process, consumers and carers should be consulted and have some influence on the services provided for them.

Moreover, where provision is offered on a group basis (day hospital, day care centre) simple representational forms should be developed to tap the opinion and seek the support of consumers.

Even where services or provision are highly individualised, attempts should be made to canvas general opinion. Examples might be the use of surveys to judge, say, how many/all consumers feel about the meals service; or the inclusion of consumers on interview panels for staff appointment.

In all these ways, it is hoped to draw consumers more fully into the fabric of provision, and to close the gap between professional and lay person.

Partnership

This mode of consumer responsiveness requires, in many cases, changes in the ethos of the providing bodies, both social services department and actual service agencies, where these are distinct. Care management and care staff must share equally with consumers and carers a genuine commitment to that mood of provider/consumer partnership and friendliness, the more so as, in reality, shortage of funds and resources will sometimes press hard on any system of care.

Amongst several elements that need to be addressed in this respect, the following are considered vital:

Consultation

- The need to sustain a high quality of information and its dissemination, and to maintain excellent consultative processes. This might include the use of consumers and carers in the training of staff so that this and other consumer-oriented approaches are emphasised.
- The need to ensure there is compliance with agreements.
- The need to involve staff, for example through a watch on training and by acknowledgement of trade union involvement.
- The need to include *all* staff, not just 'front-line' staff in attempts to fulfil these general aims.
- The need to encourage management and staff to understand and co-operate in complaints procedures.
- The need to encourage the development of independent representation and advocacy on behalf of consumers, particularly by bearing in mind the needs of those from ethnic minorities or severely disabled people.
- The need to guarantee, all in all, the centrality of the consumer. For example:
  - the way a worker is introduced into the consumer's home
  - the right of the consumer, without demur (subject to legislation referring to race and sex discrimination), to refuse a worker who is unacceptable
  - the expectation that work is done in a reasonable manner at a reasonable time
  - a ready appreciation of that complex relationship between providing worker and consumer, especially in the more complicated instance where a carer is involved.

Complaints procedure

The social services department should develop a complaints procedure which enshrines the following principles:

Prompt informed resolution   One suggestion is that the appointment of a consumer rights or customer relations officer might be made to encourage first-stage problem-solving.

Reasonable progress   One suggestion is that one officer be administratively associated with each case, staying in touch with the complaint, gathering the provider's response, and generally acting as progress chaser.

Advocacy   One suggestion is that consumers should be permitted representation.

Fair-minded investigation   One suggestion is that an investigative officer should be appointed for the quick and fair-minded scrutiny of complaints. Another suggestion is that the social services department should organise a complaints procedure panel to assess such issues, including, if possible, either consumer and/or independent representation. Where complaints are made, at senior level, against the social services department, arrangements to deploy investigating officers from another authority should be included.

Channel of appeal   One suggestion would be the creation, where necessary, of a separate appeal panel, but again including consumer and/or independent membership.

A Charter for Citizens' Rights. Harlow Council has drawn together the following set of principles which sum up all of its policies and projects.

Harlow Council believes that all Citizens have inalienable rights and in exercising these rights deserve to be treated with the respect due to them both as individuals and as members of the community.

To this end Harlow Council will positively assist all Citizens to exercise their rights in relation to the Council and wherever possible with other agencies.

All citizens, irrespective of age, sex, sexuality, race, disability or income, have the right:

To be heard and listened to in a respectful manner

This means that all Citizens have the right to have their interests and concerns weighed by the Council. It is about consultation and inviting comment, about unsolicited comment, but also about taking the Citizens' opinions into account and giving clear answers even if in some cases a particular standpoint does not prevail.

Of access to the authoirity and all those who speak on behalf of the authority

This is the ability to debate and discuss issues before the Council; for the Citizen's voice to be heard on these issues and those that should be before the Council.

To clear and unambiguous information

Citizens need to have clear understandable information about decisions and policies and the reason for these, as well as information about services offered to which they are entitled.

To fairness, equity, honesty and justice

Citizens should know what their rights are and how they can exercise them. All citizens will be treated fairly and equally when exercising their rights.

To be actively involved in the governing of the local community

All Citizens have the right to participate in the decision-making process and to mould the work of the Council – and to vote.

To advocacy in upholding these rights

Provisions for advocacy will be made available to all Citizens as of right. This includes Councillors' surgeries, welfare rights, consumer advice, community development and other forms of advocacy such as a community architect.

30

Human Need and the Moral Right to Optimal Community Care

LEN DOYAL

The report on community care by Griffiths in 1988 and the White Paper presented in 1989 both emphasise the importance of needs assessment and implicitly accept the entitlement of individuals to needs satisfaction (Griffiths, 1988; Department of Health, 1989). In these documents and elsewhere it is argued that through participating in, rather than being excluded from, their local communities, individuals will optimise their self-sufficiency and their ability to contribute to the finance of their own care. In so doing they will realise or recover their self-respect as citizens.

Case work, it is suggested, should focus on such 'empowerment' as its goal, with clients and community care workers becoming much clearer about their specific rights and duties (Meteyard, 1990, section 1). For similar reasons, a shift is recommended from care within large institutions to care within the community, which will also lead to increases in need satisfaction (Murphy, 1991, pp. 1064–5). Other proposed changes in social service administration and finance are justified in the same terms.

While these proposals sound good, their practical feasibility has been questioned, with much of this criticism focused on under-capitalisation (Langan, 1990). However, more adequate funding would not resolve another problem that jeopardises the potential success of the new policies: the absence of a clear and detailed theory of human need on which accurate needs assessment can be based. Which needs must be satisfied in order to enable optimal social participation, and why do individuals have a right to those goods and services identified as necessary for this purpose? The answers to both of these questions are hotly disputed.

On the one hand, social service bureaucracies tend to perceive the identification of need as the province of experts versed in the generation of orthodox social and epidemiological statistics. Yet increasingly such orthodoxies are called into question. Both community activists and clients themselves demand more say in identifying local need, but the insularity of bureaucratic perception can be more than matched by lack of clarity within communities about how to differentiate real needs from mere preferences.

On the other hand, there is a tendency for carers and clients – like doctors and patients – simply to assume that the right to need satisfaction exists through justifications that amount to little more than the expression of emotional conviction. Such sentiments stand little chance of success against the articulate arguments of neo-liberals who deny the existence of welfare rights, who grudgingly tolerate a minimal welfare state and who constantly seek to reduce its size.

Unless these problems are adequately resolved, approaches to community care that attempt to combine elements of both decentralisation and centralisation stand little chance of real success. Without a coherent and properly operationalised theory of need, their results will be eclectic and difficult to assess. It is also more likely that the political argument for the expenditure necessary to finance more than just minimal levels of care will be lost.

This chapter will briefly outline a theory of human need developed by myself and Ian Gough which addresses the issue of how human needs should be conceptualised and argues that individuals have a right to their optimal and not just minimal satisfaction (Doyal and Gough, 1991).[1] This theory, I will argue, can provide the moral foundation for what is best about the new proposals for community care while at the same time revealing the political and economic circumstances under which they will inevitably fail.

30.1 What are the basic human needs and why?

Let us begin by returning to the importance played on social participation in all the proposals for change in community care provision. There is no doubt about the correctness of this emphasis on the quantity and quality of interaction with others for the objective welfare of the individual. We discover who we are through learning from others what we can do. Others remind us – as we do them – of our individual narratives, of the goals we have tried to achieve in our everyday lives and the degree of success we have had in the process. They help us to remember what we have done and what we might reasonably try to do in the future.

Social participation thus empowers us by providing the space for practising old skills or acquiring new ones, which we and others identify as 'ours'. If we lack the capacity for such participation, we are seriously and objectively harmed as a result – disabled with respect to continuing to express ourselves through performing our present skills, learning new ones and reinforcing others in their attempts to do the same.

Identifying significant personal harm with seriously impaired social participation provides the key with which to identify universal and objective human needs. For these will be the necessary conditions that everyone must meet – wherever they may live and whatever their culture: to avoid such harm through being able to participate in society with as little serious impairment as their genetic or acquired state allows. These conditions are the personal attributes of physical survival/health and individual autonomy.

As regards the first basic need, without physical survival individuals can clearly do nothing whatever. Reduced physical health disables social participation by hindering an individual's scope of action and interaction. The specific ways in which this can occur are described by the physical consequences of diseases catalogued by the biomedical model. 'Illness' – the phenomenological experience of physical disease – can take a variety of forms, but provided that the associated disease is serious, so will be the illness to which it leads. The result will be disablement, and thus significant harm as defined above. Those who are suffering from the disease of, and are ill with, severe heart disease, for example, are objectively more impaired in their social participation than those who are not.

There are, of course, ways of identifying and treating disease other than those outlined by orthodox medicine. However, all international organisations with the aim of finding ways of improving physical health on a global scale embrace both its diagnostic categories and therapeutic technologies. For this reason, the weaknesses of biomedicine – which are many – should never be allowed to cloud its strengths. If you have a burst appendix then you need appropriate surgical and medical care, whoever and wherever you are. The same applies to the treatment of infectious diseases and to our complete understanding of how they are best prevented. We cannot treat cholera as successfully as we might or understand why clean water is so important in its prevention, without the understanding provided by the biomedical model (Doyal, 1987).

Aside from physical health, the other basic human need is individual autonomy. In order successfully to participate in any form of life, actors require more than just physical health. They also require the capacity to formulate aims about what to try to achieve and beliefs about how to do this – the ability to reason and to act on the basis of reasons. These attributes create the unique human potential to choose future goals and actions, to plan one's life. Autonomy is the exercise of such reasoned choice and individuals are thus able to participate in their form of life in proportion to their possession of autonomy.

So, like physical health, one's basic need for autonomy may be satisfied to a greater or lesser extent. The degree of satisfaction will depend on the value of the three component variables of autonomy: degree of understanding; emotional capacity; and social opportunity. Let us examine each in turn.

Actors do not make up their own reasons for action – they are not intellectually self-sufficient. They must learn to use language to communicate and to act in ways that are normatively and vocationally appropriate to the rules of their social environment. Even though much of what we do and say may seem essentially private in character, the fact is that our actions and communication derive much of their meaning from such rules and their specific configurations in different social institutions. Clearly, we must learn these rules from others and once our correct understanding of them is confirmed, we inevitably become teachers ourselves. Robinson Crusoe, that archetype of so-called self-sufficiency, had to learn from others the skills that enabled him to survive before he was shipwrecked alone.

Further, autonomous individuals who have learned the manual and mental skills to participate within their form of life must have the emotional wherewithal so to do. This will depend on the absence of *serious* mental illness. As with physical disease, there is much we understand about the symptoms of such illness, even though its aetiology is much more contentious. Serious mental illness entails, for example, a sustained lack of capacity for intellectual understanding, for consistent reasoning, for confidence to try to interact with others, for the recognition of responsibility for action and for the empirical constraints that the physical and social environment place upon it.

Of course, serious mental illness varies both in its severity and in the way in which associated disabilities are conceptualised in different cultures. What does not vary, however, is the universality of its symptoms or the objectivity of the personal harm to which they lead. For no matter how culturally valued the idiosyncratic expression of any of these symptoms, the fact remains that they describe the contours of personal experience which, if sustained, will seriously impair participation in any form of life. For example, what is referred to in orthodox psychiatry as 'psychotic depression' entails severe harm in precisely these terms.

Finally, the autonomy of individuals can be measured in proportion to the *social opportunities* they enjoy to exercise their cognitive and emotional capacities – their freedom to interact with their fellow citizens in pursuit of individual or common goals. Human freedom has negative and positive dimensions. Negatively, it is the ability to act without being prevented from doing so or physically and/or psychologically forced to do otherwise than one chooses. Under such circumstances, the fact that you are physically healthy, educated and not suffering from severe mental illness will obviously not enable you to participate socially in ways that you choose.

Positive freedom is having access to the goods and services necessary to achieve the goals that we set for ourselves, always against the background of our social environment. Without such access, our efforts will be limited, no matter how much we are left alone by others or how many opportunities exist for social participation. Political liberty, for example, will mean little to those whose daily labour is so focused on keeping body and soul together that they do not have the time or energy for active involvement in democratic decision-making, even if the formal opportunity exists for them to do so!

If survival/physical health and autonomy are necessary conditions for all humans to participate in their form of life, what universal satisfiers or 'intermediate needs' must everyone have access to for these universal needs to be met satisfactorily? Generally speaking, the answer is clear.

Optimal physical health requires nutritional food and water, protective housing, a non-hazardous work environment, a non-hazardous physical environment and access to appropriate health care if physical disease develops through, among other things, lack of access to these intermediate needs.

Optimal autonomy *within* a culture demands security in childhood, significant primary relationships, physical security, economic security, basic education and, for women, safe birth control and child-bearing. Even greater levels of 'critical autonomy' will depend on the ability of the individual to make choices not only within cultures but between them. Here, the extent of cross-cultural education and opportunity for cross-cultural choice become crucial variables.

Again, each of the preceding intermediate needs are universal (for example nutrition), although the ways in which satisfaction for each is achieved (for example different culinary traditions) are not. It follows that one can accept the universality of our theory of need, without questioning the importance and viability of different cultural approaches to need satisfaction. It equally follows that its acceptance does not deflect emphasis from the needs of particular groups within a single culture.

For example, specific types of permanent physical disability (such as paraplegia) demand particular, and often similar, types of satisfiers in order to optimise individual opportunities for social participation (such as relevant technologies for mobility and access) and to minimise the handicap they cause. Physical disabilities that are correctable (such as poor vision) or might be correctable (such as some forms of chronic disease) make similar demands for appropriate satisfiers. In the case of the former, the demand is for a known correcting technology that works in practice. As regards the latter, it is for research into technologies that might work in practice.

How much of each satisfier an individual requires – the degree to which the basic need for physical health and autonomy should be satisfied – is both an empirical and normative question. Empirically, individuals need what is necessary for them to participate in their forms of life to specified levels. From this perspective, most individuals in underdeveloped nations or poor communities within developed nations might be argued to need less than those from more wealthy environments. Normatively, however, the issue is not whether or not such inequalities exist but whether it is possible to provide a convincing moral justification of them. It will now be argued that this cannot be done.

30.2 The right to optimal need satisfaction

To argue that an individual has a right to something is to make a very serious claim. It is to maintain that an entitlement exists which others have a strict duty to provide whether they want to or not. In other words, if we really believe that a person has a right, say, to good community care, then doing what we can to provide it is not simply a matter of altruism or charity. This is why there should be no social stigma attached to the receipt of such care.

Private property is a good example. To the extent that we believe that we have a right to use and dispense with our property as we see fit – provided that we harm no one else in the process – then we impose a duty on others not to interfere with our exercise in it. We also impose a duty on ourselves to take seriously their rights to do the same with their property. Otherwise, the social institution of private property would be called into doubt and there would be no reason why others should take seriously our beliefs about our own rights. Of course, if others believe themselves to have identical rights as well, they in turn impose identical reciprocal duties. Empirically speaking, beliefs in the existence of rights correspond to beliefs in the existence of corresponding duties.

As we have seen, all individuals mature in their self-awareness and social skills against the background of rules – a normative environment that explicitly or implicitly postulates a *vision of the moral good*. Such environments can differ even within the same society. The substance of the visions of the good that they embody can vary widely, some being quite similar and others dramatically in conflict.

Yet, logically speaking, different forms of social life implicitly or explicitly share a common theory of good citizenship, despite any moral conflict that might otherwise exist between them. The good citizen is the individual who does her or his duty, as prescribed by the values of the culture or subculture of which they are a part. This is as much the case in Manchester as it is in Mecca.

In Britain, for example, the good citizen is supposed to do and not to do a variety of things relating to home, employment, recreation and politics. Of course, there are huge variations on the general theme, depending on things such as class, gender, race, region, religion and so on. But, leaving aside subcultures that positively endorse criminality, there is still a consensus that everyone should do their best to work within the law to optimise their well-being and to be as economically self-sufficient as possible. Certainly, the Conservative government in Britain has a very pronounced moral vision of the good, which takes this model of self-sufficiency to its limit. In short, no one who takes morality seriously can question the reality of duties as such, although they might and do disagree about their content.

The imputation of duties of good citizenship entails at least two things on the part of those who impose them. First, they must believe that those on whom these duties are imposed have the right to basic need satisfaction – of access to culturally acceptable satisfiers of those intermediate needs that must be satisfied for physical health and autonomy themselves to be sustained. In Britain this means, for example, the right of access to certain types of food and certain types of education. To be consistent, those who impute duties on others must also assume some responsibility for ensuring their access to basic need satisfaction, through, say, paying taxes for this purpose.

Otherwise, potential good citizens will not necessarily be able to do what is expected of them. This inability will be due to the disablement they suffer as a result of disabling physical, educational, emotional or social deprivation from which there is no escape. The imputation of duties of citizenship without the right to basic need satisfaction thus becomes meaningless. In other words, 'ought' implies 'can', and the belief that others should be good in our terms commits us to do what we can to help them to obtain the basic need satisfaction that is necessary for them to be so.

Second, if the imputation of strict moral duties on others entails their right to basic need satisfaction, the question remains of *how much satisfaction* is required for this right to be met. The simple answer is as much as is available for citizens to do their *best*. If a government expects less than the best of its citizens, through not providing them with access to the basic need satisfaction necessary for them to do their best, then this reflects badly on its own commitment to the vision of the good that it imposes on others. The professed good would not be that good after all! Another way of putting it is that to the extent that the state neglects the optimal objective welfare of its citizens, it potentially creates a group of moral outcasts who may well decide that since they cannot live up to the moral expectations of the state, they will ignore them (Harris, 1991).

So the belief in the duty of good citizenship entails a further belief in the right not just to minimal levels of need satisfaction but to optimal levels as well, recognising that optimal levels may differ in proportion to unavoidable practical constraints imposed by different levels of national scarcity. As far as community care is concerned, this means specific types of goods and services and as many of them as are necessary for individuals to achieve optimal levels of physical health and autonomy. It is the achievement of this aim that must be at the heart of good community care and organisation, provision and training for it. Not surprisingly, it is an aim reflected in the detail of much contemporary literature in community care.

Therefore, governments that impute visions of good citizenship cannot then consistently argue for a minimal welfare state. It is just contradictory to claim that citizens who for whatever reason cannot do their best should still do so. The continuation of this contradiction through the perpetuation of political policies that embody it reveals either lack of awareness or, more likely, irrational self-interest.

This does not mean, of course, that citizens should not be responsible for as much of their own need satisfaction as they can be, and it may be difficult as a worker in community care to know where to draw the line. Yet decisions should always err in favour of the client. The worst thing that can happen if a mistake is made is that an already badly off client may get slightly more than they deserve, given their meagre personal resources. This is well worth the risk since, as we have seen, it will ensure that they are optimally able to accept their designated responsibilities in the future.

30.3   Putting principle into practice

We have seen that good community care demands access to those goods and services that are necessary for the satisfaction of the basic human needs for health and autonomy. Unless these needs are optimally met, individuals will be unable to do their best to flourish as persons and as good citizens. In principle, many of the proposals of the Griffith Report and the related White Paper are steps in this direction.

However, none of these aims can or will be achieved in practice unless sufficient capital is made available to finance them. Thus far this has not been forthcoming and there are good arguments for believing that it will not be forthcoming in the future. The problem of under-capitalisation is a major one in welfare provision in Britain, the National Health Service being the other obvious example. The advantage of linking basic need satisfaction to the rights that the duties of good citizenship entail is that this offers a cogent argument for their inclusion in a constitutional bill of rights. It is only then – when the state will allow itself to be taken to court for doing otherwise – that the human right to optimal community care will be seen to be taken seriously in the UK.

This said, problems still remain. So far we have outlined the substantive needs of citizens and linked them to their right to optimal community care. However, we have not faced the dilemma of how to proceed when there is dispute about what constitutes the optimal level of related need satisfaction and how the detail of such satisfaction should be addressed in specific circumstances. In other words, for it to be a feasible moral foundation for the formulation of welfare policy, we must further link our substantive theory of needs and rights to a procedural theory of need. This must outline the necessary conditions for optimising the rationality of debate about community care on a micro- and macro-level.

The success of such debate will depend on its 'communicative competence' – the commitment of those involved to structure it in ways that optimise its rationality. Even when there may be no absolutely 'right' answer, and when policies that are agreed are seen to be compromises between competing interests, it is all the more important to arrive at solutions to problems concerning need satisfaction that can be supported in the local community by workers and clients alike. This means that those participating in policy formation must include representatives of all parties with a legitimate interest in the dispute. These will include, on the one hand, case workers, managers and researchers with codified expertise about the problem under consideration and, on the other hand, clients and community representatives with experientially based understanding of what the problem entails in practice.

Only then will the best technical and experientially based information be available on which rational decisions can be based. Further, debates themselves must be monitored to ensure that their outcomes are not determined by the arbitrary power and vested interest of individuals or representatives in either group. And finally, when steps are taken to implement policies that have been established, they must be subject to regular review to ensure that what has been agreed in principle is followed through in practice. Many of the examples of how social planning in the past had negative effects on community care have been due to the absence of one or more of these conditions.

There will always be a tension in the theory and practice of community care, as there is in politics generally, between those who opt for decision-making from providers and those who do the same for recipients. The fact is that here, as in all other areas of public policy, we need the participation of both – a dual strategy for community care and for welfare provision in general. This will entail as much centralisation in administration, provision and expertise as is necessary for the efficient delivery of appropriate goods and services to those in need. Also required is as much decentralisation as is compatible with this aim, with the right of clients to participate in the processes of planning and execution also being guaranteed as a matter of legal right.

30.4 Conclusion

Thus through effective representation, participation and co-operation, all grounded in rational communication, providers and recipients of care can work together to ensure good community care through the optimisation of basic need satisfaction. If the procedures to ensure this possibility are not incorporated in the final shape of community care provision within the UK – along with the capitalisation sufficient for the right of the individual to optimal need satisfaction to be respected – then it will fail.

This will be a tragedy for those who are deprived in the process. For they will be unable to do their best when they demand it of themselves and it is demanded by others of them. Yet the tragedy also applies to all of those who remain aloof from such deprivation while having the wherewithal to help to bring it down to acceptable levels. For in not doing so they participate in undermining the moral foundation of the very values in which they purport to believe, with potentially destructive consequences both for themselves and the rest of society.

We know how to solve the major problems confronting community care. What is required is the political will.

Note

1. Much of this chapter is an outline of arguments developed in this book where further detail and extensive bibliographical references for all of the arguments are included.

References

Department of Health (1989) *Caring for People: Community Care in the Next Decade and Beyond*, Cm 849, HMSO, London.
Doyal, L. and Gough, I. (1991) *A Theory of Human Need*, Macmillan, London.
Doyal, L. (1987) 'Health, Underdevelopment and Traditional Medicine', *Holistic Medicine*, Vol. 2.

Griffiths, R. (1988) *Community Care: Agenda for Action*, HMSO, London.

Harris, J. (1991) 'Equity in health care', talk given at the Royal Institute on Public Health and Hygiene, London.

Langan, M. (1990) 'Community care in the 1990s: the community care White Paper: "Caring for People"', *Critical Social Policy*, Vol. 29.

Meteyard, B. (1990) *Community Care Keyworker Manual*, Longman, Harlow.

Murphy, E. (1991) 'Community mental health services: a vision for the future', *British Medical Journal*, Vol. 302.

31

Markets, Contracts and Social Care Services: Prospects and Problems

LESLEY HOYES and ROBIN MEANS

31.1 Introduction

The introduction of the concept of 'markets' into social care services has gained momentum in recent years and is now embodied in the National Health Service and Community Care Act 1990, which incorporates the main recommendations of *Caring for People* (Department of Health, 1989), the White Paper on community care. This legislation represents a response to what is seen as the many years of failure to develop an adequate legislative and financial framework for community care services.

Local authority social services departments have been given the lead role in community care planning. However, their role at the client level will increasingly be confined to the assessment of need, the designing of care arrangements to meet that need by appointed 'care managers', and the provision of funds to finance those arrangements. They are discouraged from directly providing all care services themselves; instead, services are to be provided increasingly by a 'mixed economy' based largely on the private and voluntary sectors. Local authorities are to become 'enablers' through the allocation of funds; they will have a declining role in service provision.

This chapter discusses the main implications of introducing markets and contracts in social care provision. First, however, we look at the development of 'quasi-markets'.

31.2 The arrival of the quasi-market

Despite the 'new right' rhetoric of the post-1979 Conservative governments, much of the welfare state remained untouched in the late 1980s.
However, LeGrand (1990, p. 1) has argued that 1988–9 saw 'a major
offensive against the basic structure of welfare provision'. Radical
changes in the legislative basis of the provision of education, housing
and the National Health Service have been enacted alongside those in
community care, representing the most significant shift in British social
policy since the 1940s.

The contracting out of core services to other agencies and other
reforms introduced following the White Paper and legislation have one
common feature: the introduction of what might be termed 'quasi-
markets' into the delivery of welfare services (LeGrand, 1990). In each
case the state ceases to be both the funder and provider of services.
Instead it becomes primarily a funder, with services being provided by a
variety of private, voluntary and public suppliers, all operating in
competition with each other. The method of funding also changes.
Instead of resources being allocated directly by bureaucrats to providers,
a budget or 'voucher' is given directly to the consumer, or to someone
acting on his or her behalf (such as a care manager), who then allocates
the budget between competing suppliers.

Quasi-markets are 'markets' because they replace state provision with
more competitive, independent services. They are 'quasi' because they
differ from conventional markets in a number of important respects. The
differences are on both the supply and the demand sides. On the supply
side, as with conventional markets, there is competition between service
suppliers. However, in contrast to conventional markets, these organisations (for example residential homes) are not necessarily privately
owned, nor are they necessarily out to maximise their profits. On the
demand side, consumer purchasing power is not expressed in terms of
cash, but in the form of a budget confined to the purchase of a specific
service. Also, the immediate consumer may not be the one who exercises the choices concerning purchasing decisions; instead these may be
delegated to a third party, such as a care manager.

31.3 Developing quasi-markets in social care

Hoyes and LeGrand (1991) argue that the role of the local authority in the
successful introduction of a market-led pattern of services must not be
underestimated. It is at least as important that the authority be prepared
to generate supply as to purchase services, and the way in which

authorities choose to award contracts may in itself have a profound effect upon the local market structure (Flynn, 1990a). The existing market structure varies enormously between areas; the uneven distribution of private and voluntary residential homes, with a concentration in seaside resorts, has been graphically demonstrated (Audit Commission, 1986). The independent market in domiciliary services is far less developed, with few large suppliers and many small ones; local authorities have little experience of contracting out in this field although, if future services are to be based on individual packages of care for people in their own homes, these are likely to assume greater importance (Flynn and Common, 1990; Booth and Phillips, 1990).

Stimulating new and diversified markets may not be easy. The voluntary sector has expressed fears about losing autonomy and flexibility, and compromising its advocacy and campaigning roles; smaller groups in particular may not feel up to the demands of bidding for and fulfilling contracts (Gutch, 1990; Flynn, 1990b). The government recognises the need for authorities to continue to provide core grant funding to voluntary organisations to underpin administrative infrastructure and development work, but it is questionable whether social services authorities will choose to spend their limited resources on this rather than the purchase of particular services.

If a local authority is to stimulate a market, it will need to do more than contract out its residential care. Flynn has listed a range of other interventions on both the supply and demand sides which social services could engage in to encourage alternative suppliers of services (Flynn, 1990b). These include, on the supply side, help with business development; grants, subsidies and credit for start-up and working capital; training; and licensing and regulation. On the demand side, care managers need to operate more as brokers and advisers rather than as agents making all the decisions.

In addition to authorities' ability to stimulate alternative provision, they will also have scope for manipulating the markets to operate efficiently; perfect competition requires that there should be neither a monopoly (one or a few suppliers) nor a monopsony (one or few purchasers) situation. It is likely that in some areas for some services the social services department will be the only purchaser. Whilst this may make it easier for the authority to dictate terms, it may also deter potential suppliers from entering a market where they will be dependent on a single buyer. On the other hand, if an authority, for the sake of administrative convenience or economy, chooses to enter into block contracts with one or two suppliers, they risk squeezing out other smaller suppliers and will find themselves faced with a monopoly and in a very weak position.

31.4 Managing contracts

The successful introduction of quasi-markets into social care services
may depend ultimately on whether or not local authorities are able to
specify, write, manage and monitor contracts that ensure a quality
service. Each of these tasks presents difficulties because of the nature of
social care and the importance of high standards. These issues will need
to be addressed, whether the main form of service provision is expected
to be via internal markets based on splitting the purchasing branch of a
department from its service delivery or provider arm, or through the
award of external contracts to independent service providers.

31.4.1 Internal markets and the purchaser/provider split

The introduction of a 'contract culture' into social care services will have
a profound effect upon the management structures of social services
authorities. The most significant changes are likely to be in the separation of the purchaser and provider functions within departments
(Department of Health, 1989, p. 23).

The purpose of the proposed split appeared to be twofold: to ensure
equality of treatment for alternative suppliers and the authorities' own
services, so as to increase consumer choice; and the identification of
service provision costs, so that choices can be fair. However, it is not at
all clear that a structural split will always be the only or the best way of
achieving the ultimate goal of enhanced choice (Claridge and Outran,
1990). Where there are no alternative suppliers, for example for respite
care for highly dependent people, the need is for the identification of
costs, and this can be achieved by improved accounting. Where there
are alternative suppliers, a split will only be necessary at the point of
purchase, at care manager level, and will then only be effective if
accompanied by real scope for care managers and clients to exercise
choice.

The formalisation of relations between purchasers and providers will
not only effect local authority internal arrangements but will change the
nature of the relationship between authorities and suppliers (Association of Metropolitan Authorities, 1990). Flynn has argued that the total
separation of budget management from service delivery may constrain
financial flexibility within local authorities, making them less willing to
tie up all their budget at the beginning of the year; this may in turn make
the voluntary sector's income less predictable and its involvement more
risky (Flynn, 1990c).

31.4.2 Selecting external providers

Where local authorities seek to contract out services to private or voluntary sector providers, they are faced with the problem of deciding which organisations to enter into arrangements with and on what contractual basis. Much will depend upon the ability of purchasers to select providers of good-quality services. This requires them to be able to observe and collect accurate information on all potential suppliers. If the characteristics of the supplier cannot be observed, 'adverse selection' may result; that is, the purchaser selects a poor-quality supplier because he or she cannot tell a good from a bad producer. It is likely that some authorities will attempt to avoid adverse selection by purchasing only from well-known, established suppliers. However, this strategy distorts the conditions for efficient market operation, namely that there should be many providers supplying services to many purchasers.

Policy guidance from the Department of Health lists options available to authorities for selecting service providers; these include open tendering, select list tendering, direct negotiation with one or more suppliers or setting up a new organisation, for example management/worker buy-outs (Department of Health, 1991). Flynn and Common (1990) conclude that tendering may be appropriate for 'going concerns', but only where price is not the sole criterion; management/worker buy-outs are found to offer no additional consumer choice. The view of the Association of Metropolitan authorities is that competitive tendering for social care services is impractical and not in the best interests of social care provision; there are not enough local agencies and the process would inevitably emphasise costs over quality (Association of Metropolitan Authorities, 1990). Moreover, competitive tendering will bring contracts under the provision of the Local Government Act 1988, which prohibits contract conditions that are non-commercial, including terms and conditions of employment and composition of the workforce. This would not necessarily exclude considerations of genuine occupational qualifications and an organisation's ability to recruit and retain staff if these can be justified as on commercial grounds. However, it may well prove difficult for an authority, even where committed to non-exploitation of employees and to equal opportunities, to build such factors into contracts.

31.4.3 Specifications and contracts

The main debate about contracts in social care services centres on how 'tight' or 'loose' they should be. A 'tight', formal contract might facilitate compliance, but it might also leave loopholes which the providers can exploit to their own advantage. On the other hand, a service might be provided by a highly trusted supplier who is known to share the authorities' objectives, in which case there may be seen to be no need for a contract at all. Between these two extremes will lie a whole range of situations which will influence the decision on the most appropriate arrangement.

In the field of social care services, the use of specifications and contracts as a means of ensuring services of a high standard is problematic. Specifications describe what is to be provided and contracts set out the terms under which the purchaser and provider agree to achieve compliance. Many social services departments would have difficulty in describing in detail the characteristics and costs of the services they provide directly now. Such descriptions would need to reflect outcomes and processes as well as inputs. They may have even greater difficulty in describing the standards they are meeting. Services such as those involved in community care are difficult to describe and define since it is often the less tangible and less equaliy quantified aspects that are of most importance to the consumers. Yet when the potential risks to those consumers of poor-quality services are too serious, standards must be defined. If specifications are flexible to permit provider initiative, what happens when a decision is taken with which the purchaser disagrees?

It is clearly important that authorities should think about and write down the standards of services that they will expect from providers (Barnes and Miller, 1988). Quality assurance is not just about inspection in the narrow sense of correcting a service which is badly provided, but should be a means of ensuring that services are high quality from the start. Specifications will need to include inputs, since it is on these that costings are based. Nevertheless, contracts that are couched in general terms and emphasise the desired outcomes can have the details defined by negotiation between the purchaser and provider in a collaborative effort.

31.5 Will markets in social care work?

The claims made in *Caring for People* (Department of Health, 1989) for markets and contracts are substantial and varied, and these claims need to be evaluated. The major justification made for change is that markets generate competition and hence they are more efficient and effective than the bureaucratic systems they are replacing. But this is open to question. The indeterminacy of the relevant organisations' objectives (profits, turnover, social welfare) makes it difficult to predict how they will respond to market incentives. Also, consumers of community care, even if aided by a care manager, may find it difficult to shop around to find the best 'value for money'; once in a residential home, for example, it is difficult for elderly persons to convince those responsible for their welfare that they should be moved.

A second set of questions concerns choice. Another important justification for the introduction of quasi-market arrangements is that to do so increases both the range and the quality of consumer choice. But again this could be challenged. To what extent is the consumer able to choose what he or she actually wants and to what extent is service access dependent upon the assessment and negotiation skills of a professional? How much choice does the client of a care manager have? Can they choose their care manager? Will there be enough independent providers to provide an adequate range of choice in all cases?

A third set of questions concerns equity (see chapter 23). The White Paper is harshly critical at the failure of the previous community care system to target resources at those in greatest need, and this is backed up by extensive research evidence (Davies and Knapp, 1988). And yet an equally common criticism of conventional markets (Foster, 1983) is that they create inequalities and therefore inequities. Will quasi-markets have similar effects? Will residential care providers compete for healthy elderly people, while ignoring those suffering from dementia and incontinence? Will the poor – constrained by lack of resources – be particularly disadvantaged?

The importance of market-making and developing a clear contract strategy have already been emphasised, and how this is tackled by individual authorities will have a major impact upon outcomes. An implementation problem faced by nearly all authorities will be the paucity of their information and financial management systems. Technological change opens up the prospect of tight–loose systems of public sector management (Hoggett, 1990, 1991), but many social services departments are woefully short of both the information technology hardware and the officer expertise required to operate such systems. This could become a major stumbling-block to the effective implementation of quasi-markets and contracts into the British social care system (Miller, 1991).

Finally, it is important not to lose sight of the question: success or failure for whom? The research of Smith and Cantley (1985) on psychogeriatric day services underlines that there are different interest groups (officers, managers, field-level staff, clients and carers) in any policy initiative and each stakeholder group will have different ideas about what will represent 'success' or 'failure' in any policy change. If the implementation of markets and contracts into social care services acheives efficiency in the narrow terms of cost minimalisation, this may represent 'success' for many had-pressed senior managers faced with a growing gap between demand and available resources. However, this might be achieved at the expense of a major deterioration in the employment conditions of many social care staff (residential staff, home helps, meals deliverers) since some elements of the private and even the voluntary sector may offer lower salaries than the public sector and be reluctant to recognise pension, holiday and trade union rights. Thus, the changes could represent a disaster for some already low-paid social care staff. Equally, a central focus on costs may reduce choice for the individual consumer since expensive but preferred care options may be dismissed or ignored by the care manager, although it could equally be argued that such an approach ensures the maximum number of clients can be helped for any given amount of resources.

Our own view is that the changes will have failed if they do not lead to the provision of flexible care packages that are perceived as appropriate and high quality by consumers and their carers. A good test of this will be the experience of clients from minority ethnic groups. Such individuals should receive services appropriate to their needs, not only when they happen to live in local authorities where a significant proportion of the population is from such groups, but also when they represent an isolated household in a largely all-white community.

References

Association of Metropolitan Authorities (1990) *Contracts for Social Care: the Local Authority View*, AMA, London.

Audit Commission (1986) *Making a Reality of Community Care*, HMSO, London.

Barnes, M. and Miller, N. (eds) (1988) 'Performance measurement in personal social services', *Research, Policy and Planning*, Vol. 6. No. 2, pp. 1–47.

Booth, T. and Phillips, D. (1990) *Contracting Arrangements for Domiciliary Care*, Report of a National Survey by the Joint Unit for Social Services Research, Sheffield, University of Sheffield, National Council for Domiciliary Care Services.

Claridge, D. and Outran, C. (1990) 'A potential thrust for change', *Insight*, 28 March.

Davies, B. and Knapp, M. (1988) 'Costs and residential care', in Sinclair, I. (ed.) *Residential Care: the Research Reviewed*, HMSO, London.

Department of Health (1989) *Caring for People: Community Care in the Next Decade and Beyond*, HMSO, London.

Department of Health (1991) *Community Care in the Next Decade and Beyond: Policy Guidance*, HMSO, London.

Flynn, N. (1990a) 'Maintaining the monopoly', *Insight*, 11 April.

Flynn, N. (1990b) 'Stirring up supply', *Insight*, 23 May.

Flynn, N. (1990c) 'Seasonal business', *Insight*, 10 October.

Flynn, N. and Common, R. (1990) 'Contracts for community care', *Caring for People: Implementation Documents*, HMSO, London.

Foster, P. (1983) *Access to Welfare: an Introduction to Welfare Rationing*, Macmillan, London.

Gutch, R. (1990) 'The contract culture: the challenge for voluntary organisations', in *Contracting: In or Out?*, No. 4, National Council for Voluntary Organisations.

Hoggett, P. (1990) *Modernisation, Political Strategy and the Welfare state: an Organisational Perspective*, School for Advanced Urban studies, Bristol.

Hoggett, P. (1991), 'The new public sector management', *Policy and Politics*, Vol. 19, No. 4, pp. 243–56.

Hoyes, L. and LeGrand, J. (1991) *Markets in Social Care: a Resource Pack*, School for Advanced Urban studies.

LeGrand, J. (1990) *Quasi-Markets and Social Policy*, School for Advanced Urban studies, Bristol.

Miller, C. (1991), 'Hungry for megabytes', *Social Work Today*, 4 April.

Smith, G. and Cantley, C. (1985) *Asesssing Health Care: a Study in Organisational Evaluation*, Open University Press, Milton Keynes.

32

*Key Workers for Elderly People in the Community**

TIM DANT and BRIAN GEARING

32.1 The case manager project

In the United Kingdom three innovatory schemes have borrowed aspects of 'case management' and applied them in different ways. The Case Manager Project (CMP), has explored the use of case management with physically disabled people. As in the United States examples, CMP was set up as a special project, independent of existing bureaucracies and was funded as an experiment by the King's Fund. In the CMP the case manager was accountable to a Project Steering Committee but took as paramount the client's interests and acted in accord with their wishes. Initially there was an assessment by the case manager (who was a qualified and experienced social worker) of the needs of the client. Those needs were transformed into an agreement between the case manager and the client about what might be done. The case manager then acted on the client's behalf in trying to realise the goals. In the CMP these goals included securing rehabilitative therapy, getting appropriate equipment installed or obtaining suitable housing.

Advocacy was a strong feature of the CMP and an important reason why professionals referred their cases to the Project (Pilling, 1988, p. 33). The case manager negotiated with representatives of the agencies providing the services (doctors, nurses, social workers, occupational therapists, housing officers), arguing the client's case, producing reasons for requests to be met, countering reasons why they should not

*This is an abridged version of a paper that was first published in *Journal of Social Policy*, Vol. 19, No. 3, pp. 331–360.

be. It is a significant skill to be able to understand the procedures of these agencies and to speak the language of their representatives.

The skill of the case managers meant that they were able to represent their clients' interests better than the client. Their 'unattached' status meant that they were free to complain and be forceful in a way that social workers conscious of hierarchy, authority policy and the interests of Council members could not. On occasion, the case managers were able to call case conferences to sort out the role of various professionals and agencies in their clients' cases. Through using advocacy skills the case managers began to exercise authority without having any direct control over resources; professionals accepted their assessment of their client's need for resources or services.

The case manager approach demonstrated in the CMP depends on the plurality of services and the complexity facing the consumer. But they did not only act like 'brokers', merely connecting people to services to meet their needs. The active, advocate role was necessary because services and resources needed to be negotiated, even fought for – and not always successfully. This suggests limitations in the services: their scarcity and lack of accessibility to people who needed them.

32.2 Kent Community Care Scheme

The Kent Community Care Scheme (KCCS) is perhaps the best known example of applying the principles of case management to community care in the United Kingdom (see chapter 22). In the KCCS the keyworker operated from within a statutorily constituted bureaucracy and had direct control over the resources that would provide care. The case manager not only had control over the management of social services resources (social work, home care, occupational therapy, short-term residential care) but also had a budget with which to buy care in the form of local, paid helpers. This direct control over resources led to a level of control over the outcome of care not available to the case manager in the CMP.

The KCCS has been well documented (Challis and Davies, 1986; Davis and Challis, 1986) but some features of the case manager approach are worth emphasising. The case managers were qualified social workers with experience of working with elderly people, who were set up in a special team to provide a community care alternative for people who were seeking or considered to be in need of residential care. Referrals came mainly from an area social work team but also from local GPs and community nurses. The case managers were a separate team, partly managed by the university researchers from outside the social services department. Their work was focused on a single client group in the manner of very specialised practitioners – but they still had power and authority equivalent to colleagues in other teams.

With smaller caseloads than area team colleagues and a single client group, the case managers were able to use a systematic assessment procedure (Challis and Davis, 1986, pp. 43–4). This drew on other professional assessments (geriatricians, occupational therapists) as well as taking into account what existing services and information support was being provided. The procedure was based on assessment, monitoring and review documents designed partly as research tools and partly as monitoring devices. In the KCCS, assessment was not seen as a one-off event but as the first stage in an on-going monitoring of the client's needs and how they were being met. The case manager had a commitment to managing the package of care by regular monitoring – daily if necessary. The documentation enabled the team of case managers to reflect both on their work with individual clients and on the work of the team (Challis and Chesterman, 1985).

The package of care concept is central to the case manager approach exemplified in the KCCS. The scheme utilised existing resources (aids and equipment, meals on wheels, home care, domiciliary nursing, respite care) but supplemented these with care from local people. Support from local people was partly formalised by offering payment for services and by a letter stating what the services would be. These various components were fitted into a package that could support the person in their own home, designed to suit the individual, while meeting their needs within the resources available. If, for example, the nutritional needs of an elderly person could not be met through the domiciliary meals services – perhaps because the person refused them – a local helper would be recruited to provide meals. A future of the package of care approach was the interweaving of informal care (perhaps relatives willing to manage finances) with semi-formal care (for example, a helper paid to visit daily) and formal, statutory services (a district nurse, visiting weekly) so that not too much burden was placed on one source of support. Flexibility meant that one source of care could be substituted for another (for example, local paid helper for home care assistance) when the caring relationship was no longer working.

The goal of the package of care established by the case manager in the KCCS was to avoid the need for residential care – although it is clear that the wishes of the elderly person were central. However, there was a strong commitment to controlling the expenditure of resources and the case managers were given a target budget of two-thirds of the cost of residential care per person. They were allowed to be flexible on the cost of a plan for individuals provided that the total cost of the team's clients met the budget criteria. The managers spent their budget in two ways –

either by expending social services resources or by paying non-social services staff, the paid helpers, to provide services.

32.2 Gloucester Care for Elderly People at Home project

The Care for Elderly People at Home (CEPH) project was set up in 1986 and was based around three 'care co-ordinators' who took on the role of keyworkers with elderly people. The design of the CEPH project owed much to work done elsewhere that derived from case management – notably the Kent Community Care Scheme (see Carley *et al.*, 1987).

The CEPH project was, however, different in a number of respects from the schemes already considered. First, the project was set up in collaboration with Gloucester Health Authority which employed the care co-ordinators in its community unit. Second, the care co-ordinators were located in three primary health care teams. Third, not only were they not located in social services offices, they were not professionally oriented to social work. The three people were chosen for personal skills and abilities and formal qualifications not necessarily related to the post (degrees, teaching and nursing qualifications).

Unlike the case managers in the CMP, the care co-ordinators worked daily alongside the same team of professional staff responsible for the same group of people – elderly people at risk who were on the patient list of the primary health care team. Not only were they accountable to this group of colleagues, they were also accountable to their employers who were a public body. Unlike the case managers in the KCCS the care co-ordinators in the CEPH project had no direct control over any resources. They had a budget but it was specifically not for buying in care. The budget was a small amount of immediate cash to facilitate their work with clients, for example by providing 'tasters' of different services or buying urgently needed items.

Despite these differences the care co-ordinators worked as keyworkers for elderly people in the community. Their work could be described as 'social work', at least as Goldberg and Connelly (1982) would like to see it. Their role could also be understood as 'case management' in the terms used by Ballew and Mink (1986) or Capitman *et al.*, (1986).

The rare co-ordinators were not set up as a model service. The aim of the project was to use their experience both to understand the needs of elderly people at risk and at home and to explore the different ways that they might be supported. They were not trained or instructed to perform the role of care co-ordination in any particular way but they were encouraged to:

(i) become expert in the availability of local services for elderly people;
(ii) explore new ways of helping elderly people that did not necessarily rely on the existing statutory services;
(iii) attend to the needs of carers, recognising that supporting elderly people in remaining at home often means supporting their personal carers.

As the care co-ordinators developed their role through experience over a period of two years, they included in it all the features listed for the various keyworkers discussed in previous sections. The development of the role was, of course, under the gaze of a research team who passed on experiences from elsewhere learnt through the literature. To show how the care co-ordinators' role operated, various aspects of their work with elderly people can be described under 10 headings derived from the various lists of tasks featured in the literature on social work and case management considered earlier.

Engagement: Initial referrals came mainly from GPs and community nurses who were asked to identify, in the course of their work, elderly people at risk of failing to cope in their own homes. One hundred and seventy-two such referrals were taken on as cases. Some referrals were not accepted as cases, for example when the person only needed 'one-off' help and did not have multiple problems that required co-ordination. Referrals were also taken from sheltered housing wardens, social services staff, vicars, volunteers and directly from elderly people and their carers.

The response to a referral was usually to make an initial home visit, but there was seldom an immediate move to assessing need. Some people had refused services, others did not have a clear perception of what support they needed. The care co-ordinator took time to get to know the person, using a biographical approach to understand their present needs in the context of their past life (see Johnson *et al.*, 1988; Boulton *et al.*, 1989).

Assessment: An assessment 'checklist' was used to ensure that sufficient, appropriate information had been gathered during the initial meetings. Together, the record of the biographical interviews and the checklist formed the basis of record keeping on cases in the project. The checklist ensured that information about the elderly person's current situation was recorded as were needs that could be met and had been agreed with the person. The information on the checklist was coded so that it could be stored on a computer and all the care co-ordinators' cases could be considered on a comparable basis. The checklist was designed in the light of the case review system originally developed by Goldberg and Warburton (see Dant *et al.*, 1987).

Care planning: The care co-ordinators worked with an elderly person towards a plan for a package of care that would help that person remain at home. They worked as a member of the primary health care team and established close working relationships with social service and health authority staff who provided services in the community. They learnt how the main statutory services operated and how best to use them but they also gathered detailed information on local services (luncheon clubs, people willing to do gardening, decorating and private domestic help).

Setting up a package of care: Packages of care incorporated statutory, voluntary and private services with local informal paid and unpaid care. No component of the package was set up without the prior agreement of the elderly person. There were no typical or pre-formed pacakges; each was specific to the individual and their situation (for case studies see Dant, 1988; Boulton *et al.*, 1989; Dant *et al.*, 1989). While home care from social services was an important part of many packages it was by no means always present. A substantial part of the care co-ordinators' work was in liaising with service providers.

Monitoring-reviewing: Maintaining the package of care was a continuous process although inevitably some cases were more active at some times than at others. People's needs change; sometimes a need that has been obscured comes to the fore; sometimes a component in the package of care breaks down and needs replacing. As well as this continuous monitoring, the care co-ordinators reassessed each case at six-monthly intervals using the original checklist. Assessments and reassessments were recorded on the same form so that changes in the person's situation could be reviewed and variations in support monitored.

Community work: Considerable emphasis was placed on work with local groups early in the project. Even though emphasis later shifted more to work with individuals, the care co-ordinators continued to be involved with carers' groups, luncheon clubs, keep-fit groups and the local volunteer forum throughout the project.

Counselling: It was originally anticipated that the care co-ordinators would co-ordinate services rather than provide them directly. However, the difficulty in arranging counselling support for elderly people and their carers combined with the contact that the care co-ordinators had with elderly people meant this developed as part of their own role. Many people who needed counselling support were unable to attend counselling services; they needed the support in their own home. The trust and rapport that derived from the care co-ordinators getting to know people first, before addressing their problems and needs, means that a natural counselling relationship developed with a number of people. In many cases 'counselling' in a formal sense did not take place but a good initial relationship meant that the complex feelings about need for practical help could be communicated. It was then an easy progression for feelings and concerns to become the object of support if that was what was needed.

The care co-ordinators received a small amount of in-service training to help with the demands on them as counsellors as well as support from a clinical psychologist. They found that the most difficult counselling situations were where the elderly person and a personal carer were expressing differing needs.

Advocacy: It also became apparent early on that many elderly people needed advice, support and advocacy in dealing with welfare rights and benefits. While maximising the person's income was often a part of establishing a package of care, the care co-ordinators also acted, on occasion, as advocates in negotiations with solicitors and housing departments. Most of their 'advocacy' work was actually arranging things on behalf of the elderly person – filling in forms, arranging holidays, asking for servies. This sort of work had to be done with the old person, both so that their wishes were always respected and so that they did as much of it as they were willing and able to.

Resource person: Their specialist knowledge about the problems facing elderly people and the range of services available to help them meant the care co-ordinators became a resource to elderly people, their carers and other workers. In an ideal system, information would be available in booklets or a database, especially for use by other workers. During the project, however, the care co-ordinators were the resource and spent a significant proportion of their time passing on information to other professionals.

Disengagement: A feature of the care co-ordinators' work with people was that it was likely to involve long-term support. The people referred to them were at risk of 'failing to cope in their own homes' and therefore of institutionalisation. This meant that while they remained at home they were likely to continue to need a package of care to support them and the package required constant maintenance as circumstances altered. The care co-ordinators did 'disengage' from some cases in the sense of supporting elderly people when they moved into residential care and supporting carers when an elderly person died.

References

Ballew, R. and Mink, G. (1986) *Case Management in the Human services*, Charles C. Thomas, Springfield, Ill.

Boulton, J., Gully, V., Matthews, L. and Gearing, B. (1989) *Developing the Biographical Approach in Practice with Older People*, Care for Elderly People at Home, Project Paper 7, Open University, Milton Keynes.

Capitman, j. A., Haskins, B. and Bernstein, J. (1986) 'Case management approaches in coordinated community oriented care demonstrations', *The Gerontologist*, Vol. 2814, pp. 398–404.

Carley, M., Dant, T., Gearing, B. and Johnson, M. (1987) *Care for Elderly People in the Community: a Review of the Issues and the Research*, Care for Elderly People at Home; Project Paper 1, Open University, Milton Keynes.

Challis, D. and Chesterman, J. (1985) 'A system for monitoring social work activity with the frail elderly', *British Journal of Social Work*, Vol. 15, pp. 115–132.

Challis, D. and Davies, B. (1986) *Case Management in Community Care*, Gower, Aldershot.

Dant, T. (1988) 'Old, poor and at home: social security and elderly people in the community', in Baldwin, S., Parker, G. and Walker, R. (eds) *Social Security and Community Care*, Avebury, Aldershot.

Dant, T., Carley, M., Gearing, B. and Johnson, M. (1987) *Identifying, Assessing and Monitoring the Needs of Elderly People at Home*, Care for Elderly People at Home, Project Paper 2, Open University, Milton Keynes.

Dant, T., Carley, M., Gearing, B. and Johnson, M. (1989) *Co-ordinating Care: the Final Report of the Care for Elderly People at Home Project, Gloucester*, Open University, Milton Keynes.

Davies, B. and Challis. D. (1986) *Matching Needs to Resources*, Gower, Aldershot.

Goldberg, E. M., and Connelly, N. (1982) *The Effectiveness of Social Care for the Elderly*, Heinemann, London.

Goldberg, E. M., and Warburton, R. W. (1979) *Ends and Means in Social Work*, Allen and Unwin, London.

Johnson, M., Gearing, B., Carley, M. and Dant, T. (1988) *A Biographically Based Health and Social Diagnostic Technique: a Research Report*, Care for Elderly People at Home, Project Paper 4, Open University, Milton Keynes.

Pilling, D. (1988) *The Case Manager Project: Report of the Evaluation*, Rehabilitation Resource Centre, Department of Systems Science, City University, London.

33

Hurdles for Social Workers

SUSAN GOFF

My experience of putting together a package of care for an elderly, high dependent woman who suffers from senile dementia may be useful to those currently considering the White Paper on community care. The confused financial arrangements and general lack of alignment between services make the role of co-ordinator very time-consuming (and therefore costly) and fail, at the end of day, to meet the client's needs adequately. The issue of 'choice' is complex, influenced as it is by others and by the availability of services.

October 1988: Mrs G is referred to the social services department (SSD), having recently been discharged from hospital with a broken hip. She is confused and suffers poor mobility. She lives in a warden-controlled local authority flat, and has a married son. She wants to remain in her own flat. Mrs G is offered day care at one of the local authority's residential homes. She does not accept this as her husband died there. She does accept an introduction to day care at the Over 60s' Club. She starts this for a few weeks but when another elderly confused lady joins, there are behavioural difficulties and she is stopped from attending.

November 1988: Mrs G is awarded attendance allowance and offered Part 2½ accommodation by the housing department. (This is North Hertfordshire District Council's term for accommodation which is one step up from sheltered housing. Residents still receive care services but are semi-independent in that they have their own front door.) This would enable her to have her own flat, very similar to the one she currently has, where her attendance allowance would be used to pay a service charge for carers that are provided.

This might have been acceptable to Mrs G but her son feels she should

---

This chapter was first published in *Community Care*, 18 January, 1990.

live with him. He wishes to claim invalid care allowance. This would enable him to continue claiming income support without needing to be available for work. There is concern that his house is physically unsuitable and he and his wife might not be able to cope with caring for his mother.

Christmas 1988: Her condition deteriorates to such an extent that she is unable to get herself a drink, is at times doubly incontinent and has an erratic sleep pattern. Her confusion varies. Often she's unaware of where she is or who her son is.

January 1989: Mr G decides that he cannot cope with caring for his mother but the offer of the Part 2½ accommodation has gone. He and his wife decide to care for Mrs G at her flat for 35 hours a week for no more than five days a week. Mr G is to claim invalid care allowance. Care on the other two days is covered by the housing department's staff and the social services, home helps and domiciliary care assistants.

February 1989: Mr G finds he cannot cope with the stress of caring for his mother. SSD's support services increase and an application is made to the Independent Living Fund, who offered to help with the cost of 30 hours care a week (less attendance allowance and severe disability premium). Initially, Mr G is reluctant to take up this offer using his mother's attendance allowance and severe disability premium.

April 1989: Mr G withdraws from caring for his mother and agrees to me making inquiries to find carers that may be employed privately. I contact about six different nursing and care agencies but none are operating in this area. I eventually find two carers on the grapevine and through Aunties, a new small, local business which makes introductions to carers but does not act as an agency.

We arrange 15 hours of care and there is a noticeable improvement in Mrs G when she has more company and her sleep pattern is re-established. The rota now uses four Independent Living Fund funded carers, domiciliary care assistants, home helps and housing department staff. The administration of the finances is complicated and now handled by a social work assistant.

Mrs G agrees to residential care. Many people have been encouraging her to accept this. The SSD within the area has no vacancies. The local elderly forum is aware of a vacancy in a private residential home which is registered for caring for the mentally ill.

This is explored and visited with Mr G and later with Mrs G. Mrs G is initially very positive as her brother used to live in the same road. However, when it comes to offering her an assessment place Mrs G decides to remain in her flat. Although confused on many issues, she seems quite clear about the decision that she is making and about not wishing to go to the residential home.

There are also many administrative problems arising out of placing Mrs G in a private residential home. The residential home charges are higher than her DSS entitlement. The residential home agrees to take her at this lower amount on the condition that I try to obtain the top-up £35 per week through charities. I endeavour to do this.

Further, the private residential home ask for a sponsorship form to be signed. It does not seem appropriate for Mr G to be asked to sign this and this department has reservations about doing so.

After Mrs G has decided not to accept the private residential home, I discover that the SSD registration officer visited the home three weeks ago and was not happy with its standards. Some weeks later the situation is clarified. It is acceptable to use this home.

June 1989: We are able to increase the Independent Living Fund funded care to 24 hours, but the rota system remains erratic, especially as it is summer and carers go on holiday. Gaps are filled by the domiciliary care assistant who pops in for 15 minutes where an Independent Living Fund funded carer may stay up to three hours. There are difficult delays in receiving carers' wages from the fund.

Attempts are made again to introduce Mrs G to day care as a way of reducing her anxiety about residential care. She will need one of her carers to go in a taxi with her to the home, stay there with her and bring her back. From this she may move on to respite care and, if a place becomes available, accept residential care. We would use one of the carers funded by the Independent Living Fund for care at home but this carer would have to be funded by SSD for this task. Waiting some weeks to see if this is possible.

We aim to continue to enable Mrs G to live as she wishes at home, while hoping to introduce her to residential care in a way that might reduce fears she may have of it.

We have tried to maximise all available resources.

I have over-simplified the details of this case. I have not, for instance, mentioned that this department [the SSD] decided to become appointee of Mrs G's financial affairs and the associated administrative problems this entailed. I have not talked of the lack of procedures for employing carers privately on Mrs G's behalf, or the lack of information and the difficulties of meeting these carers' needs as employees. I have not given vent to the frustrations I have felt in my role of trying to make all this work.

The idea of enabling people to live in the community for as long as they may wish to do so is correct. The concern has to be that lack of suitable available resources, the influence of others and a system which lacks coherence means that choice is not a reality. The current system might be entitled 'hurdles for social workers' but once on the track there appears to be no end to the obstacles to be overcome.

34

*Involving People With Learning Difficulties in Meetings**

ANDREA WHITTAKER

The meeting had been in progress for twenty minutes. There was a knock on the door and in came the last member of the committee. He was empty-handed. He glanced rather uncertainly around the room. He was greeted briefly and invited to take a seat. Discussion on the current agenda item continued. After a while, the latecomer began to join in: some comments were relevant to the topic – some were not. Now and then, the latecomer would take up a point enthusiastically and talk at length in a way which appeared to the rest of the committee to bear little or no relation to the subject under discussion.

Nothing particularly unusual in that brief scenario you might say. We all know people who come to meetings late, have forgotten their meeting papers, and who waste everyone else's time by waffling on about their own particular hobby-horse! However, what made that scene different from dozens of similar occasions was that the latecomer happened to be a person with learning difficulties (former term: 'mental handicap').

It is now quite common for policy and planning documents about services for people with learning difficulties to include statements about the importance of service users participating directly in service planning and delivery. Unfortunately though, these are often no more than general statements of intent and nothing is said about how these intentions will be turned into action.

This chapter discusses one way in which service users can participate in the development of services, looking at how people with learning

---

*This chapter was first published in *Power to the People*, Winn, L. (ed) (King's Fund Centre, London, 1990) pp. 41–48.

difficulties can play an effective part in meetings. It focuses on meetings specifically because, however much we may complain about their frequency or question their usefulness, they remain an important and often-used method of communication in service-providing agencies such as health authorities or social services departments.

This chapter focuses on people with learning difficulties, partly because of the author's experience (as advisor to the self-advocacy organisation People First)[1] and partly because general progress towards participation by service users in Britain is more widely developed amongst people with learning difficulties than amongst other groups such as people with physical disabilities or mental health service users. Through membership of student or trainee committees in day centres and the activities of groups such as People First, many people with learning difficulties have become skilled at speaking up for themselves and identifying what they want from services.

To return to the scenario described at the beginning of this chapter. A keen observer of the scene might have noticed other ways in which people were behaving differently. Most contributions to the discussion would be acknowledged in some way by others present – by a nod of the head, murmurs of agreement (or disagreement), by eye contact; in these small ways, individual contributions would be woven into the general ebb and flow of the discussion. But comments from the person with learning difficulties seemed to be handled differently. Sometimes they were passed over – almost ignored. If the comment seemed irrelevant then silence descended and people seemed to be feeling rather uneasy. On the other hand, sometimes he was given the floor and allowed to talk at considerable length, unchecked by fellow committee members or by the chairperson. But when he stopped, discussion among the rest resumed as if he had not spoken at all.

This story illustrates several key issues which need to be considered when thinking about how to involve service users most appropriately in meetings.

34.1 Professionals with problems with participation

One of the most important points to emerge from the story is that it isn't only service users who may lack the necessary skills. Even when professionals are committed to the idea of participation, they may still find it difficult. The fact that someone may have worked with people with learning difficulties for many years may not mean that they find this sort of communication easy. For some people, moving up the career ladder may mean they end up spending little or no time in face-to-face contact with service users. But even when people do work on a daily basis with users they may still never really get to know the people they work alongside.

Genuine participation in situations like the one described above means involving service users as real partners. Services do not tend to foster that sort of equality of relationship. People with learning difficulties are used to a much more passive role, to being on the receiving end of services which have been planned and shaped by other people who have decided that they know what is best for them.

As a result of all this, people may feel uncertain about how to react or even how to talk to a service user in a group. They may feel impatient if the pace of the meeting seems to be slowing down; or frustrated by the need to explain or clarify more often than usual. Whatever the reason, it is not unusual for profesionals to be anxious about the idea of working with a person with learning difficulties on the basis of participation and partnership.

34.2 People with learning difficulties as participants

People with learning difficulties have demonstrated time and again that they can make extremely effective contributions to all types of discussions – as conference speakers or in meetings or in small group discussions; the growth of self-advocacy has provided many more opportunities for people to express themselves. A person with learning difficulties will often say something which gives fresh insight to the discussion. Listening to someone speaking of their own direct experience can be a most effective way of keeping the real world in our minds. It can help prevent discussion drifting off into the realms of theory and help everyone present focus on people – rather than beds, buildings, service structures and systems.

Nevertheless, when it comes to being involved in meetings, it is unlikely that the service user will have the same level of skills as others in the group. Most members of the group will be used to attending meetings – usually as a regular part of their working life, but often as a part of their social and leisure activities too. They will have little difficulty in holding conversations on a one-to-one basis as well as taking part in group discussions. Most people with learning difficulties, however, have not had the opportunities to develop and practise these skills.

There are various reasons for this, most of which are the result of the way other people have acted towards them. For a start, people with learning difficulties have not been expected to have opinions or ideas of their own – or not ones which were worth discussing with other people.

In many cases they will have spent most of their waking hours in an environment where other people told them what to do and where to go. Responding to these sorts of 'orders' doesn't really require any verbal response at all. Even questions can usually be answered with a brief 'yes' or 'no'. A person's latent abilities may have remained hidden because of the low expectations of those around them.

It is not surprising, therefore, that the service user who joins a committee or working group may have some catching up to do in terms of learning new skills and may need special support in order to contribute effectively to the discussions. There are several ways in which the group as a whole can offer that support.

34.3 Commitment

Without the commitment of a majority of people in a group involving service users, their involvement is unlikely to be more than tokenistic, failing to develop into a real partnership and sharing of power.

Real commitment is about more than a written statement of intent (although that may be a useful starting-point). It means individual group members believing that service users have a right to be involved and that they have a valued contribution to make. At the start, it is unlikely that everyone will have the same degree of commitment or hold the same views on participation. Some may be for it, some against and others may be willing to give it a try. Sometimes user participation may have been 'imposed' on the group by more senior colleagues, causing possible resentment.

So, before service users become involved, the group needs to talk through how they feel about the idea, being as frank and honest as they can. A brief discussion at one meeting may be all that's needed – but it may take longer than that. Take your time – but take care that discussion doesn't become an excuse for inaction!

The best way of breaking down barriers and prejudices is to get to know people as individuals. Think about where the potential service-user members of your committee or working group are likely to come from; it might be a local self-advocacy group or a student/trainee committee at a day centre. Invite a few people from that group to meet your group; this gives both sides the chance to explore whether they want to work together.

One way to arrange a meeting would be to write to the group, asking if they would be willing to meet members of your group. The letter should state clearly and simply why you would like a meeting, including perhaps one or two very practical examples of issues you would like to work on with service users. This meeting might form part of the agenda of one of your meetings, or the service users might like some of your group to attend one of their meetings.

When the Independent Development Council (IDC)[2] decided it wanted to involve people with learning difficulties as members of the Council, it invited representative of People First to attend one of its meetings as observers. These observers then reported back to their colleagues in People First and the group was then able to decide whether they actually wanted to become more involved with the IDC.

Whatever you decide to do – keep it simple! Avoid lengthy letters and complicated enclosures. Avoid large gatherings of people. This is all about getting to know people as individuals – as potential working partners. As in other situations, a few people meeting together over a meal may do more to increase understanding and commitment to collaboration than any amount of formal education or training.

34.4 The importance of language

A chairperson was summing up at the end of a day's workshop. The day had begun with a contribution from two people with learning difficulties who had advocated passionately for the abolition of the term 'mental handicap'. This had obviously affected the majority of participants who made considerable efforts throughout the day to remember not to use that term. The chairperson commented on this, ending with 'We have learnt that we must watch our language – at least in the presence of people with handicaps'.

A joke? Or a sad reflection of how shallow our commitment and understanding can be? The way we speak about people with disabilities says a great deal about how we value – or devalue – people and how serious we are about working with them as partners in planning and developing services. A lifetime of being labelled has made labels a major issue[3] and learning to use descriptive terms which are acceptable to people with learning difficulties is an important issue.

But it is also important to think more generally about the language we use – particularly in meetings. We need to talk clearly and simply and avoid jargon. If a service user does not seem to be following the discussion in a meeting it is all too easy to assume that that is part of being handicapped. It may be that the discussion is not particularly meaningful or clear to others either. The onus is on everyone present to make the discussion comprehensible. This can be challenging at times but is likely to result in greater clarity and understanding not only for the person with learning difficulties but for all those present.

34.5 Listening

Listening is something we tend to do automatically, without thinking consciously about it, particularly when we are with people of similar interests and background who 'speak our langauge'; it rarely occurs to us that we might need to develop our listening skills; but if we did, some of us might become better listeners!

When we join a group such as a committee or working party, however, it can take time for the group to become comfortable in communicating with one another. So really listening to someone who is a newcomer to the group, and whose opportunities to develop conversational skills, think logically and get a message across clearly may have been severely limited, requires a deliberate effort on our part and even the development of new skills.

For example, the person with learning difficulties may say something which seems to be way off the point. But a good listener will often be able to detect a link. It might be the last word said by another person present. The person with learning difficulties has picked this up and related it to his own experience in some way. Other members of the group need to discover what this link might be – building on it to draw out something meaningful to the rest of the discussion – perhaps also helping to lead the service user 'back on to the track' and fostering his involvement in the group.

The baseline must always be 'Have we explained this carefully enough?' or 'Have we provided all the support that this person needs in order to participate in the discussions?' It should never be 'Oh, he can't be expected to understand that idea or that document'.

This type of listening needs time, patience and practice. But it is crucial if we are to enable service users to be effective participants.

34.6 Remember the usual pitfalls of meetings

It is useful to remember what happens ordinarily at meetings; there are people who talk too much while others may say virtually nothing; some people stick to the topic while others are inclined to wander off it. If the group is really committed to participation, they will want to do all they can to ensure that the service user feels involved with what is going on. But this does not mean making the service user into some sort of 'special' member of the group, entitled to 'special' treatment. As the story at the beginning illustrates, there is a danger that concessions may be made for the service user which are not applied to any other members of the group. On the other hand, the service-user member should not be expected to act as a 'super-participant' – never straying off the topic, never left alone, and expected to contribute to every single agenda item!

In short, although he or she may need extra help to become a real part of the group, the service user should be treated as far as possible like any other member of the group. There is a very important balance to be struck here – and it is not always easy – but a good chairperson should be able to ensure that this is achieved.

34.7 The fear of tokenism

Many people express concern about the dangers of tokenism, citing examples of people with learning difficulties being used as the token consumer. This can happen in a number of ways and for a variety of reasons. Service users may have words put into their mouths, or be asked questions in a way which allows only the answer the questioner wants to hear '(Don't you think we ought to . . .' or 'Wouldn't it be a good idea if . . .'). They may be 'paraded' in front of an audience like some sort of special exhibit, their presence, in some way, making professionals 'feel good' about themselves. Lastly, they may be asked leading questions which take advantage of the service user's inexperience at handling impromptu questioning.

These sort of concerns are valid, and these practices unacceptable and exploitative. But they can also become reasons – or excuses – for not doing anything about participation.

Although it is likely that someone joining a committee or working party as a service user representative will already have some of the skills needed to participate, there may well be times when that person appears not to be making any contribution. We need to consider carefully, though, whether that person makes a contribution simply by being there. The presence of a service user can say something positive about what we believe about that person's right to be involved. If we are committed to participation, then our awareness of that person's presence should have a positive effect on the outcome of discussions. If the issues discussed in this chapter have been understood and worked through, then tokenism should not be a real danger.

34.8 Providing additional support

It may be helpful if someone is appointed to attend meetings as a supporter for the service user – either for an initial period, or perhaps on a more permanent basis (although that may not be necessary if the service-user representative becomes more skilled and comfortable in meetings).

It is important that the supporter is independent of other members of the group, to avoid any conflict of interest. For example, if the supporter is already a member of the committee or working group, then he or she will almost certainly find there are times when loyalty to the group will clash with loyalty to the service user.

In a meeting of residential care managers, it may seem logical and convenient for service-user members to be supported by one of the staff from their group home. But will that staff member always be able to put the wishes and needs of the service user first, or will they sometimes find they are supporting the wishes of their employers?

In the case of the IDC quoted above, it might have been thought practical for the People First group's advisor to be the supporter. However, the advisor also happens to be a member of the IDC so someone with no connection with IDC was appointed.

The supporter's job might include: helping the person get to the meeting on time, checking that they have the right papers, helping them read and digest papers before meetings, and reinforcing and developing the service user's group discussion skills.

During the meeting it is important that the supporter doesn't 'take over'. The supporter's role is to facilitate not to participate directly, to support and not supplant. It's very much a 'back-seat' role with as little intervention as possible.

However, although the supporter is there primarily to support the service user, he or she may also have a role in helping other members of the group – for example, asking for simpler language, asking for clarification on particular points. Gradually, though, the service user should be gaining the confidence to make those requests directly.

It is important for the supporter's role to be clearly understood by all members of the committee or working group. It might be helpful to write brief guidelines – a very simple 'contract' – so that everyone knows the ground rules within which the supporter will work and their relationship with the service user.

34.9 In conclusion

In spite of all that has been written and said about 'consumer participation', when it comes to involving people with disabilities directly in the development of services, we are all beginners. Participation requires us to think about people in new ways. It challenges long-held beliefs and long-standing practices. This chapter has been concerned with how we deal with some of these issues, moment by moment, during the course of a meeting.

Perhaps the two most important words in the chapter are 'commitment' and 'listening'. Without commitment, participation is unlikely to get started. Without skilled listening, it is unlikely to develop in a way which will lead to the ultimate goal of participation – real changes for the better in the lives of people with disabilities.

Notes

1 People First, Oxford House, Derbyshire Street, London E2 6HG, tel. 071 739 3890.
2 IDC, Independent Development Council, 126 Albert Street, London, NW1 7NF.
3 Bill Worrell, *People First: Advice to Advisors*, National People First Project, Ontario, Canada. For information on availability in UK please contact People First, London (see above).

35

Elfrida Rathbone Islington: An Experience of Contracting

CHRISTINA SCHWABENLAND

35.1 Background

Elfrida Rathbone Islington is a registered charity and limited company that for over 70 years has developed and run services for people in Islington with moderate learning difficulties. Prior to negotiating a new contract with the London Borough of Islington we ran three community education projects: an under fives' unit; a literacy unit; and a groupwork and activities unit (the latter for adults). We had three housing projects: a registered hostel for 12 residents and seven staff; and two houses with housing projects: a registered hostel for 12 residents and seven staff; and two houses with bedsits and flats and minimal support. We also run Elfrida's Cafe – a training scheme in catering and employment skills. We work with approximately 2,000 users per year.

In June 1989 we were approached by the local authority and asked if we would be interested in taking over the social-services-run local hostel for 21 people with moderate learning difficulties. The impetus came from social security and there was never any question of competitive tendering. It was easy to see why Islington approached us. We are the largest voluntary organisation working with people with learning difficulties in the borough, we had an established track record and the work of our other hostel was well respected. We have an equal opportunities policy and trade union recognition – both important factors to the local authority, which has gone on record as saying that it will not contract out its existing services to the private sector, or to voluntary organisations without good employment policies.

Islington's motives were primarily financial. The government had created a loophole whereby a resident who lives in a hostel run by the voluntary or private sector is entitled to claim a Department of Social Security (DSS) benefit called board-and-lodgings money. If they live in a hostel run by the local authority or health authority, however, they are not entitled to this benefit and the authority has to pick up most of the costs. Therefore, simply by transferring ownership of the hostel from one sector to another, a large amount of central government money would be attracted into the borough.

The government has created this anomaly because it believes that the independent sector can run services better, because of smaller size, flexibility and closer proximity to service users. Islington never publicly said that they shared this belief or that it was a motivating factor. However, it was occasionally hinted at privately and for us it had to be an important concern. We would not have wanted to take over the hostel if we did not think we could run it at least as well, and preferably better, than the local authority.

This was *our* main reason for agreeing to begin the process of negotiations. Our primary interest had to be that of providing the best possible service for people with learning difficulties. But we also had pragmatic reasons – the security of a contract which meant that the local authority, our primary funder, needed us as much as we need them, was very attractive.

35.2 The process of the negotiations

From the initial approach to the day we formally took over the hostel was a period of over 18 months. After we told the local authority that we were tentatively interested in proceeding we heard very little for about six months. Meetings were to be scheduled but somehow never happened. We used the time to find out as much as possible about any received wisdom in the great big world outside about contracting. The director (me!) took it on herself to do most of the leg work, especially in the early stages, and this took up a substantial amount of time. I went on courses about contracting and rang up everyone I knew who was involved in contracts. I made contact with the London Voluntary Service Council, the National Council of Voluntary Organisations and the Association of Residential Care. I discovered that a lot was being talked about, concerning the contracting out of existing services, but very little had, as yet, really happened, so there was little real experience on which to draw.

However, everyone I spoke to agreed that the most important element in negotiating a contract is to agree a statement of claims and objectives, because these will provide a firm base for negotiating all the day-to-day bits and pieces. (The other important thing to do right at the beginning is the preliminary costings – but more of that later!)

For us this highlighted a major deficiency in our own organisation: we didn't have a clearly written statement of aims. So, because we needed to have one in place by the time negotiations began, we convened a small working party consisting of staff and management committee members, and drew up a statement of values and aims and objectives for the agency as a whole.

35.2.1 Negotiations begin

In January 1990 the first meeting with the leader of the council and ourselves took place and the negotiations suddenly got underway. We put our aims and objectives item at the top of the agenda; very little time was actually spent discussing them – about five minutes! The rest of the meeting concentrated on the practical issues that had to be resolved and a reasonable timetable was established.

All of a sudden there seemed to be vast numbers of meetings happening, nearly every week. Specific meetings were set up to deal with all the separate issues – the contract, the residents, staffing, finance, building works. I went to all of them. The local authority, of course, fielded different people for different meetings and no single officer was required to match the time commitment needed from us. Elfrida Rathbone established a sub-committee of management committee members who met regularly to talk through the issues that were coming up, and to give me support.

In March, nine months after the initial approach, we drafted a provisional working budget based on what was known about the current hostel budget and also on our experience of running our other hostel. Many costs were not known, as the local authority was not, at this stage, able to completely cost its services. We presented it to the leader of the council and a handful of other members and officers, and immediately sparks began to fly. Our initial budget gave the local authority only a very small saving on the current running costs of the hostel. The councillors were extremely unhappy and ordered us to go away and come back with something better. This was the first time that anyone had had a serious look at the finances.

The reasons why our budget seemed so high were various. First, we allowed for management costs and various services that the local authority provide in house and do not charge to individual projects. Second, our estimates for various unknown factors, such as building maintenance, were quite high because we wanted to minimise the risk factor. Third, our other hostel cares for a younger and more rumbustious group of people and our wear-and-tear costs are higher there.

So there was some scope for trimming costs. However, what horrified us was the tone of the discussions at that and subsequent meetings. We felt that we had been harangued and browbeaten, and sent away to do better. Previous meetings had been conducted as if we were equals, each needing something from the other, and each prepared to negotiate and occasionally compromise. We had broad agreement on basic principles and a shared aim. But the finance meetings felt different. The underlying assumption suddenly seemed to be that our status was that of a rather junior department of the council that wasn't doing what it was supposed to do. Veiled and unclear threats were implied as to what might happen to our current grant aid if we did not produce a 'better' budget – one that would guarantee a higher level of savings for the council.

This was the most unpleasant and uncomfortable stage of the entire negotiation. We sat down with the officers of the finance department and eventually produced a compromise budget which we felt we could probably live with, and which produced a higher level of estimated savings to the council. We reduced our management costs a little, and lowered our assumptions about repairs and maintenance. The council increased their assumptions about staffing levels. In the end, the negotiations continued.

35.2.2 Different understandings

But several significant things had emerged. One was about the difference in approach between the council and ourselves. We prepared budgets based on real assumptions about real costs. We are a smallish organisation with few resources, and our working budgets have to be as accurate as possible. The council used a lot of formulae, such as budgeting for a 10 per cent vacancy rate in staffing costs, which are just not appropriate for a small organisation. The council assumed a much lower rate of inflation than we did. Their approach seemed to be to underestimate costs and hope for the best, while ours was to get them as accurate as possible and build in a slight margin of error for unforeseen emergencies. Needless to say, we didn't entirely see eye to eye!

More importantly, there was no shared understanding of our status; this only emerged when we had a disagreement, and, of course, money was the issue over which that disagreement was most marked. We view ourselves as an autonomous organisation accountable to our management committee and our users. I think the local authority would broadly agree with that view, but they are our primary funders and expect us to satisfy certain criteria in order to receive funding from them. And it felt to us as though beneath the finance negotiations the assumptions of the councillors were that we were there to help them out of a fix, and of the finance officers, that we were obliged to manage the budget set for us. And indeed there seems to be no objective clarity to be had about these issues. We are constituted as an independent organisation. The council is our primary funder and can withdraw funding tomorrow if it wishes. We set our own budget for our hostels, but the local authority has to approve the level of the fee. The relationship is unclear and it seems to me that it can only be managed by some degree of consent about a shared interpretation of these difficult areas. And what emerged from this phase of the negotiations was that this consent and this understanding is partial. A negotiation like this involves so many disparate arms of the council; there may be shared understanding with a handful of officers in the social services department, but does that extend to the legal department, the buildings and maintenance?

In the end obviously the negotiations continued and we papered over the cracks in our shared understanding. There were some negative sides to it – we did feel a little intimidated, and unsure of what would happen if we pulled out. We weren't sure the budget we ended up with would allow us to manage the hostel as we wanted to. And we didn't quite know at what point the power balance had shifted, nor at what point we had become committed to the hostel takeover. Up till this time we had thought that we could simply pull out of the negotiations if they didn't go as we wanted, but that no longer felt possible.

However, the other reasons for getting involved still remained; at this time we also met the residents and their families for the first time, and that provided more impetus to continue. A series of meetings was organised between ourselves, the residents and their carers to discuss the transfer. On the whole these went well, but it was rather distressing that many of the residents were deeply concerned about losing the current staff and worried about who the new staff would be, and there was no obvious way of allaying that concern before the new staff were appointed.

Meanwhile the draft contract was written, primarily by us. Initially there were joint meetings to discuss its content but we took on the task of drafting it, primarily to save time. This proved to be very fortuitous as we were able to write it as we wanted and to ensure that it contained everything that we wanted it to have.

In the early days of the negotiations various options about staffing were suggested, but we decided almost immediately that we ourselves would like to interview anyone who was to become an employee of Elfrida Rathbone, and that we didn't want to inherit staff whom we had had no part in selecting. The local authority unions NALGO and NUPE were involved in negotiations with the council, and they asked that we offer preferential interviews to anyone from the old staff team who would be interested in applying to work for Elfrida Rathbone. The unions were interested in seeing a contract of employment and in comparing terms and conditions between the two agencies. There are some differences: salaries are on the same grades, but our sickness benefit is not as good as the local authority's. When the time to recruit the staff drew near, we asked the previous staff to let us know if they wanted preferential interviews. By 'preferential' we meant that we would interview them on their own ahead of any other applicants and offer them the jobs if they met the specification; we would only advertise externally if we still had vacancies. But none of them applied for the jobs. The local authority has had a guaranteed redeployment policy, so all of the staff either took voluntary early retirement or were redeployed on their existing terms and conditions.

I have no idea whether any staff considered applying to work for us or not. I do know that the staff felt unhappy about the transfer and that the group became quite a powerful source of support for the individuals within it; and I speculate that it would have been hard indeed to break ranks! Also, of course, they had all applied for jobs working for a local authority, and didn't have any commitment or any real understanding of the voluntary sector. They kept referring to the transfer as a 'privatisation'. The unions did circulate a press release, fairly early on, hoping to mobilise support to stop the transfer, but only our local paper picked it up, and it didn't have any repercussions. After that, the staff and unions co-operated with the negotiations, although they made it clear that they did not think the idea was a good one.

One point they raised against the transfer, which I think is valid, is that the local authority would lose the ability to be flexible and innovative with their resources. The funding agreement with us is very tightly circumscribed – we have to take only residents who can claim board-and-lodgings money, etc. Whereas had the local authority kept the hostel, in theory they could have changed its function and been more flexible about whom they took in. In theory they could have decided to change its use completely and, say, turn it into a home for the elderly instead. Whereas we are limited by the financial constraints and also by our own constitution – we only work with people with learning difficulties. I think this is an interesting point. However, in our case we pressed to have the contract limited to five years and it will only be renewed after a very thorough review.

35.2.3 Under new management

A steering committee was established by the local authority – chaired by the Assistant Director of Social Services and the Principal Assistant, and having input from the finance, legal and architects' departments and from the Registration Officer. We established a timetable for a provisional takeover in mid- to late autumn 1990.

35.2.4 Delays and stress

Several things happened to delay it. First, we discovered that although the hostel normally had 22 spaces, only 16 people were currently resident, and six of those were due to move out before we took over. We had done the budget on the basis of a minimum of 17 people and instead there were only likely to be 10! We sent three mailings to all the social workers in the department to drum up new referrals, and two months later we had only two names. It became clear at this point that we had all done very little long-term strategic thinking about what the need in Islington really was for this unit. No one really knew why the take-up of places was initially so poor and it seemed risky making long-term plans without that information.

After much discussion we decided to go ahead on the basis of a smaller staff team and smaller numbers of residents and to retain the option of increasing numbers at a later date if the need was there. But the overall lack of strategic planning is an issue for both agencies to address.

The last six months have been spent planning the actual takeover, staffing issues, building works, etc. The building did not meet the standard laid down in the 1984 Registered Homes Act. It is still the case that homes run by the voluntary or private sector need to meet much more stringent criteria than those run by statutory authorities. Islington agreed to fund and carry out all the essential building works, but delays of over six months in the building schedule meant that we had to change our plans. We decided to go ahead with the takeover and move in before the building works were completed because the delays were proving so stressful for the residents, and unmanageable for the staff teams. Several months later, the finance needed to complete the building works was still awaiting committee approval.

We negotiated a two-week handover between our new staff team and the outgoing team, who were being relocated into other jobs by the local authority. The handover went reasonably successfully but was clearly a stressful time for all concerned, as the residents were unsettled. The previous staff team were feeling a lot of antagonism towards us, and our new staff team felt somewhat overwhelmed by the amount of information they needed to learn quickly. We organised one day of team-building for them with an outside facilitator, which helped to give them a sense of identity. It proved very difficult for everyone to manage the boundaries between their obligations to the residents and loyalties to each other, and we discovered that some crucial pieces of information about residents had not been given to us because they involved disciplinary issues within the council. There were no clear guidelines about what we did and didn't need to know, and of course again there was no shared understanding of whether we were insiders or outsiders. This confusion was even reflected in such mundane questions as whether or not we should have access to the controls of the central heating system, normally restricted to only certain council employees. This is such a new situation with so little precedent that there is no blueprint for working through issues such as these.

35.2.5 The contract

The contract, however, does make the relationship between us fairly explicit, and it has proved a very relevant and valuable basis for negotiations. But its status, too, has not been straightforward. Having produced the original draft, with which social services officers, councillors and ourselves were happy, it was then sent off to the council's legal department to be turned into a legally binding document. And here again, we had problems. The lawyers came up with the proposal that the basic agreement between us should be in the form of a lease, with an appendix containing the operating policy of the hostel. We said that, to us, an operational policy was a practice document about the day-to-day running of the hostel, and that it didn't need to be legally drawn up. What was needed was some sort of management agreement between us. The legal department didn't understand what we meant; we were to be managing the hostel, so what might the agreement need to be about? It soon emerged that the legal department were blissfully (or not so blissfully!) unaware of all the recent discussions in the world at large about contracting. They didn't know what contracts, in the sense that the word is now being used, were all about.

This debate continued for several months until we finally gave them a book recently published by the NCVO entitled *12 Charity Contracts*, which proved that it could be done! From that point on things progressed quickly. Our original document was unearthed, and, nearly a year after it was originally written, it came back barely changed, ready for official signatures.

35.2.6 Partnerships

On 11 February 1991 we finally took over the hostel. At the time of writing the building works are unfinished, the lease of contract still needs some fine tuning and we are daily uncovering things that need resolution – such as who maintains the burglar alarm, and the boiler, especially if the boiler belongs to a leasing company rather than to the council? But these problems are all manageable, if infuriating. The new staff have a great deal of enthusiasm and, generally speaking, the residents have adjusted to the change remarkably well. We have started regular residents' meetings so they have a formal forum for planning with us how the hostel wil be run in the future.

On the whole we feel quite optimistic about the future, but we have some reservations. The financial arrangements carry some risk: the local authority has not guaranteed to maintain a fixed number of spaces, and as the budget is worked out on the basis of a per capita fee, we need to make sure we have enough residents to be financially viable. The question of the need for this kind of hostel in the long term still remains. We have established a review group, which will meet quarterly in the first year and six-monthly during the next four years; its function will be to monitor both the work on the ground and also the terms of the partnership agreement, so I hope this will be a forum where these and many other questions can be raised.

35.3 Impact on Elfrida Rathbone Islington

Looking back over the last 18 months I think that these negotiations have had a very significant effect on our agency.

Time. The negotiations have taken up an incalculable amount of time and energy. The management committee have regularly had extra meetings. The finance officer has spent weeks drawing up new budgets, looking at the knock-on financial effects for the agency as a whole, cash-flow projection, yet more budgets, inventories, new petty cash systems, DSS liaison, etc. The social work co-ordinator was seconded to the hostel for two months to get it up and running. The administrator handled the staff recruitment side – mailing application forms, photo-copy, postage – our advertisements brought a response of over 400 enquiries about the jobs. And for all of these months I have made this project my top priority and couldn't begin to calculate the time spent on it. The solicitor's bills haven't yet arrived either, but they will be horrendous.

Mangement systems. The negotiations have exposed all sorts of problems with our internal management systems. I've already mentioned one – our previous lack of a defined statement of aims and objectives. Many other things were thrown up during these months: a lack of clarity about who our clients were; differentials in pay scales throughout the agency; and a lack of clarity about decision-making processes and who does or doesn't get consulted. I personally view this as a wholly positive side-effect, and have found it incredibly useful to have had so many issues exposed, but it may not be a process that smaller organisations are prepared for, or are able to respond to.

Growth. Elfrida Rathbone is now the single largest provider of residential services for people with learning difficulties in Islington. This has happened by default and we haven't yet really thought through what this might mean in the future.

35.4 Conclusions

The issues that cause us concern are the element of financial risk and the unclear nature of our relationship that caused the lack of clarity – it was there all along and has only been exposed by the process of negotiating the contract. All the contract does is to define expectations more precisely than the terms of grant aid. Clear expectations can be liberating or constricting depending on how you look at them. But there are deeper confusions about the identity and role and autonomy of the voluntary sector and these are now 'solved' by having a contract.

Also, although it is not particularly an issue for us, the government's aims of creating a market-place are not met simply by transferring services from one existing provider to another. There is no more choice for Islington residents with learning difficulties than there was before. I think we are offering them a better service than they had before, but there is still only one choice and one service. And there is an irony in the fact that because of the financial incentive most of the new initiatives around contracting are securing the future of residential institutions, *not* community-based services!

On the plus side, we have welcomed the opportunity to take over a new (for us) and challenging project. We enjoy the work! We are glad that it offers us a measure of security that we didn't have before, and we want to be able to develop a more influential role in planning for the future of residential and community services in Islington for people with learning difficulties. And I have enjoyed the challenge and the questions that have been raised for us by taking this on.

36

Community Development and Community Care: A Strategic Approach

PAUL HENDERSON and JOHN ARMSTRONG

In this chapter we identify six areas of experience, knowledge, skills and methods that we believe community development can contribute to community care policy development and practice. In giving consideration to this theme it is important to relate it to what we know about informal and formal networks in communities, self-help groups, and the idea of community capacity: the existing and potential resources that are contained in communities, and the abilities of people to organise and take action for themselves.

It is this last point that is the most significant element of any definition of community development. Encouraging and enabling people, usually on a neighbourhood basis, is at the core of community development practice. High value is placed on people working together: collective action as opposed to action taken by individuals on their own behalf, and collective action that normally is taken on behalf of a broad constituency, not solely for members of a particular group. A community centre committee, for example, acts for an array of users and supporters.

Given the close association historically between community development and social work (see Thomas, 1983) the relative paucity of written material that makes the connections between community development and community care is surprising. Yet the potential benefits of using a community development approach as part of implementing community care policies is, we suggest, considerable. There is evidence for this in a limited number of social services and social work departments. For example, an audit of practice in Strathclyde Social Work Department, carried out in 1989, showed that over 10 per cent of groups that community workers were supporting were concerned directly with the needs of elderly or disabled people, or with carers. And a lot of work aimed at providing resources to support local groups is directly relevant to community care consumers. It will be seen too that the following six themes relate as much to the role and skills of professional staff as they do to communities, community groups and informal networks.

36.1 Alerting community care planners to community strengths

The word 'community' can often remain an abstraction. It can carry little or no meaning, especially for the dependent or vulnerable. Yet it is difficult to conceive how professional staff who are responsible for community care – the community care managers and planners in local authorities – will be able to work effectively unless they have the ability to analyse community needs and resources accurately and with skill.

This will involve them in knowing which groups and organisations exist in any neighbourhood. In this way they can build up a map or profile of how local people relate to each other. They can find out about the informal caring that is going on, and about the work of volunteers and community groups that relates to the needs of those people in need of care.

It is crucial for comunity care planners and managers to avoid holding presuppositions about communities, whether of a 'labelled' inner-city council estate or an idyllic rural village. Equally, their agencies cannot be committed to community policies such as community care without equipping their staff with the ability to intervene effectively and sensitively in neighbourhoods. At a policy level, a weakness of the Barclay Report (1982) was that its recommendations for community social work were insufficiently rooted in the complexities and conflicts of interest to be found in many communities.

By understanding and 'getting inside' communities, community care planners wil be in a position to work in partnership with community groups and small voluntary organisations. They can be introduced to the experiences accumulated by community development workers over the last 20 years.

36.2 Helping communities prepare for community care

Have government and local authorities paid sufficient attention to peparing communities for receiving more dependent people, explaining the reasons for the government's community care policy, and minimising fears and uncertainties? One rarely hears the words 'adult education' in the context of community care debates. Yet work done, for example, by Flynn (1987) shows the high social and personal costs that some people with learning difficulties pay for living independently, including not just failure to integrate with the community but being actively victimised by some members of it.

There is an educative task to be undertaken to explain the origins and purposes of the community care policy, its partnership proposals, and the financial arrangements. The language and jargon surrounding these matters need to be interpreted, and related to people's experiences. In the community setting, this means making use of community development and informal adult education methods.

Furthermore, it means working with community groups in addition to setting up specific forums or conferences focused on the issue of community care. This is an important distinction. With the former, professionals will need to negotiate with groups as to how the issue will be discussed, and often it is at that point that a community worker can be very useful, because he or she will be in close contact with groups. With the latter, the educational and information-giving agenda is more in the hands of professionals. But if their agencies genuinely want to support community care at a local, grassroots level, then here too they will need to spend time in finding ways to acheive broad-based participation in conferences and forums that speak to variety and differences in society: black and white; men and women; carers and persons cared for.

There is important experience showing how community development and adult education methods can be used together in work with community groups. Two useful source books are those of Lovett (1982) and, in the rural context, the handbook on community development course by Scott *et al.* (1989). The pre-condition, however, must be for community care policy-makers to recognise the need for communities to be helped to prepare for the impact of the community care policy. Otherwise one fears that local authorities may be surprised by the extent of local reaction to the policy, hostility that might be avoided, or at least minimised, through community development and adult education programmes.

36.3 Empowerment

Evidence suggests that care by the community will place immense additional pressures on care by family members, who can be damaged by the experience. Accordingly, it is essential to find more effective ways of supporting them. Increasing numbers of carers' groups and networks are being formed, and this is a welcome development. A workshop on carers at a Scottish conference emphasised the position of carers 'as being caught in a poverty trap, being effectively house-bound, and gradually losing social contact and self-esteem' (Godridge, 1990), thereby making it extremely difficult to organise carers on a community development basis. It is important to win their confidence, and help them build strong groups, which are rooted in, and supported by, community networks and community groups.

We see potential not only for self-help groups but also for campaigning groups – of both carers and persons cared for/consumers. Community development has mainly focused on work with carers, and it is important for its work with care consumers to be undertaken with considerable skill and in partnership with others. How this is done will vary with client groups. For example, there are more examples of physically disabled people taking action on their own behalf than there are of people with learning difficulties doing so.

But there can be no doubt of the need to strengthen the capacity of both carers and those they care for to speak to themselves. They are clearly the weaker partners, in terms of power and the holding of resources, compared with the local authority. Hence the understandable concern to promote advocacy and self-advocacy. In addition, care groups are likely to have put increasing amounts of energy into talking and negotiating with neighbours and community groups. Community development skills and techniques of organizing groups can usefully be harnessed by such groups. They include questions such as how to increase or maintain levels of participation in groups, leadership of groups, and accountability. These are bread-and-butter matters for community workers, the core of organising in the community.

The other experience of organising that community development can bring to community care is from its support of community enterprises. The growth of community business and community enterprise over the last 15 years has not been strong in the community care field compared, for example, with the emphasis on community shops. Experience of nursery and crèche provision, run on an enterprise basis, are nearest to community care.

There is evidence to suggest that the community development aspects of developing community enterprises have often been a crucial factor (see Henderson, 1991). This experience can be drawn upon by social services agencies when interest in community enterprises begins to grow. Such initiatives, which combine social and economic objectives, have the advantage of providing services to people in their area, and the providers would be likely to know and relate to the consumers. Problems of capitalisation of community businesses suggests that projects with low start-up costs are likely to be most feasible: domiciliary and day care may have more potential than residential care. Respite care schemes, where a community enterprise co-ordinates the use of respite provision in people's own homes in the locality, thus avoiding capital costs for premises, may be particularly appropriate.

36.4 Enhancing community support and networks

It is difficult to see how the problems faced by severely disabled people outside institutions can be met by community development. However, when one considers less severely disabled people, community development methods become more relevant. Essentially we are talking of ways of integrating dependent people as far as possible into 'normal' community life.

The creation of community-run lunch clubs, adult education classes, various recreational activities, voluntary visiting schemes, self-help groups of people with specific disabilities; all of these can result in the strengthening of the general capacity of a community to care, and a greater sense of well-being among people in need of support and care. Such community resources are the key to the Audit Commission's statement that 'the objective of any changes should be to create an environment in which locally integrated community care can flourish' (*Audit Commission*, 1986). The overlap between self-help groups, whereby 'young' elderly people, less severely disabled people, HIV-positive people, recovered alcoholics, etc., form and control their own groups, with community groups, is something to be welcomed. They can exist alongside each other, support each other, or a self-help group can join or become a community group. Whichever practice model is chosen, the aim should be to oppose any semblance of 'apartheid' between people who are seen to be so different that links are not forged with them.

Community development aimed at enhancing mutual support and networks may be particularly relevant in some disadvantaged communities: in particular, inner-city areas from which younger people with famlies have moved away, leaving a high proportion of elderly people in the population; areas where the pressures on people's lives, especially poverty and fear of crime, are already considerable. Historically it is these areas where one might have found strong support systems of neighbours for the vulnerable and dependent. All the more reason, therefore, for agencies to make special efforts to support community development there.

We emphasise, however, that groups and networks do not necessarily have a benign attitude to those people in need of care. It may be important to combine community development methods with small-group work techniques and conflict resolution/mediation.

A more ambitious scenario would suggest that community development can put forward 'structural' argument concerning the needs and rights of vulnerable people in relation to society – arguments that are increasingly articulated by the disabled people's movement. Rights to employment, access to public buildings and transport are the tangible gains that are being sought. Behind them is the viewpoint that it is society that needs to change its attitudes and assumptions towards dependent and vulnerable people. To date, there is little evidence of those involved in community development work opening up this debate. That does not mean, however, that it should not be on their agenda. Potentially, the contribution of community development to the structural debate is considerable.

36.5 Contracting

We have raised already the case for community enterprises to expand into the care field, and this would entail them having contracts with local authorities. Many voluntary organisations are preparing themselves for the contract culture too. There is a justifiable concern that local authorities will find it easier and more efficient to contract almost entirely with the visible, relatively well-resourced part of the voluntary sector, thereby denying community groups opportunities for involvement in care schemes. Accordingly, community workers and others have a role to play in providing training and development support to community groups that wish to supply services. They need also to advocate in policy areas for there to be small-scale contracts, and contracts that recognise differences between communities, not blueprints. Inseparable from such debates is the question of how contracts will be monitored, and the need for consumer involvement in the monitoring.

All of this is very difficult territory. Entering the contract culture may radically alter the nature of the organisations doing so, including community groups. There is also the contrast of scale between small, neighbourhood-based groups entering the world of finance, objectives and monitoring, etc., and large organisations, which can call upon different kinds of expertise. Some would argue that community groups should not risk joining the contract culture. Others advise that they should seek to do so as consortia, coalitions of groups that together can assemble strength and expertise whilst each retains individual autonomy.

Smallness and localness may eventually prove to be important cards for community groups to play, because it will be these characteristics that will enable the purchasers of community care to reach people. The risk being run at present by policy-makers within both central and local government is of community care failing to connect with the grassroots. It could end up being a very partialised, even distorted, programme. We believe that community development can provide a significant counter to this potential weakness.

36.6 Training for Social Services staff

In addition to community care planners and managers learning about communities (see 36.1 above), attention may also need to be given to training them and their staff to work with community groups and small voluntary organisations. The tasks will involve not only utilising existing provision, but creating it. One set of training needs exists around the skills of working in communities: knowing how community groups function; being able to win their trust and co-operation; respecting their independence; offering them support – in other words, a host of skills that are at the fingertips of good community workers (see Henderson and Thomas, 1987).

A second set of training needs relates to supporting carers in the community, the networks of paid and unpaid support that are needed if people severely at risk are to be assisted to stay in the community. There is surely a role here for the Carers' National Association and community development agencies such as the Community Development Foundation, for the scope is considerable. It will be important for the training content and materials to relate directly to the priorities of community care managers and other staff. Indeed, they could be important in suggesting ways in which the priorities could change.

36.7 Concluding comments

Few community workers would argue that they should work exclusively with local people, in the sense of direct, face-to-face contact with them. That is certainly the engine-room of community development, and it would be very strange to move far away from it. Yet by itself it is unlikely to help communities obtain the resources and services they need. Work has to be done within agencies and within policy arenas, thereby helping local people indirectly. The area of training highlighted above illustrates how community workers have a role within their agencies as well as in the community.

It also points to the way in which the community development contribution to community care can take place at a number of levels: practice and policy; neighbourhood and city-wide; case studies of practice; and the articulation of ideas. We believe that it will be by encouraging such a multi-layered strategy that alternative models of practising and delivering community care can evolve. We have sought to show that this need not be dependent on the employment of more community workers, because it is possible for a range of professional staff to learn to use community development methods and skills. Thus the potential for giving a new dimension to the implementation of community care is enormous.

References

Audit Commission (1986) *Making a Reality of Community Care*, HMSO, London.
Barclay Report (1982) *Social Workers: Their Role and Tasks*, National Institute for Social Work Bedford Square Press, London.
Flynn, M. (1987) 'Independent living arrangements for adults who are mentally handicapped', Martin, N. (ed.) in *Re-assessing Community Care*, Croom Helm, London.
Godridge, C. (1990) *Community Development and Community Care*, Report of Scottish Community Development Residential School.
Lovett, T. (1982) *Adult Education, Community Development and the Working Class*, University of Nottingham.
Scott, I., Denman, J. and Lane, B. (1989) *Doing by Learning*, Action with Communities in Rural England, Cirencester.
Henderson, P. and Thomas, D. N. (1987) *Skills in Neighbourhood work*, 2nd edn, Unwin Hyman, London.
Thomas, D. N. (1983) *The Making of Community Work*, Unwin Hyman, London.

37

The Right to Make Choices*

ANN MACFARLANE

The personal assistant is someone every successful company director commands along with a Filofax. A personal assistant makes each day organised and more bearable, and adds those touches which humanise lifestyles. Until recently they have remained almost entirely within the province of the business community, but now the personal assistant is coming to change the lifestyles of disabled people.

In April 1988, Jane and I, both disabled people, sought a meeting with the Director of Social Services in Kingston-upon-Thames to enlist support for the development of our own personal assistance packages. It was crucial that we went together and supported each other as so often disabled people seek assistance in isolation and are marginalised and rejected or ignored.

Two disabled people who were able to identify and present similar requirements to the director resulted in recognition and, in April 1989, a pilot project was ready to go before members of the social services committee.

Meanwhile, in Strasbourg, disabled people were holding an independent living conference where it was resolved: 'Personal assistance services are a human and civil right which must be provided at no cost to the user'.

Following our initial meeting, the diector of social services suggested that Jane and I should prepare a document setting out our requirements. Coincidentally our draft personal assistance package proposals were similar in principle and content to the Strasbourg recommendations so we felt we were on course.

It took Jane and I, who are both professional business women, five months to produce the document. Although we were clear about what

---

*This paper was first published in *Community Care*, 1 November 1990.

assistance we were seeking, it was, nevertheless, a painful process progressing our personal and financial self-assessments while 'laying bare' our private lives to establish what should be a basic human right. At the time of our applications, Jane requested 35 hours' assistance each week; I applied for 14.

We sat through the tensions of the Social Services committee. We have different experiences and backgrounds, mine mainly institutionalised, and the thought of committee members discussing our basic human needs, when probably none of them had ever experienced institutionalisation and never lacked control over their own lives, overwhelmed me.

Most of all I wanted flexible support which would enable me to work and socialise and it had already taken a great deal of confidence and organisation to a return to the business world because of the difficulty in getting support when needed.

The pilot project was approved unanimously without further invasion of our privacy. The scheme was initially agreed for one year starting in April 1989 with a progress report presented to committee members in the November.

The packages would allow each of us to arrange our own system of obtaining personal support, employing the personal assistants directly and controlling their conditions of service. In this way we would retain full control over our day-to-day living. It was to be a free service with the money paid directly into separate bank accounts which we would set up.

The job description requested that personal assistants be responsible for all or some of the following tasks: bathing, dressing, toileting, hair care, cooking, bedmaking, laundry, shopping, light gardening, sorting papers, books, files, maintaining electric wheelchairs, plus any other tasks which come within a personal or domestic situation.

The implementation of this unique initiative would include the appointment of a liaison officer between the two of us and the Department of Social Services, acceptance of the self-assessment procedure, as well as acknowledgement of our own understanding of our capabilities and need for assistance with the professional's role as that of adviser and listener.

Jane and I live within 200 yards of each other and planned to advertise the posts and interview applicants together. We had previously decided that it would be cost- and time-effective to share some of the personal assistants, perhaps employing one main assistant each as there are differences in our age and personalities.

We advertised in local newsagents as it was relatively inexpensive and hoped it would bring more responses from the area. We found a suitable number of applicants to set up the project by June.

Each employee was given a basic contract which included: 'You will be expected to respect each home and confidentiality, be a good time-keeper, and be responsible for your own insurance and tax.' It was important that Jane and I checked with our own insurance companies to ensure we were covered for people working on our premises. We were surprised that, in an area with low unemployment, it had been relatively easy to find people to cover early mornings and late evenings. We also selected people who had very few hours to give but who were willing to undertake just one of the tasks.

However, applicants were encouraged to undertake any task and it was decided to implement the project only partially for Jane and I to get used to being employers and to absorb a number of different personalities into our lives. I found this easier than I had anticipated and perhaps this was enhanced by the fact that I went from a state which 'imprisoned' to one which 'liberated'.

Between us Jane and I employ 10 personal assistants to undertake 49 hours each week. We keep our own records of when assistants work and we have retained all the assistants we initially engaged except one who has now returned to her homeland.

The pilot project is now growing out of its embryonic state and the word has spread to other disabled people. Jane and I feel that the scheme's success lies in the coherent way in which it was established.

There is a commitment to expand our pilot project to involve two or three other disabled people while developing new schemes for disabled people who are not yet ready or who do not want to take on the role and responsibility of employer. As we begin to empower disabled people they will demand flexible support services. With lifestyles in our control we will truly be contributors to the national economy, and not the 'burdens' we are so often accused of being.

Every disabled person has the right to make choices and decisions over their own lives and Jane and I are determined that we will be part of the momentum for demanding more personal assistant packages and other flexible support services from which disabled people can make informed choices.

Currently an information pack and short training video is being produced based on this project which will enable disabled people and service providers to develop their own individual and personal scheme.

Index